A Clinician's Guide to Antibiotics

A Clinician's Guide to Antibiotics

Edited by Clancy Knightley

hayle medical
New York

Hayle Medical,
750 Third Avenue, 9th Floor,
New York, NY 10017, USA

Visit us on the World Wide Web at:
www.haylemedical.com

ISBN: 978-1-63241-790-9

Cataloging-in-Publication Data

A clinician's guide to antibiotics / edited by Clancy Knightley.
p. cm.
Includes bibliographical references and index.
ISBN 978-1-63241-790-9
1. Antibiotics. 2. Antibiosis. 3. Pharmaceutical microbiology.
I. Knightley, Clancy.
RM267 .C55 2019
615.792 2--dc23

Table of Contents

Preface

The antimicrobial substances which are active against bacteria are called antibiotics. They are most commonly used in treating and preventing bacterial infections as they kill and inhibit the growth of bacteria. Penicillin antibiotics are considered to be the first antibiotics which were found to be effective against several bacterial infections. Antibiotics play a significant role in empiric therapy and definitive therapy. Empiric therapy involves the use of a broad-spectrum antibiotic for the management of an infection for which the causative pathogen has not been identified. Definitive therapy is a therapy involving the use of a narrow-spectrum antibiotic. It is used in cases where the responsible pathogenic microorganism has already been identified. This book includes some of the vital pieces of work being conducted across the world, on various topics related to antibiotics. It will also provide interesting topics for research which interested readers can take up. The readers would gain knowledge that would broaden their perspective about antibiotics.

The researches compiled throughout the book are authentic and of high quality, combining several disciplines and from very diverse regions from around the world. Drawing on the contributions of many researchers from diverse countries, the book's objective is to provide the readers with the latest achievements in the area of research. This book will surely be a source of knowledge to all interested and researching the field.

In the end, I would like to express my deep sense of gratitude to all the authors for meeting the set deadlines in completing and submitting their research chapters. I would also like to thank the publisher for the support offered to us throughout the course of the book. Finally, I extend my sincere thanks to my family for being a constant source of inspiration and encouragement.

Editor

1

Pectocin M1 (PcaM1) Inhibits *Escherichia coli* Cell Growth and Peptidoglycan Biosynthesis through Periplasmic Expression

Dimitri Chérier, Sean Giacomucci †, Delphine Patin, Ahmed Bouhss ‡, Thierry Touzé, Didier Blanot, Dominique Mengin-Lecreulx and Hélène Barreteau *

Institute for Integrative Biology of the Cell (I2BC), CEA, CNRS, Univ Paris-Sud, Université Paris-Saclay, Gif-sur-Yvette 91198, France; dimitri.cherier@i2bc.paris-saclay.fr (D.C.); sean.giacomucci@umontreal.ca (S.G.); delphine.patin@i2bc.paris-saclay.fr (D.P.); ahmed.bouhss@univ-evry.fr (A.B.); thierry.touze@i2bc.paris-saclay.fr (T.T.); didier.blanot@gmail.com (D.B.); dominique.mengin-lecreulx@i2bc.paris-saclay.fr (D.M.-L.)

* Correspondence: helene.barreteau@i2bc.paris-saclay.fr

† Present address: Department of Microbiology, Infectiology and Immunology, Université de Montréal, Montréal, QC H3T 1J4, Canada.

‡ Present address: Laboratoire Structure-Activité des Biomolécules Normales et Pathologiques, INSERM UMRS 1204 and Université Evry-Val d'Essonne, Evry 91025, France.

Academic Editor: Christopher Butler

Abstract: Colicins are bacterial toxins produced by some *Escherichia coli* strains. They exhibit either enzymatic or pore-forming activity towards a very limited number of bacterial species, due to the high specificity of their reception and translocation systems. Yet, we succeeded in making the colicin M homologue from *Pectobacterium carotovorum*, pectocin M1 (PcaM1), capable of inhibiting *E. coli* cell growth by bypassing these reception and translocation steps. This goal was achieved through periplasmic expression of this pectocin. Indeed, when appropriately addressed to the periplasm of *E. coli*, this pectocin could exert its deleterious effects, i.e., the enzymatic degradation of the peptidoglycan lipid II precursor, which resulted in the arrest of the biosynthesis of this essential cell wall polymer, dramatic morphological changes and, ultimately, cell lysis. This result leads to the conclusion that colicin M and its various orthologues constitute powerful antibacterial molecules able to kill any kind of bacterium, once they can reach their lipid II target. They thus have to be seriously considered as promising alternatives to antibiotics.

Keywords: pectocin M1; peptidoglycan; bacteriocin; colicin; periplasmic expression

---

1. Introduction

Colicins are bacterial toxins produced by some *Escherichia coli* strains in order to kill susceptible strains of *E. coli* and related species. Among the ca. twenty colicins identified to date [1], colicin M (ColM) is unique as it is the only one interfering with bacterial peptidoglycan biosynthesis. ColM acts by cleavage of the last precursor of this essential metabolic pathway, thereby causing cell death. Indeed, it was shown ten years ago, both in vivo and in vitro, that ColM was an enzyme catalyzing specifically the hydrolysis of the peptidoglycan lipid intermediate C_{55}-PP-MurNAc(pentapeptide)-GlcNAc (lipid II), by cleaving between the prenyl chain (C_{55}-) and the pyrophosphoryl group of this precursor [2]. The two reaction products, undecaprenol and 1-PP-MurNAc(pentapeptide)-GlcNAc, that do not normally exist in *E. coli* growing cells, were accumulated in the ColM-treated cells. These products cannot be reused into peptidoglycan metabolism or be recycled, thereby leading to cell lysis.

ColM develops its bacteriolytic activity in three sequential steps deeply linked to its structural organization in three domains and parasitizes proteins from the targeted cell to enter the periplasm. Accordingly, the ColM central domain first binds to an outer membrane receptor for siderophores, FhuA [3]. Subsequently, it is translocated towards the periplasm by using the proton-motive force, through the interaction of its N-terminal domain with the TonB machinery system comprising the TonB, ExbB and ExbD proteins [4]. Finally, once shuttled into the periplasm of the targeted cell, ColM is maturated by the ubiquitous chaperone protein FkpA, so that its C-terminal domain can display its cytotoxic effect on lipid II [5,6].

As this is the case for many bacteriocins, ColM-producing cells are protected against the lethal effect of their own colicin by the concomitant synthesis of an immunity protein, named ImM (or Cmi). Although the latter protein has been structurally characterized [7,8], the mechanism of protection of the bacterial cell from lysis is still unknown. However, non-producing cells can also protect themselves against the action of ColM by mutation or deletion of genes encoding proteins involved in ColM reception/translocation/maturation processes [9,10].

During the last few years, several ColM orthologues have been identified, by sequence alignments of their C-terminal domains, in some other bacterial genera, such as *Pseudomonas*, *Burkholderia* and *Pectobacterium* species, and several of them have been both biochemically and structurally characterized [11–15]. All of the purified ColM orthologues displayed the same enzymatic activity of cleavage of lipid II and a bacteriolytic (or at least bacteriostatic) activity [11,12]. Yet, despite their similarities in terms of enzymatic activity, these orthologues did not share the same 3D structure, especially in their N-terminal domains. On the one hand, ColM shared a very compact structure with PaeM and syringacin M (also named PsyM), i.e., its orthologues from *Pseudomonas aeruginosa* and *Pseudomonas syringae*, respectively, where the usual three structural domains did not form distinct entities [12,13]. On the other hand, the structure of pectocin M2 from *Pectobacterium carotovorum* and probably also that of pectocin M1, since it has been strongly suggested that both pectocins M1 and M2 used the same outer membrane receptor on *Pectobacterium* spp. [14], presented an atypical translocation domain, where the helical receptor-domain and unstructured N-terminus were replaced by a single globular plant-like [2Fe-2S] ferredoxin domain, directly connected to the cytotoxic one through a small α-helix linker [15]. Moreover, while numerous receptors for colicins and closely-related pyocins were Tol- or TonB-dependent, these ferredoxin-containing pectocins presumably used a bacterial ferredoxin uptake mechanism to cross the outer membrane, without any evidence for Tol or TonB complex requirements [15].

The cytotoxicity of all of these ColM-like bacteriocins has been previously demonstrated to be pointed towards a limited number of bacterial species. The specificity of their receptor-binding and translocation domains presumably prevents them from targeting a broad range of bacteria. It thus seems that, if reaching the target constitutes a crucial step for the colicin cytotoxicity, it is also the limiting one. Yet, ways allowing the bypass of this specific and limiting step do exist. Indeed, the use of an osmotic shock was shown to be efficient to make extracellular proteins enter the periplasm of Gram-negative bacteria without loss of cell integrity [16,17]. Another efficient means to send proteins into the periplasm of a target cell was the use of fusion proteins between the bacteriocin of interest and a signal sequence. This strategy was particularly used to study the pore formation by colicin A [18,19]. According to the latter methodology, we describe in the present paper how we managed to evaluate the antibacterial activity of pectocin M1 (that will be named PcaM1 throughout this work, following the nomenclature we previously used [11]) and some of its variants on *E. coli* cells by triggering their periplasmic expression. We show that when addressed to the periplasm of *E. coli*, the PcaM1 protein, as well as its isolated activity domain could catalyze the degradation of the peptidoglycan lipid II precursor, which leads to the arrest of the biosynthesis of this essential cell wall component and, consequently, to cell lysis. It is also shown that, contrary to ColM, this pectocin does not depend on the presence of the host FkpA chaperone protein to exert its deleterious toxic effects.

2. Results

2.1. Design, Production and Purification of Wild-Type and Mutant PcaM1

The gene encoding PcaM1 was amplified from the *P. carotovorum* ssp. *carotovorum* strain PC1 and cloned into a pET expression vector allowing the production of a C-terminal His_6-tagged protein. The catalytic point mutant (D222A) in which Asp222 is replaced by Ala, which was previously reported to be devoid of cytotoxic activity [14], was also produced as a C-terminal His_6-tagged protein.

According to SDS-PAGE analysis of the crude extracts, the best recovery yields of both wild-type and mutant proteins were obtained following overnight IPTG-induced expression at 22 °C. Thereafter, the proteins were purified by affinity chromatography with an overall yield of about 10 mg per liter of culture, and their purity, as judged by SDS-PAGE, was about 95%. Subsequent gel filtration analysis showed that both wild-type and mutant forms of PcaM1 mainly eluted as monomers. No protein aggregates were observed, confirming that the proteins were homogeneous (Supplementary Materials Figure S1). As previously described, both wild-type and mutant purified recombinant proteins had a red-brown color and displayed absorption spectrum maxima at 329, 423 and 467 nm [14]. It should be noted that when protein samples were not boiled before SDS-PAGE analysis, two slightly differently-migrating protein bands of the expected molecular mass for PcaM1 were observed (Supplementary Materials Figure S1). The fast migrating species could represent a more compact and, thus, a more SDS-resistant form of the protein. It is tempting to link this observation to the two protein populations (compact and extended forms) that have been previously revealed by SAXS experiments on pectocin M2 by Grinter and collaborators [15]. MALDI-TOF mass spectrometry analyses of the wild-type PcaM1 revealed only one major peak at *m/z* 30,266 Da for the $[M + H]^+$ ion, which is in agreement with the theoretical mass of 30,401 Da calculated for the His_6-tagged protein and with the loss of the N-terminal methionine residue (Supplementary Materials Figure S2).

2.2. Enzymatic Properties of PcaM1

Pure wild-type PcaM1 was tested for its capacity to hydrolyze the peptidoglycan intermediate lipid II in vitro, as previously shown for ColM and its homologues from *Pseudomonas* species [2,11]. The peptidoglycan composition of the genus *Pectobacterium* is not known to date, but as this genus belongs to the *Enterobacteriaceae*, a classical diaminopimelic acid (A_2pm)-containing peptidoglycan structure is likely present in this bacterium [20]. Therefore, the corresponding lipid II was synthesized by using *E. coli* MraY and MurG enzymes to be used as a substrate in our assays [2]. PcaM1 was able to convert the radiolabeled [^{14}C]lipid II substrate to a reaction product migrating with a lower R_f (0.3 vs. 0.7 for lipid II) on TLC plates (Figure 1A,B), confirming the enzymatic nature of this protein and its similarity with ColM and the *Pseudomonas* orthologues [2,11].

Under the standard assay conditions used, the specific activity of PcaM1 was 0.53 nmol/min/mg of protein, which is quite similar to that previously determined for ColM (0.4 nmol/min/mg) [2]. The K_m value of wild-type PcaM1 for *meso*-A_2pm-containing lipid II was determined to be 55 μM, which is also in the usual range of other ColM-orthologues [11].

The ability of the D222A PcaM1 mutant to hydrolyze lipid II was also tested in the same conditions. As expected, this catalytic point mutant did not exhibit any in vitro activity of degradation of the lipid II (Figure 1C), even when high amounts of proteins were used (up to 15 μg per assay).

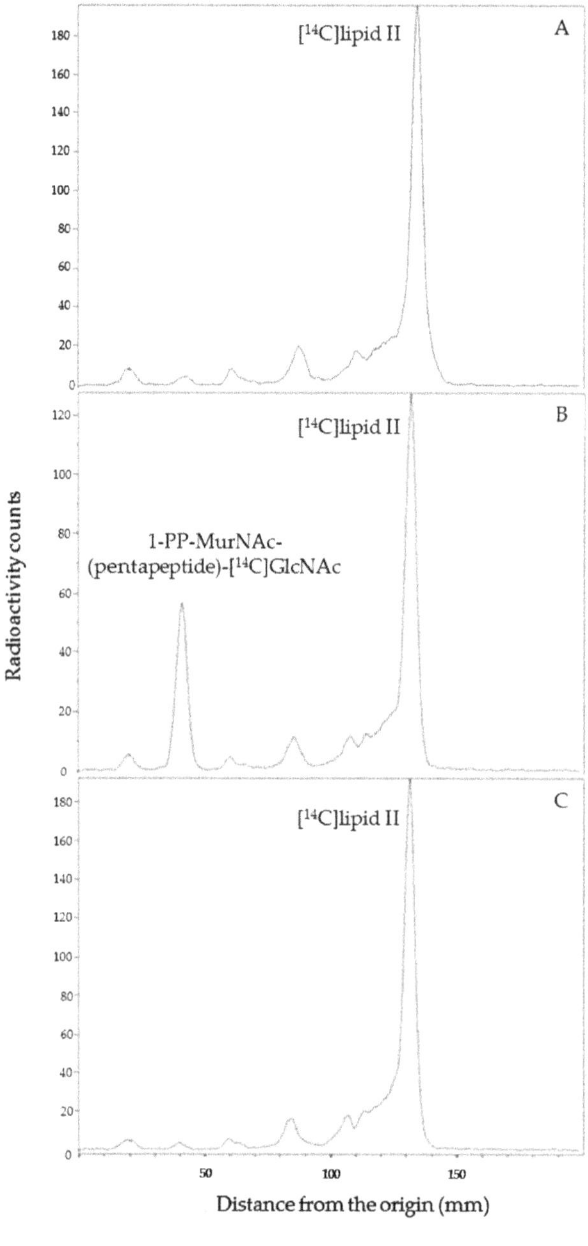

Figure 1. In vitro degradation of lipid II by PcaM1. Conditions that result in ca. 20% hydrolysis of radiolabeled lipid II were used. Purified [^{14}C]lipid II radiolabeled in the GlcNAc moiety (140 Bq) was incubated without (**A**) or with 1.2 μg of wild-type (**B**) or D222A mutant (**C**) PcaM1. The substrate and reaction product were separated by TLC (solvent system: 1-propanol/ammonium hydroxide/water; 6:3:1; v/v/v), and the corresponding spots were detected with a radioactivity scanner, as detailed in the text (R_f = 0.7 and 0.3 for lipid II and 1-PP-MurNAc(pentapeptide)-GlcNAc, respectively).

2.3. Cytotoxicity of PcaM1 and Its Variants

Purified PcaM1 was tested on agar plates for its cytotoxic activity against various wild-type *E. coli* strains (DH5α, BW25113, FB8), and it was found to be totally inactive, as expected. Then, in order to bypass the receptor and translocation machineries, the potential cytotoxicity of PcaM1 was highlighted on the *E. coli* FB8 strain by using the pASK-IBA4 vector, which allowed a controlled expression and subsequent export towards the periplasm of this bacteriocin thanks to its fusion to the OmpA protein signal sequence. Indeed, the addition of anhydrotetracycline triggered the expression of PcaM1 and induced a rapid lysis of *E. coli* FB8 cells (Figure 2). To the best of our knowledge, this is the first time that a bypass of the species specificity following periplasmic expression was described for a member of the ColM family, whose members have been reported to possess a narrow antibacterial spectrum.

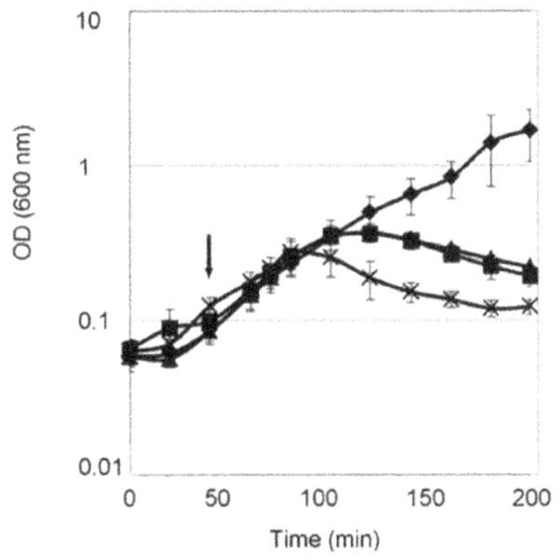

Figure 2. Effects of the periplasmic expression of PcaM1 variants on the growth of *E. coli*. FB8 cells were grown at 37 °C in 2YT medium and the expression of the PcaM1 variants was induced by the addition of anhydrotetracycline (arrow). Growth curves observed for the FB8 strain carrying the pASK-IBA4 empty vector or pASK plasmids expressing the wild-type PcaM1, the D222A mutant or the isolated activity domain (Δ1-107 PcaM1) are shown by diamonds, squares, triangles and crosses, respectively. Four independent experiments were performed for each strain.

We then designed two variants of PcaM1: the same catalytic point mutant (D222A), which had been expressed in the pET vector, and a truncated form deleted of the 107 first N-terminal amino-acid residues (which corresponds to the isolated activity domain). Both variants were tested for their potential toxicity in the *E. coli* FB8 strain background. An identical lytic phenotype was observed following induction of the periplasmic expression of these two proteins (Figure 2).

Such a phenomenon was somewhat expected for the strain expressing the truncated form of PcaM1, considering that isolated ColM and PaeM catalytic domains generated by protein dissection experiments were previously demonstrated to be enzymatically active [13,21]. In contrast, data obtained with the strain expressing the PcaM1 D222A mutant were more surprising, as it was previously shown that the mutation (D226N) of the corresponding catalytic residue of ColM completely abolished the enzymatic activity and toxicity of the latter colicin when exported into the periplasm [22].

As the P_{tet} promoter from the pASK-IBA4 vector is known to be a reasonably strong promoter, we checked whether the lytic phenotype observed for strains expressing wild-type and mutant PcaM1 proteins was not due to a non-specific protein overexpression effect, but rather to the intrinsic toxicity of the PcaM1 activity. Decreasing the concentration of the inducer anhydrotetracycline (30–200 ng/mL range) and, consequently, of PcaM1 expression led to the same growth defect and lytic behavior for both strains (Supplementary Materials Figure S3). Then, to confirm that the decrease of the optical density of the cultures indeed reflected a loss of viability and cell lysis, the experiments of growth monitoring were repeated at the anhydrotetracycline concentration of 200 ng/mL, and colony forming unit counting was performed in parallel to determine the survival ratio in each case (Supplementary Materials Figure S4). These experiments revealed that cell lethality occurred in both cases, as we observed a three-log decrease in CFU for the strain expressing wild-type PcaM1 ca. 30 min after the anhydrotetracycline was added, but only a two-log decrease in CFU after the same time for the strain expressing the D222A PcaM1 mutant, thus showing a less pronounced loss of viability effect for the mutant.

Our data thus demonstrated that the PcaM1 and its derivatives were able to bypass the biological "partners" needed for internalization of a regular exogenous bacteriocin, that is the receptor and translocation machineries. Then, to address a possible role of the maturation chaperone protein FkpA in the activity of PcaM1, the same type of experiment was performed in the *E. coli* BW25113 Δ*fkpA* mutant strain (Supplementary Materials Figure S5). Unlike ColM, whose toxicity of the full-length protein and isolated catalytic domain was found to be FkpA-dependent and independent, respectively, a lytic phenotype was similarly observed here with all of the PcaM1 variants in a Δ*fkpA* genetic background. PcaM1 and its two variants thus did not need a maturation process by FkpA to be active in vivo, once delivered in the *E. coli* periplasm. This result was quite interesting, as only the truncated form of ColM was reported to date to be FkpA-independent [22].

2.4. Consequences of the Periplasmic Expression of PcaM1 and Its Derivatives on Peptidoglycan Metabolism in E. coli

To better understand the effects of the periplasmic expression of these enzymes in *E. coli*, microscopic examination of FB8 cells expressing wild-type and mutant forms of PcaM1 was performed. As compared to control cells that were relatively small and presented a smooth surface (Figure 3A), wild-type, as well as mutant PcaM1-expressing cells appeared elongated and displayed multiple swelling zones on their surface (Figure 3B–D,C–E, respectively). Some of these cells also exhibited amazing membrane protuberances (Figure 3D,E) that ultimately burst. These observations demonstrated that both wild-type and mutant forms of PcaM1 similarly affected *E. coli* cell growth and morphology, a phenotype that was consistent with a perturbation of their peptidoglycan metabolism.

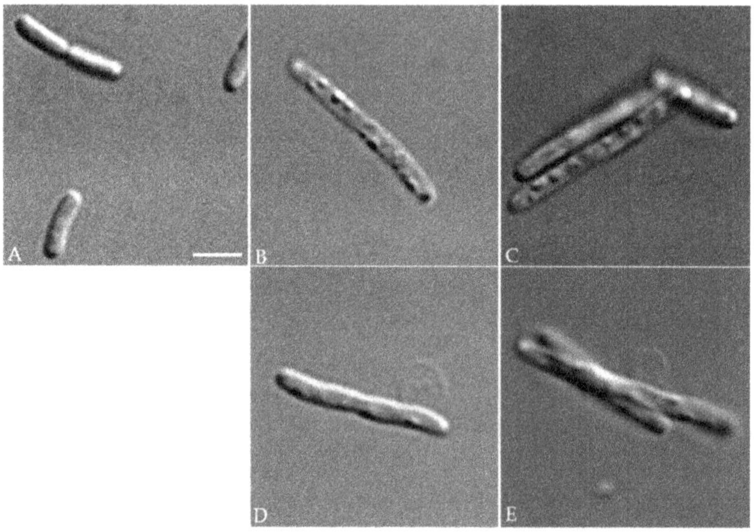

Figure 3. Morphology of *E. coli* strains. Optical micrographs of exponentially-growing control FB8 cells (**A**) and of cells expressing either the wild-type (**B**,**D**) or the D222A mutant (**C**,**E**) PcaM1. As compared to control cells, those expressing either form of PcaM1 in the periplasm appeared elongated, presented swellings on their surface (**B**,**C**), and some of them were blebbing (**D**,**E**). The scale bar shown is 3 μm.

To test this hypothesis further, the pool levels of the carrier lipid undecaprenyl phosphate (C_{55}-P) and of its two derivatives undecaprenyl pyrophosphate (C_{55}-PP) and undecaprenol (C_{55}-OH) were determined in membranes of *E. coli* cells expressing the three PcaM1 variants, using previously-described procedures [23]. Indeed, ColM is known to provoke the cleavage of lipid II into C_{55}-OH, thereby blocking the recycling of the carrier lipid C_{55}-P and peptidoglycan synthesis [2]. Following the expression of PcaM1 and its resulting growth defect, a pool of the isoprenoid C_{55}-OH was thus expected to appear. The results of the isoprenoid HPLC analysis and quantification are presented in Figure 4 and Table 1.

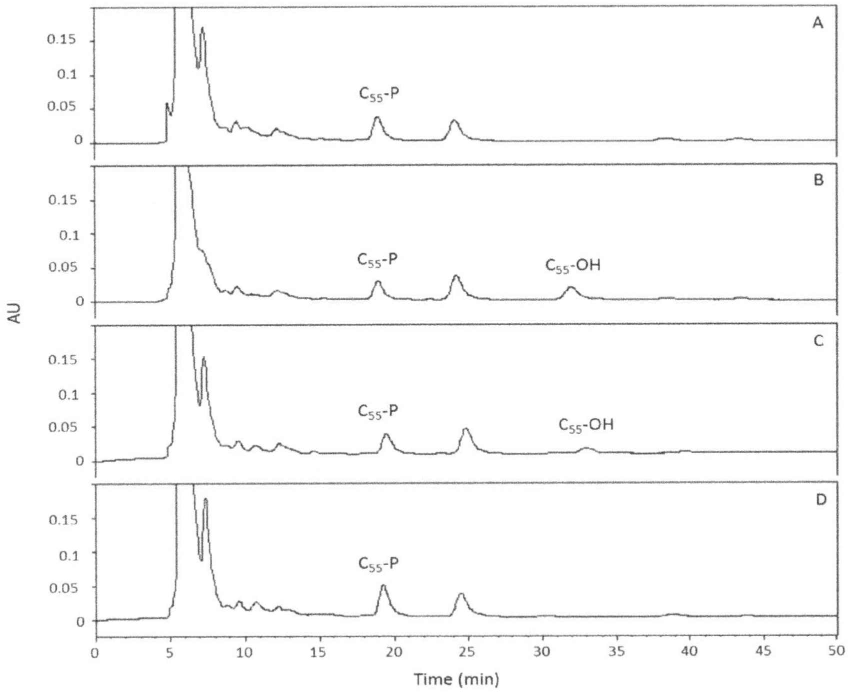

Figure 4. HPLC analysis of membrane extracts (Bligh and Dyer procedure) prepared from *E. coli* FB8 cells carrying either the empty pASK vector (**A**) or pASK plasmids expressing the wild-type PcaM1 (**B**), its isolated cytotoxic domain (**C**) or the D222A mutant (**D**), respectively. Cells were grown exponentially in 2YT medium, and PcaM1 variants' expression was induced at OD_{600} = 0.2 by the addition of anhydrotetracycline. Cells were harvested just before the onset of lysis and treated by sonication. Membrane extracts were prepared and isoprenoids extracted and analyzed by HPLC as described in the text.

Table 1. Pool levels of C_{55}-isoprenoids in *E. coli* FB8 cells following periplasmic expression of PcaM1 and its variants.

Periplasm-Expressed Protein	**Pool Level (nmol/g (Dry Weight) of Bacteria) [a]**			
	C_{55}-PP	**C_{55}-P**	**C_{55}-OH**	**Total**
Control	57 ± 28	77 ± 7	ND	134 ± 31
PcaM1	0 ± 1	68 ± 10	52 ± 18	120 ± 25
Δ1-107 PcaM1	4 ± 7	80 ± 11	27 ± 12	110 ± 15
D222A PcaM1	13 ± 20	127 ± 12	ND	140 ± 20

FB8 cells carrying the pASK-IBA4 empty vector (control) or pASK plasmids expressing the wild-type PcaM1, the D222A mutant or the isolated cytotoxic domain (Δ1-107) were grown exponentially in 2YT medium, and anhydrotetracycline was added when the OD_{600} reached 0.2. Cultures were continued until an arrest of growth was observed and cells were harvested before the onset of cell lysis. The pools of isoprenoids were extracted and quantified as described in the text. [a] Mean ± SD of 5 independent experiments. ND, not detectable.

These experiments allowed us to detect the appearance and accumulation of C_{55}-OH in membranes of *E. coli* cells expressing wild-type and truncated forms of PcaM1 (Figure 4), which was expected considering the lytic effect of this bacteriocin in liquid culture conditions and was reminiscent of previous data observed with ColM [2,23]. This C_{55}-OH pool represented between one third and a half of the total isoprenoid pool in both *E. coli* strains. Another interesting trait was the total isoprenoid content that remained generally quite similar, irrespective of the strain considered (Table 1). In both the full-length and truncated PcaM1-expressing strains, this effect is likely due to the fact that the C_{55}-PP pool was depleted to maintain the C_{55}-P pool at a standard level of about 75 nmol/g of dry cell weight, as previously described for *E. coli* [23].

However, the *E. coli* strain expressing the D222A mutant form of PcaM1 did not show the same pattern of isoprenoids. Surprisingly indeed, although this mutant also provoked *E. coli* cell lysis in liquid culture conditions, membranes of the latter strain did not contain any detectable C_{55}-OH. Here too, the pool of C_{55}-PP was significantly depleted, but a ca. 60% increase of the C_{55}-P pool was observed in these conditions. As will be discussed later, these findings suggested that the D222A enzymatically-inactive mutant also inhibited the same step of the peptidoglycan synthesis pathway, without displaying any lipid II-degrading activity.

To unambiguously demonstrate that the observed cell lysis was the consequence of an arrest of peptidoglycan synthesis and to investigate why the strain expressing the catalytic mutant form of PcaM1 also lysed, cell labeling experiments were performed, in which radiolabeled *meso*-[^{14}C]A_2pm was used as a specific marker of peptidoglycan biosynthesis. To ensure a specific and optimal labeling of peptidoglycan, an *E. coli* FB8 Δ*lysA* mutant strain was used and grown in minimal medium conditions, as previously described [2,24]. In this way, we were able to follow the specific incorporation of *meso*-[^{14}C]A_2pm into the peptidoglycan macromolecule of *E. coli* cells expressing wild-type and mutant forms of PcaM1, compared to a control strain (Figure 5).

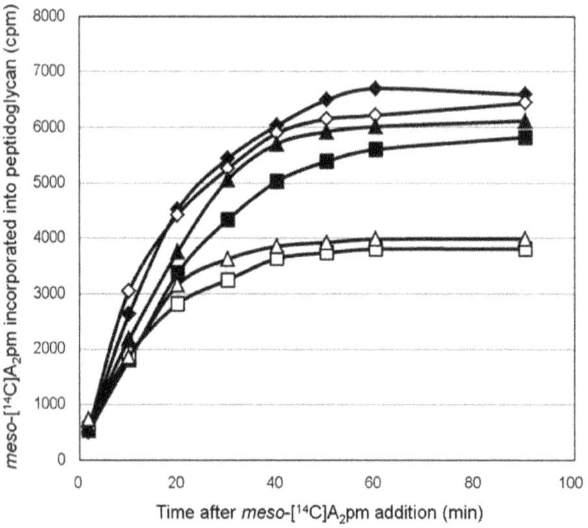

Figure 5. Effect of the periplasmic expression of wild-type and mutant forms of PcaM1 on *meso*-[^{14}C]A_2pm incorporation into peptidoglycan. Cells were grown in M63-glucose minimum medium supplemented with lysine, threonine and methionine. When the OD_{600} reached 0.2, anhydrotetracycline was added, or not, and *meso*-[^{14}C]A_2pm was added 10 min thereafter. The incorporation of radioactivity into the peptidoglycan (trichloroacetic acid (TCA)-insoluble material) was then followed as described in the text. Symbols: diamonds, strain carrying the pASK-IBA4 empty vector; squares and triangles, strains expressing the wild-type and D222A mutant PcaM1, respectively. Open and closed symbols represent cultures treated or not with anhydrotetracycline, respectively.

As shown in Figure 5, *meso*-[^{14}C]A_2pm was rapidly incorporated into the peptidoglycan polymer after its addition to the culture medium. When anhydrotetracycline was added, this incorporation was rapidly blocked in strains expressing either the wild-type or the D222A mutant form of PcaM1, but not in the control strain carrying the empty vector pASK-IBA4. This arrest of incorporation happened about 30 min after *meso*-[^{14}C]A_2pm addition to the culture medium. As observed in Figure 2, *E. coli* cell lysis started about 40 min after addition of anhydrotetracycline. The observed lytic phenotype was thus clearly correlated to an arrest of peptidoglycan synthesis.

We then investigated the cellular distribution of the radioactive material in cells expressing PcaM1 variants. Radioactivity counts recovered in the soluble and insoluble cell fractions from both strains are presented in Table 2, compared to control cells.

Table 2. Effects of PcaM1 variants on the cellular distribution of *meso*-[^{14}C]A_2pm incorporated into *E. coli* cells.

E. coli cells	Radioactivity (counts per min)		
	Soluble Fraction	Insoluble Fraction	Total
Control cells	40,240 (100%)	271,130 (100%)	311,370
+ wild-type PcaM1	168,100 (417%)	104,210 (38%)	272,310
+ D222A PcaM1	163,950 (407%)	112,420 (41%)	276,370

FB8 *lysA* cells (50 mL cultures) were grown in M63-glucose minimum medium supplemented with lysine, threonine and methionine. At an OD_{600} of 0.2, anhydrotetracycline was added and *meso*-[^{14}C]A_2pm (0.2 kBq/mL) 20 min thereafter. Cells were harvested after 30 min of labeling, just before the onset of cell lysis and were treated with boiling water. Suspensions were ultracentrifuged, and the radioactivity present in the supernatant (soluble) and pellet (insoluble) fractions was measured. The distribution of the radioactivity in these fractions (peptidoglycan and its different intermediate precursors) was then analyzed using appropriate analytical procedures, as described in the text.

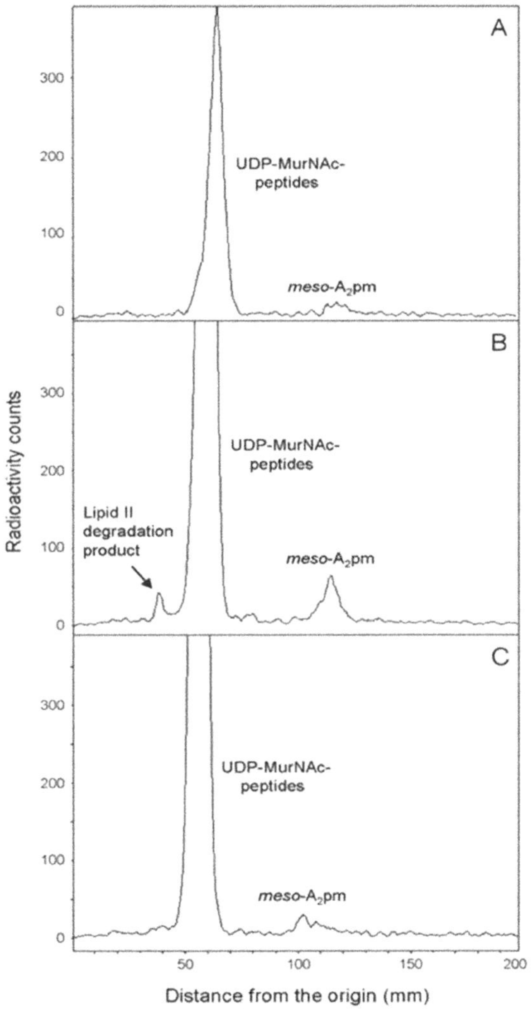

Figure 6. TLC analysis of the soluble fractions from *E. coli* FB8 *lysA* cells expressing (**B**,**C**) or not (**A**) the wild-type and D222A mutant forms of PcaM1, respectively. The peak corresponding to UDP-MurNAc-peptides was shown to contain essentially UDP-MurNAc-pentapeptide (>95%) and low amounts of UDP-MurNAc-tripeptide by HPLC analysis. A peak of radiolabeled lipid II degradation product 1-PP-MurNAc(pentapeptide)-GlcNAc was only observed in cells expressing the wild-type form of PcaM1.

These data first showed that the total radioactivity incorporated in the three *E. coli* strains was similar, ca. 300,000 counts per min in the typical experiment shown, indicating that the expression of the PcaM1 variants did not affect the *meso*-[^{14}C]A_2pm uptake. Expression of PcaM1 was shown to result in a 60% decrease of incorporated radioactivity in the insoluble fraction, which contains peptidoglycan (mainly) and lipids I and II intermediates (Table 2), consistent with our previous data shown in Figure 3. As a result, the "missing" radioactivity that has not been incorporated in the polymer was found to be accumulated in the soluble fraction, which is known to contain *meso*-[^{14}C]A_2pm and the peptidoglycan nucleotide precursors as the main labeled compounds. Chromatography (TLC) analysis of these fractions (Figure 6) confirmed the decrease of radioactivity counts incorporated in the polymer and the significant (four-fold) accumulation of the UDP-MurNAc-pentapeptide precursor as the main soluble radiolabeled compound, as expected for an inhibition of the membrane steps of this pathway. Moreover, an additional peak of radiolabeled compound was observed (R_f of 0.3), specifically when soluble extracts from the strain expressing the wild-type PcaM1 were analyzed (Figure 6). This peak, which was also observed in ColM-treated cells, had been earlier identified as the lipid II-degradation product 1-PP-MurNAc(pentapeptide)-GlcNAc [2]. The absence of this peak in extracts from cells expressing the D222A variant was perfectly consistent with the absence of a detectable pool of C_{55}-OH in these cells, as well as with the inactivity of this mutant protein.

3. Discussion

In this work, we focused our investigations on PcaM1, one of the two ColM-like orthologues produced by *P. carotovorum*. We first revisited the results previously published by Grinter and collaborators in 2012 by producing the wild-type and catalytic point mutant D222A PcaM1 proteins. We thus confirmed, on the one hand, the enzymatic activity of lipid II degradation by the wild-type PcaM1, whereas the mutant was inactive, and on the other hand, the absence of cytotoxic activity of PcaM1 preparation on *E. coli* cells, as no growth inhibition zone was detected when up to 57 μg of this protein were spotted on *E. coli* BW25113-inoculated agar plates.

Although PcaM1, as well as the other ColM orthologues [11] did not display any cytotoxic activity against *E. coli* cells, we recently showed that the application of an osmotic shock treatment to *E. coli* cells allowed the *P. aeruginosa* ColM orthologue (PaeM) to bypass the outer membrane reception and translocation steps, reach its lipid II target and thus exert its deleterious activity [13]. This allowed us to demonstrate that PaeM, as well as its isolated catalytic domain, was able to kill *E. coli* cells. It was the first example of a ColM-like protein capable of killing another bacterial species.

Another way to get access to the *E. coli* periplasmic space was to fuse ColM to the OmpA protein signal sequence. In these conditions, the hybrid ColM was directly exported from the cytoplasm to the periplasm of the producing cells and was then demonstrated to be toxic [22]. Therefore, to check whether another ColM orthologue would be able to kill *E. coli* cells by this approach, we fused the PcaM1 to OmpA signal sequence and expressed the hybrid protein in *E. coli*. In this way, we visualized that PcaM1 was toxic for *E. coli* cells, as the controlled induction of its expression led to cell lysis. To the best of our knowledge, this is the first example of cell lysis due to periplasmic expression of a ColM-like orthologue. A hybrid protein obtained by fusion of the PcaM1 variant truncated of its 107 first amino acids to the OmpA signal sequence led to the same lytic phenotype, as also did the D222A point mutant PcaM1. That the expression of the isolated catalytic domain of PcaM1 yielded cell lysis in these conditions was somewhat expected, as this had been observed also with the catalytic domain of ColM [22]. However, the lytic effect exhibited by the D222A variant was much more surprising. Indeed, as described above, no enzymatic activity of in vitro degradation of lipid II was reported for this mutant protein. The Asp222 residue from PcaM1 corresponds to Asp226 in ColM, which has been previously demonstrated to be essential for the catalytic activity and, consequently, for the cytotoxicity of ColM [21]. Moreover, it was previously shown that the D226N mutant of ColM did not display any toxic activity when exported to the periplasm [22]. The lytic phenotype of the *E. coli* strain expressing the D222A PcaM1 mutant was thus intriguing. Cell lysis was observed even at low doses of anhydrotetracycline, suggesting that toxicity is due to an effect of mutant PcaM1 per se and not to a potential toxicity of protein overexpressed (Figures S3 and S4).

As the induction of periplasmic PcaM1 expression triggered *E. coli* cell lysis whatever the PcaM1 variant expressed, we investigated whether this phenotype was indeed the consequence of an arrest of peptidoglycan biosynthesis. Accordingly, ColM and its orthologue PaeM were previously shown to exhibit bacteriolytic and bacteriostatic effects on their specific *E. coli* and *Pseudomonas* targeted species, respectively, that were in both cases correlated to an inhibition of peptidoglycan biosynthesis [2,11]. In this respect, optical microscopy analyses showed that PcaM1-producing cells displayed greatly altered, elongated and bloated morphologies that are characteristic of an impaired cell wall biogenesis. The arrest of peptidoglycan synthesis in these cells was clearly demonstrated by (i) radiolabeling experiments, using *meso*-[^{14}C]A_2pm as a specific marker, that revealed the accumulation of the cytoplasmic UDP-MurNAc-pentapeptide precursor and the concomitant arrest of the synthesis of the polymer, as well as the presence of the lipid II degradation product; (ii) analyses of isoprenoid pool levels in membranes, which revealed the appearance and accumulation of C_{55}-OH, which normally do not exist in *E. coli* cells. Quite interestingly, although the D222A PcaM1 mutant did not show detectable lipid II-degrading enzymatic activity, either in vitro (enzymatic assays) or in vivo (no C_{55}-OH or 1-PP-MurNAc(pentapeptide)-GlcNAc detected in the cell content), its expression in the periplasm led to the same and specific dramatic morphological changes and arrest of peptidoglycan synthesis that have been observed with the functional wild-type PcaM1. This intriguing result could be interpreted in several ways. For instance, the D222A mutant whose lipid II hydrolase activity is abolished likely conserved its ability to interact with this substrate. A sequestration of the lipid II by the mutant protein could thus be envisaged, which would result in an inhibition of peptidoglycan polymerization steps catalyzed by the penicillin-binding proteins (PBP). Validation of such a hypothesis would need to precisely determine the relative numbers of lipid II and PcaM1 molecules present in the periplasmic space of *E. coli* in these conditions, as well as to develop in vitro analyses of these protein-substrate interactions. Further work is thus needed to elucidate by which mechanism this inactive variant of PcaM1 could still interfere so efficiently with the peptidoglycan synthesis pathway.

In this study, we also tested the periplasmic expression of the three PcaM1 variants in an *E. coli* strain carrying a deletion of the FkpA chaperone-encoding gene. Contrary to what was previously observed with periplasmic variants of ColM, i.e., that the full-length ColM protein and its isolated catalytic domain were FkpA-dependent and -independent, respectively [22], all of the PcaM1 variants constructed here were able to induce *E. coli* cell lysis in the absence of FkpA, meaning that no maturation process, at least by this chaperone, was needed for them to be toxic in *E. coli*. It thus seems that the PcaM1 protein was produced right away in an active form in these particular conditions of heterologous expression.

This work thus clearly demonstrates that the limiting reception and translocation steps usually required for colicin cytotoxic activity can be bypassed. We already knew that ColM-like orthologues were able to hydrolyze in vitro peptidoglycan lipid II intermediates of various composition and structure originating from major pathogenic bacteria (*Staphylococcus aureus*, *Enterococcus faecium*, *E. faecalis*) [25], and we confirmed that they could potentially do it also in vivo, as soon as they can reach the periplasmic space of the targeted bacterial species. In *E. coli*, the ColM immunity protein, Cmi (or ImM), that prevents ColM toxicity effect is located in this compartment. A gene coding for a Cmi homologue has been identified in the genome of *P. carotovorum* PC1, which likely confers immunity towards PcaM1 in this species [14]. As these enzymatic colicins clearly constitute powerful molecules with great potential as non-conventional antimicrobial agents, we now consider engineering them in order to design chimera colicins able to exhibit a broader spectrum of antibacterial activity.

4. Materials and Methods

4.1. Bacterial Strains, Plasmids and Growth Conditions

The *E. coli* strains DH5α (Bethesda Research Laboratories) and C43(DE3) (Avidis) were used as the hosts for the propagation of plasmids and the production of proteins, respectively. The *E. coli* strains FB8 and BW25113 were used for bacteriolytic activity assays, while the *E. coli* FB8 Δ*lysA*::kan was used for *meso*-[^{14}C]A_2pm incorporation experiments [24]. The *Pectobacterium carotovorum* ssp. *carotovorum* strain PC1 was kindly provided by Dr. Iris Yedidia [26]. The construction of the plasmid vector pET2160, a pET21d derivative allowing the expression of proteins with a C-terminal 6× histidine tag (His_6), has been previously described [11]. The pREP4groESL plasmid allowing overexpression of the bacterial chaperones was obtained from Amrein, K., et al. [27]. The pASK-IBA4 vector was used for the export of proteins to the periplasm of *E. coli*, as described previously [22]. For cloning experiments, protein production and lysis experiments, cells were grown aerobically at 37 °C in 2YT medium [28], whereas they were grown in M63 minimum medium supplemented with 0.4% glucose and 100 μg/mL each of lysine, threonine and methionine for *meso*-[^{14}C]A_2pm incorporation experiments [2,24]. When needed, ampicillin and kanamycin were used at 100 and 50 μg/mL, respectively. Growth was monitored at 600 nm with a Shimadzu UV-1601 spectrophotometer.

4.2. Molecular Biology Techniques

Polymerase chain reaction (PCR) amplification of genes was performed in a Thermocycler 60 apparatus (Bio-Med, Guilford, CT, USA) using the Expand-Fidelity polymerase (Roche Applied Science, Indianapolis, IN, USA). DNA fragments were purified with the Wizard PCR Preps DNA purification kit (Promega, Charbonnières-les-Bains, France), and standard procedures for DNA digestion, ligation, agarose gel electrophoresis and plasmid isolations were used [29]. *E. coli* cells were transformed with plasmid DNA by the method of Dagert and Ehrlich [30] or by electroporation.

4.3. Construction of Expression Plasmids

A plasmid allowing high-level overproduction of the ColM homologue gene from *P. carotovorum* (*pcaM*) was constructed as follows: PCR primers Pcam-O1 and Pcam-O2 (Table 3) were designed to incorporate NcoI and BglII sites at the 5′ and 3′ extremities of the gene, respectively. The gene was amplified from the PC1 strain chromosome, and the DNA fragment was treated with NcoI and BglII and ligated between the same sites of the vector pET2160. The resulting plasmid, pMLD365, allowed the expression of the protein with a His_6-tag (Arg-Ser-His_6 extension) at the C-terminal extremity. To produce the D222A catalytic point mutant of PcaM1, site-directed mutagenesis of the C-terminal His_6-tagged protein was performed directly on the pMLD365 expression plasmid by using the QuikChange II XL mutagenesis kit (Stratagene, La Jolla, CA, USA), using the pair of complementary nucleotides Pcam-mut1 and Pcam-mut2. This yielded the pMLD464 plasmid.

Table 3. Oligonucleotides used in this study.

Oligonucleotides	Sequence [a]
Pcam-O1	5′-CGCG**CC<u>ATG</u>G**CTACTTATAAAATTAAAGATTTGACAGG-3′ (NcoI)
Pcam-O2	5′-CGCG**AGATCT**TAAACGCTGACCACGCCCAGAAATATC-3′ (BglII)
Pcam-O3	5′-CGCG**AAGCTT**ATAAACGCTGACCACGCCCAGAAATATC-3′ (HindIII)
Pcam-mut1	5′-GGATTCGTGCTTATAATGCTCTTTATGATGCCAATCCC-3′
Pcam-mut2	5′-GGGATTGGCATCATAAAGAGCATTATAAGCACGAATCC-3′
Pcam-Δ1-107	5′-CGCG**CC<u>ATG</u>G**GATTACTTGGTGGCAACGATTCTCCAG-3′ (NcoI)

[a] Restriction sites (in bold) introduced in oligonucleotides are indicated in parentheses, and the initiation codon of *pcaM* gene and derivatives is underlined.

Export of the PcaM protein to the periplasm of *E. coli* was obtained by fusing the sequence of this bacteriocin to that of the signal peptide of OmpA, using the pASK-IBA4 plasmid as the vector. The gene was amplified with Pcam-O1 and Pcam-O3 primers, and the fragment was cleaved by NcoI and HindIII and inserted between the same sites of pASK-IBA4, yielding the pMLD381 plasmid. Plasmid pMLD395, a pMLD381 derivative plasmid expressing the D222A PcaM1 mutant, was generated by site-directed mutagenesis using the Pcam-mut1 and Pcam-mut2 oligonucleotides. Plasmid pMLD403, a pASK-IBA4 derivative plasmid expressing an N-terminally-truncated PcaM1 variant lacking the first 107 residues, was generated as described for pMLD381, except that the oligonucleotides used for PCR gene amplification were the Pcam-Δ1-107 and Pcam-O3 primers.

4.4. Production and Purification of Wild-Type and Mutant Forms of PcaM1

For the expression of wild-type and mutant PcaM1 proteins, C43(DE3) cells were transformed with the pMLD365 or pMLD464 plasmid, respectively, as well as with the chaperone-expressing plasmid pREP4groESL. Cells were grown at 37 °C in 2YT medium supplemented with ampicillin and kanamycin (1-liter cultures), and when the optical density at 600 nm (OD_{600}) of the culture reached 0.8, isopropyl-β-D-thiogalactopyranoside (IPTG) was added at a final concentration of 1 mM and growth continued at 22 °C overnight. Then, the cells were harvested, washed with 40 mL of an 0.9% NaCl solution and finally suspended in 12 mL of Buffer A (20 mM Tris-HCl, pH 7.2, 200 mM NaCl, 0.1% 2-mercaptoethanol, 0.5 mM $MgCl_2$ and 10% glycerol). In each case, the bacterial suspension was disrupted by sonication (Bioblock Vibracell sonicator, model 72412, Fisher Scientific, Illkirch, France) and then centrifuged at 4 °C for 30 min at 200,000× *g* in a TL100 Beckman centrifuge. The wild-type or mutant PcaM1-containing supernatant was subjected to purification.

His_6-tagged wild-type and mutant forms of PcaM1 were purified first by affinity chromatography on nickel-nitrilotriacetate (Ni^{2+}-NTA)-agarose polymer (Qiagen®, Courtaboeuf, France). All procedures were performed at 4 °C. The crude soluble supernatant obtained according to the procedure described above was mixed with 2 mL of polymer pre-equilibrated with Buffer A containing 10 mM imidazole and incubated for 30 min at 4 °C according to the Qiagen® recommendations. Then, the washing and elution steps were performed with a discontinuous gradient of imidazole (20–200 mM) in Buffer A. Eluted proteins were analyzed by sodium dodecyl sulfate-polyacrylamide gel electrophoresis (SDS-PAGE). The relevant fractions were pooled, concentrated to a volume of 5 mL by centrifugation on a 10-kDa cut-off membrane (Amicon Ultra, Millipore, Molsheim, France) and then submitted to an extra purification step by gel filtration (Äkta Prime system, ©GE Healthcare, Buckinghamshire, UK) on a Hi-Load 16/600 Superdex S200 column (©GE) pre-equilibrated with one column volume of Buffer A without $MgCl_2$ and glycerol and previously calibrated with blue dextran, conalbumin, ovalbumin, carbonic anhydrase, ribonuclease, aprotinine and tyrosine. Elution was performed with the same buffer at a flow rate of 1 mL/min. The purity of the fractions corresponding to the PcaM1 elution peak was checked by SDS-PAGE, and the final protein concentration was determined by using a NanoDrop™ 1000 spectrophotometer (Thermo Scientific, Wilmington, DE, USA). The absorption spectra of purified wild-type and mutant forms of PcaM1 were determined using a Jasco V-630 spectrophotometer. Glycerol (10% v/v, final concentration) was eventually added for storage of the protein at −20 °C.

4.5. Hydrolase Activity Assays

The PcaM1 enzymatic activity was tested in a reaction mixture (10 μL) containing 100 mM Tris-HCl, pH 7.5, 20 mM $MgCl_2$, 150 mM NaCl, 10 mM 2-mercaptoethanol, 12 μM [^{14}C]radiolabeled lipid II (140 Bq) and 0.2% *n*-dodecyl-β-D-maltopyranoside (DDM), as previously described [11]. The reaction was started by the addition of the purified protein (in 5 μL of Buffer A) and incubated for 30 min at 37 °C with shaking (Thermomixer, Eppendorf, Wesseling-Berzdorf, Germany). For the determination of the Michaelis constants (K_m), assay conditions were as described above, except that the concentration of lipid II varied from 6–100 μM. The reaction was stopped by heating at 95 °C for

1 min, and mixtures were analyzed by thin-layer chromatography (TLC) on pre-coated silica gel 60 F_{254} plates (Merck, Molsheim, France) using 1-propanol/ammonium hydroxide/water (6:3:1; v/v/v) as the mobile phase. The radioactive spots corresponding to the substrate (lipid II) and product (1-PP-MurNAc [pentapeptide]-GlcNAc) were located (R_f = 0.7 and 0.3, respectively) and quantified with a radioactivity scanner (Rita Star, Raytest Isotopenmeßgeräte GmbH, Straubenhardt, Germany).

4.6. Bacteriolytic Activity Assays on E. coli

FB8, BW25113 and BW25113 Δ*fkpA E. coli* strains, carrying pASK-derived plasmids for periplasmic expression of full-length, truncated or mutant PcaM1, were grown aerobically at 37 °C in 2YT-ampicillin medium (50-mL cultures). When the OD_{600} reached 0.2, anhydrotetracycline was added at various final concentrations (from 0–400 ng/mL), and cell growth was followed by monitoring the absorbance at constant time intervals.

4.7. CFU

E. coli FB8 strains carrying the pASK plasmids allowing expression of the wild-type and D222A mutant forms of PcaM1 were grown in 2YT medium, and cultures were induced or not with 200 ng/mL of anhydrotetracycline when the OD_{600} reached 0.2. Samples were taken every 20 min and plated on 2YT agar after appropriate serial dilutions. Colonies were counted after overnight incubation at 37 °C. These experiments were performed in triplicate, for both strains and both induced and uninduced conditions.

4.8. Peptidoglycan Labeling Experiments with Radioactive meso-[^{14}C]A_2pm

To determine whether cells expressing wild-type or mutant forms of PcaM1 in the periplasm were truly impaired in peptidoglycan biosynthesis, the rate of incorporation of *meso*-[^{14}C]A_2pm into the peptidoglycan of *E. coli* FB8 Δ*lysA*::kan strain transformed with pASK-IBA4, pMLD381 or pMLD395 expression plasmid was followed. The latter strains were grown exponentially in minimum M63 medium (30-mL cultures) supplemented with 0.4% glucose and 100 μg/mL each of lysine, methionine and threonine [2,24]. In fact, only lysine is required to complement the *lysA*::kan mutation of these strains, but the addition of methionine and threonine was used here to decrease as much as possible the internal cellular pool of A_2pm, as described previously [24,31]. When the OD_{600} reached 0.2, cultures were treated with anhydrotetracycline (100 ng/mL), and *meso*-[^{14}C]A_2pm (0.2 kBq/mL) was added 10 min later. The incorporation of *meso*-[^{14}C]A_2pm into the peptidoglycan polymer was then followed as described previously [2]. Briefly, 1-mL culture samples were collected regularly over time and added to 10 mL of ice-cold 5% trichloroacetic acid (TCA). Suspensions were kept on ice for 60 min, and the TCA-insoluble radiolabeled peptidoglycan material was then filtered over Whatman GF/C glass fiber filters. The filters were washed with 5% TCA and dried, and the radioactivity was counted with a liquid scintillation spectrophotometer after their immersion in a solvent system consisting of 2 mL of water and 13 mL of Unisafe 1 scintillator (Zinsser Analytic, Maidenhead, UK).

4.9. Cellular Distribution of meso-[^{14}C]A_2pm

To identify the step in peptidoglycan synthesis that was affected following periplasmic expression of the PcaM1 variants, the cellular distribution of [^{14}C]A_2pm incorporated in these strains was analyzed in more detail. Fifty-milliliter cultures of FB8 Δ*lysA* strain transformed with pASK-IBA4, pMLD381 or pMLD395 expression plasmids were performed as above in M63-glucose minimal medium supplemented with lysine, threonine and methionine. At an OD_{600} of 0.2, anhydrotetracycline (100 ng/mL) was added and *meso*-[^{14}C]A_2pm (0.2 kBq/mL) 20 min thereafter. After 30 min of labeling, cultures were rapidly chilled to 0–4 °C, collected by centrifugation and the cell pellets suspended in 3 mL of boiling water. After 15 min at 100 °C, suspensions were chilled and centrifuged at 200,000× *g* for 20 min. The supernatant was lyophilized, and both the soluble (supernatant) and insoluble (pellet) fractions were suspended in 250 μL of water. The total radioactivity recovered in these two cell fractions was measured. The insoluble fraction is known to contain peptidoglycan and lipid intermediates I and II, as well as the soluble fraction *meso*-[^{14}C]A_2pm and the nucleotide precursors as labeled compounds [2]. Aliquots were analyzed by TLC on silica gel plates with 1-propanol/ammonium hydroxide/water (6:3:1; v/v/v) as the mobile phase. Under such conditions, peptidoglycan remains at the origin, and UDP-MurNAc-peptides, *meso*-[^{14}C]A_2pm and lipid intermediates migrated with R_f values of 0.35, 0.55 and 0.7, respectively. An additional spot (R_f of 0.3) corresponding to the lipid II degradation product 1-PP-MurNAc(pentapeptide)-GlcNAc was observed following the induction of PcaM1 expression.

4.10. Quantitation of C_{55}-P and Its Derivatives in Membranes of E. coli Strains Expressing Periplasmic PcaM1 and Derivatives

Cultures (100 mL) of *E. coli* strain FB8 expressing the different periplasmic PcaM1 variants were grown as described above, and cells were harvested just before the onset of lysis, i.e., about 40 min after the induction of protein expression by anhydrotetracycline. Isoprenoid extraction was performed from washed membrane cell pellets of the different tested strains according to two different procedures, as previously described [23]. Briefly, each culture was divided in two 50 mL samples, which were treated according to the Bligh and Dyer procedure [32] to directly quantify C_{55}-P and C_{55}-OH pool levels, or to Kato's procedure [33], to determine the C_{55}-PP pool level (through this procedure, C_{55}-PP is totally converted into C_{55}-P). The resulting isoprenoid-containing organic phases were subsequently submitted to HPLC analysis for quantitation, using an isocratic elution system (2-propanol:methanol 1:4 (v/v) containing 10 mM phosphoric acid) on a reverse-phase Nucleosil C18 column (5 μm, 250 × 4.6 mm). The flow rate was 0.6 mL/min, and the quantitation of isoprenoids, monitored at 210 nm, was performed with respect to commercial compounds previously injected as standards in the same conditions.

4.11. Optical Microscopy Analyses

Bacteria were visualized using a DMIRE2 optical microscope (Leica) equipped with a CCD camera (CoolSNAP HQ2, Roper Scientific, Martinsried, Germany).

4.12. MALDI-TOF Mass Spectrometry

MALDI-TOF mass spectra of the wild-type PcaM1 were recorded in the linear mode with delayed extraction on a PerSeptive Voyager-DE STR instrument (Applied Biosystems, Carlsbad, CA, USA) equipped with a 337-nm laser. Buffer and glycerol were removed from the samples by using a ZipTip C_4 pipette tip (Merck Millipore, Molsheim, France) according to the manufacturer's recommendations with slight modifications. Briefly, the bacteriocin was adsorbed on ZipTip, and after it was washed with 0.1% trifluoroacetic acid (TFA), the bacteriocin was eluted with 7.5 μL of 0.1% TFA in 70% acetonitrile. Subsequently, 1 μL of matrix solution (10 mg/mL sinapinic acid in 0.1% TFA-acetonitrile (70:30, v/v)) was deposited on the plate, followed by 0.3, 0.5 or 1 μL of concentrated bacteriocin. After evaporation of the solvents, spectra were recorded in the positive mode at an acceleration voltage of +25 kV and an extraction delay time of 300 ns. Carbonic anhydrase was used as an external calibrant.

4.13. Chemicals

[^{14}C]lipid II labeled in the GlcNAc moiety was prepared as described previously [2]. The lipid II used in this study was C_{55}-PP-MurNAc(L-Ala-γ-D-Glu-*meso*-A_2pm-D-Ala-D-Ala)-GlcNAc, where *meso*-A_2pm represents *meso*-diaminopimelic acid. C_{55}-PP, C_{55}-P and C_{55}-OH were purchased from the Institute of Biochemistry and Biophysics of the Polish Academy of Sciences (Warsaw, Poland) and *meso*-[^{14}C]A_2pm from the Commissariat à l'Energie Atomique (Saclay, France). *N*-Dodecyl-*β*-D-maltopyranoside (DDM) was from Anatrace (Maumee, OH, USA), isopropyl-*β*-D-thiogalactopyranoside (IPTG) from Eurogentec (Angers, France) and Ni^{2+}-nitrilotriacetate agarose from Qiagen (Courtaboeuf, France). Antibiotics and reagents were from Sigma-Aldrich (Saint-Quentin Fallavier, France). Synthesis of oligonucleotides and DNA sequencing were done by Eurofins Genomics (Ebersberg, Germany).

Acknowledgments: We thank Iris Yedidia for the PC1 strain and Magali Prigent (Station d'Imagerie, I2BC) for optical microscopy analyses. This work was supported by grants from the Centre National de la Recherche Scientifique and the University Paris-Sud (UMR 9198). We thank the Direction Générale de l'Armement (DGA) for the financial support to D.C.

Author Contributions: D.C., T.T., D.M.-L. and H.B. conceived of and designed the experiments. D.C., S.G., D.B., D.M.-L. and H.B. performed the experiments. D.C., D.M.-L., T.T. and H.B. analyzed the data. D.P., D.B. and A.B. contributed reagents/materials/analysis tools. H.B. wrote the paper with T.T.'s and D.M.-L.'s help.

Abbreviations

The following abbreviations are used in this manuscript:

PcaM1	pectocin M1
ColM	colicin M
Cmi	ColM immunity protein
meso-A_2pm	*meso*-diaminopimelic acid

References

1. Cascales, E.; Buchanan, S.K.; Duché, D.; Kleanthous, C.; Lloubès, R.; Postle, K.; Riley, M.; Slatin, S.; Cavard, D. Colicin biology. *Microbiol. Mol. Biol. Rev.* **2007**, *71*, 158–229. [CrossRef] [PubMed]
2. El Ghachi, M.; Bouhss, A.; Barreteau, H.; Touzé, T.; Auger, G.; Blanot, D.; Mengin-Lecreulx, D. Colicin M exerts its bacteriolytic effect via enzymatic degradation of undecaprenyl phosphate-linked peptidoglycan precursors. *J. Biol. Chem.* **2006**, *281*, 22761–22772. [CrossRef] [PubMed]
3. Killmann, H.; Videnov, G.; Jung, G.; Schwarz, H.; Braun, V. Identification of receptor binding sites by competitive peptide mapping: Phages T1, T5, and Φ80 and colicin M bind to the gating loop of FhuA. *J. Bacteriol.* **1995**, *177*, 694–698. [PubMed]
4. Braun, V.; Patzer, S.I.; Hantke, K. Ton-dependent colicins and microcins: Modular design and evolution. *Biochimie* **2002**, *84*, 365–380. [CrossRef]
5. Hullmann, J.; Patzer, S.I.; Römer, C.; Hantke, K.; Braun, V. Periplasmic chaperone FkpA is essential for imported colicin M toxicity. *Mol. Microbiol.* **2008**, *69*, 926–937. [CrossRef] [PubMed]
6. Helbig, S.; Patzer, S.I.; Schiene-Fischer, C.; Zeth, K.; Braun, V. Activation of colicin M by the FkpA prolyl *cis-trans* isomerase/chaperone. *J. Biol. Chem.* **2011**, *286*, 6280–6290. [CrossRef] [PubMed]
7. Gérard, F.; Brooks, M.A.; Barreteau, H.; Touzé, T.; Graille, M.; Bouhss, A.; Blanot, D.; van Tilbeurgh, H.; Mengin-Lecreulx, D. X-ray structure and site-directed mutagenesis analysis of the *Escherichia coli* colicin M immunity protein. *J. Bacteriol.* **2011**, *193*, 205–214. [CrossRef] [PubMed]
8. Usón, I.; Patzer, S.I.; Rodríguez, D.D.; Braun, V.; Zeth, K. The crystal structure of the dimeric colicin M immunity protein displays a 3D domain swap. *J. Struct. Biol.* **2012**, *178*, 45–53. [CrossRef] [PubMed]
9. Schöffler, H.; Braun, V. Transport across the outer membrane of *Escherichia coli* K12 via the FhuA receptor is regulated by the TonB protein of the cytoplasmic membrane. *Mol. Gen. Genet.* **1989**, *217*, 378–383. [CrossRef] [PubMed]
10. Pilsl, H.; Glaser, C.; Gross, P.; Killmann, H.; Olschläger, T.; Braun, V. Domains of colicin M involved in uptake and activity. *Mol. Gen. Genet.* **1993**, *240*, 103–112. [CrossRef] [PubMed]

11. Barreteau, H.; Bouhss, A.; Fourgeaud, M.; Mainardi, J.-L.; Touzé, T.; Gérard, F.; Blanot, D.; Arthur, M.; Mengin-Lecreulx, D. Human- and plant-pathogenic *Pseudomonas* species produce bacteriocins exhibiting colicin M-like hydrolase activity towards peptidoglycan precursors. *J. Bacteriol.* **2009**, *191*, 3657–3664. [CrossRef] [PubMed]
12. Grinter, R.; Roszak, A.W.; Cogdell, R.J.; Milner, J.J.; Walker, D. The crystal structure of the lipid II-degrading bacteriocin syringacin M suggests unexpected evolutionary relationships between colicin M-like bacteriocins. *J. Biol. Chem.* **2012**, *287*, 38876–38888. [CrossRef] [PubMed]
13. Barreteau, H.; Tiouajni, M.; Graille, M.; Josseaume, N.; Bouhss, A.; Patin, D.; Blanot, D.; Fourgeaud, M.; Mainardi, J.-L.; Arthur, M.; et al. Functional and structural characterization of PaeM, a colicin M-like bacteriocin produced by *Pseudomonas aeruginosa*. *J. Biol. Chem.* **2012**, *287*, 37395–37405. [CrossRef] [PubMed]
14. Grinter, R.; Milner, J.; Walker, D. Ferredoxin containing bacteriocins suggest a novel mechanism of iron uptake in *Pectobacterium* spp. *PLoS ONE* **2012**, *7*, e33033. [CrossRef] [PubMed]
15. Grinter, R.; Josts, I.; Zeth, K.; Roszak, A.W.; McCaughey, L.C.; Cogdell, R.J.; Milner, J.J.; Kelly, S.M.; Byron, O.; Walker, D. Structure of the atypical bacteriocin pectocin M2 implies a novel mechanism of protein uptake. *Mol. Microbiol.* **2014**, *93*, 234–246. [CrossRef] [PubMed]
16. Shimizu, K.; Sekiguchi, M. Introduction of an active enzyme into permeable cells of *Escherichia coli*: Acquisition of ultraviolet light resistance by uvr mutants on introduction of T4 endonuclease V. *Mol. Gen. Genet.* **1979**, *168*, 37–47. [CrossRef] [PubMed]
17. Braun, V.; Frenz, J.; Hantke, K.; Schaller, K. Penetration of colicin M into cells of *Escherichia coli*. *J. Bacteriol.* **1980**, *142*, 162–168. [PubMed]
18. Espesset, D.; Corda, Y.; Cunningham, K.; Bénedetti, H.; Lloubès, R.; Lazdunski, C.; Géli, V. The colicin A pore-forming domain fused to mitochondrial intermembrane space sorting signals can be functionally inserted into the *Escherichia coli* plasma membrane by a mechanism that bypasses the Tol proteins. *Mol. Microbiol.* **1994**, *13*, 1121–1131. [CrossRef] [PubMed]
19. Duché, D. The pore-forming domain of colicin A fused to a signal peptide: A tool for studying pore-formation and inhibition. *Biochimie* **2002**, *84*, 455–464. [CrossRef]
20. Schleifer, K.H.; Kandler, O. Peptidoglycan types of bacterial cell walls and their taxonomic implications. *Bacteriol. Rev.* **1972**, *36*, 407–477. [PubMed]
21. Barreteau, H.; Bouhss, A.; Gérard, F.; Duché, D.; Boussaid, B.; Blanot, D.; Lloubès, R.; Mengin-Lecreulx, D.; Touzé, T. Deciphering the catalytic domain of colicin M, a peptidoglycan lipid II-degrading enzyme. *J. Biol. Chem.* **2010**, *285*, 12378–12389. [CrossRef] [PubMed]
22. Barnéoud-Arnoulet, A.; Barreteau, H.; Touzé, T.; Mengin-Lecreulx, D.; Lloubès, R.; Duché, D. Toxicity of the colicin M catalytic domain exported to the periplasm is FkpA independent. *J. Bacteriol.* **2010**, *192*, 5212–5219. [CrossRef] [PubMed]
23. Barreteau, H.; Magnet, S.; El Ghachi, M.; Touzé, T.; Arthur, M.; Mengin-Lecreulx, D.; Blanot, D. Quantitative high-performance liquid chromatography analysis of the pool levels of undecaprenyl phosphate and its derivatives in bacterial membranes. *J. Chromatogr. B* **2009**, *877*, 213–220. [CrossRef] [PubMed]
24. Mengin-Lecreulx, D.; Siegel, E.; van Heijenoort, J. Variations in UDP-*N*-acetylglucosamine and UDP-*N*-acetylmuramyl-pentapeptide pools in *Escherichia coli* after inhibition of protein synthesis. *J. Bacteriol.* **1989**, *171*, 3282–3287. [PubMed]
25. Patin, D.; Barreteau, H.; Auger, G.; Magnet, S.; Crouvoisier, M.; Bouhss, A.; Touzé, T.; Arthur, M.; Mengin-Lecreulx, D.; Blanot, D. Colicin M hydrolyses branched lipids II from Gram-positive bacteria. *Biochimie* **2012**, *94*, 985–990. [CrossRef] [PubMed]
26. Yishay, M.; Burdman, S.; Valverde, A.; Luzzatto, T.; Ophir, R.; Yedidia, I. Differential pathogenicity and genetic diversity among *Pectobacterium carotovorum* ssp. *carotovorum* isolates from monocot and dicot hosts support early genomic divergence within this taxon. *Environ. Microbiol.* **2008**, *10*, 2746–2759. [PubMed]
27. Amrein, K.E.; Takacs, B.; Stieger, M.; Molnos, J.; Flint, N.A.; Burn, P. Purification and characterization of recombinant human p50^{csk} protein-tyrosine kinase from an *Escherichia coli* expression system overproducing the bacterial chaperones GroES and GroEL. *Proc. Natl. Acad. Sci. USA* **1995**, *92*, 1048–1052. [CrossRef] [PubMed]
28. Miller, J.H. *Experiments in Molecular Genetics*; Cold Spring Harbor laboratory Press: Cold Spring Harbor, New York, NY, USA, 1972.

29. Sambrook, J.; Fritsch, E.F.; Maniatis, T. *Molecular Cloning: A Laboratory Manual*, 2nd ed.; Cold Spring Harbor laboratory Press: Cold Spring Harbor, New York, NY, USA, 1989.
30. Dagert, M.; Ehrlich, S.D. Prolonged incubation in calcium chloride improves the competence of *Escherichia coli* cells. *Gene* **1979**, *6*, 23–28. [CrossRef]
31. Wientjes, F.B.; Pas, E.; Taschner, P.E.; Woldringh, C.L. Kinetics of uptake and incorporation of *meso*-diaminopimelic acid in different *Escherichia coli* strains. *J. Bacteriol.* **1985**, *164*, 331–337. [PubMed]
32. Bligh, E.G.; Dyer, W.J. A rapid method of total lipid extraction and purification. *Can. J. Biochem. Physiol.* **1959**, *37*, 911–917. [CrossRef] [PubMed]
33. Kato, J.; Fujisaki, S.; Nakajima, K.; Nishimura, Y.; Sato, M.; Nakano, A. The *Escherichia coli* homologue of yeast RER2, a key enzyme of dolichol synthesis, is essential for carrier lipid formation in bacterial cell wall synthesis. *J. Bacteriol.* **1999**, *181*, 2733–2738. [PubMed]

2

Comparison of *Staphylococcus* Phage K with Close Phage Relatives Commonly Employed in Phage Therapeutics

Jude Ajuebor [1], Colin Buttimer [1], Sara Arroyo-Moreno [1], Nina Chanishvili [2], Emma M. Gabriel [1], Jim O'Mahony [1], Olivia McAuliffe [3], Horst Neve [4], Charles Franz [4] and Aidan Coffey [1,5,*]

1. Department of Biological Sciences, Cork Institute of Technology, Bishopstown, Cork T12 P928, Ireland; jude.ajuebor@mycit.ie (J.A.); colin.buttimer@mycit.ie (C.B.); sara.arroyo-moreno@mycit.ie (S.A.-M.); emma.gabriel@mycit.ie (E.M.G.); Jim.OMahony@cit.ie (J.O.)
2. Eliava Institute of Bacteriophages, Microbiology and Virology, Tbilisi 0160, Georgia; nina.chanishvili@pha.ge
3. Teagasc, Moorepark Food Research Centre, Fermoy, Cork P61 C996, Ireland; Olivia.McAuliffe@teagasc.ie
4. Department of Microbiology and Biotechnology, Max Rubner-Institut, DE-24103 Kiel, Germany; horst.neve@mri.bund.de (H.N.); charles.franz@mri.bund.de (C.F.)
5. Alimentary Pharmabiotic Centre, University College, Cork T12 YT20, Ireland

* Correspondence: aidan.coffey@cit.ie

Abstract: The increase in antibiotic resistance in pathogenic bacteria is a public health danger requiring alternative treatment options, and this has led to renewed interest in phage therapy. In this respect, we describe the distinct host ranges of *Staphylococcus* phage K, and two other K-like phages against 23 isolates, including 21 methicillin-resistant *S. aureus* (MRSA) representative sequence types representing the Irish National MRSA Reference Laboratory collection. The two K-like phages were isolated from the *Fersisi* therapeutic phage mix from the Tbilisi Eliava Institute, and were designated B1 (vB_SauM_B1) and JA1 (vB_SauM_JA1). The sequence relatedness of B1 and JA1 to phage K was observed to be 95% and 94% respectively. In terms of host range on the 23 *Staphylococcus* isolates, B1 and JA1 infected 73.9% and 78.2% respectively, whereas K infected only 43.5%. Eleven open reading frames (ORFs) present in both phages B1 and JA1 but absent in phage K were identified by comparative genomic analysis. These ORFs were also found to be present in the genomes of phages (Team 1, vB_SauM-fRuSau02, Sb_1 and ISP) that are components of several commercial phage mixtures with reported wide host ranges. This is the first comparative study of therapeutic staphylococcal phages within the recently described genus *Kayvirus*.

Keywords: phage isolation; bacteriophage; phage resistance; MRSA; *Staphylococcus*; *Kayvirus*

---

1. Introduction

Staphylococcus aureus (*S. aureus*) is an opportunistic and important pathogen in clinical and health-care settings causing a wide variety of diseases commonly involving the skin, soft tissue, bone, and joints [1]. It is also a well-known causative agent of prosthetic joint infections (PJI), cardiac device infections, and intravascular catheter infections [1]. *S. aureus* pathogenicity is due, in part, to its ability to acquire and express a wide array of virulence factors, as well as antimicrobial resistance determinants [2], an example of which involves the acquisition of the staphylococcal cassette chromosome (SCCmec) leading to the development of methicillin resistance in *S. aureus* [3]. Methicillin-resistant *S. aureus* (MRSA) was first reported in 1961 [4], and has since been observed to cause serious infections in hospitals worldwide. Reports of MRSA clones resistant to the majority of antibiotics are a growing concern [5]. As such, new treatment options are needed.

Bacteriophages (phages) are biological entities composed of either DNA or RNA enclosed within a protein coat [6]. They are highly specific, with most phages capable of infecting only a single bacterial species [6,7], and studies on these viruses have been performed since the late 19th century [8]. The phage infection process usually begins with the recognition of the receptor on the bacterial cell surface by its receptor binding protein [9]. In natural environments bacterial hosts have evolved many mechanisms to protect themselves from phage attack to include; adsorption blocking, DNA injection blocking, restriction-modification system (R/M), abortive infection, and the clustered regularly interspaced short palindromic repeats (CRISPR)-Cas systems [10,11]. In turn, phages have evolved several strategies for overcoming these systems to ensure their survival in the phage-host co-evolutionary race [12–14].

The use of phages as therapeutics to eliminate pathogenic bacteria dates back to experiments conducted by Felix d'Herelle in 1919 at a French hospital to treat dysentery [15]. Since then, a wide range of phage therapy trials have been undertaken, many with very promising results [15,16]. Pyophage and Intesti-phage are among the commercial phage mixtures currently produced at the Eliava Institute. Metagenomic studies on these phage mixtures have been reported [17,18] and the staphylococcal phages Sb-1 and ISP are key components of Pyophage [19,20]. Other phages isolated from these commercial phages mixes have also been reported [21–24]. Phages like vB_SauM-fRuSau02 was isolated from a phage mix produced by Microgen (Moscow, Russia) [21] and Team 1 was isolated from PhageBioDerm, a wound healing preparation consisting of a biodegradable polymer impregnated with an antibiotic and lytic phages [22–24]. These phages all possess a wide host range against a number of clinically relevant *S. aureus* isolates, demonstrating the efficacy of such commercial phage mixtures in treating a range of bacterial infections [19–24].

In this paper, we employed another phage mixture from the Eliava Institute, namely the Fersisi phage mix. Fersisi is a relatively new combination developed approximately 15–20 years ago on the basis of Pyophage, although with fewer phage components. Two phages from this mix were designated B1 (vB_SauM_B1) and JA1 (vB_SauM_JA1). Phage K, on the other hand, is a well-known phage being the type phage of the recently designated genus *Kayvirus* of the subfamily *Spounavirinae* [25]. The exact origin of phage K is unknown, but descriptions of the phage are made as far back as 1949 [26,27]. An initial host range study involving this phage reported it to be ineffective against many MRSA strains [26]. Thus, phages B1 and JA1 were compared (on the basis of their host range) to phage K to explore possible host range differences and it was observed that both phages had broader host ranges. A comparative study was performed on their genomes and the genomes of similar phages from other commercial phage mixtures (Team 1, vB_SauM-fRuSau02, Sb_1 and ISP) with reported wide host ranges, to provide molecular insight into the differences in host range encountered in this study.

2. Results and Discussion

2.1. Origin of Phages B1 and JA1

Phages B1 and JA1 were isolated from the Fersisi commercial phage mixtures; batch 010112 (B1) and F-062015 (JA1). This product is used in the treatment of staphylococcal and streptococcal infections. For the isolation of B1, phage enrichment was carried out using staphylococcal host cultured from the sonicate fluid of a hospital patient suffering from PJI. DPC5246 was subsequently used as propagating host for B1, as a prophage was encountered in the PJI strain. Phage enrichment in the isolation of JA1 was done using the Cork Institute of Technology (CIT) collection strain *S. aureus* CIT281189. Both the PJI strain and CIT281189 were insensitive to phage K.

2.2. Morphology and Host Range of Phages K, B1 and JA1

Phages B1 and JA1 exhibited typical characteristics of phages belonging to the *Myoviridae* family, similar to the reported morphology of phage K [26]. All three phages possessed an A1 morphology [28], displaying an icosahedral head as well as a long contractile tail. They also contained a structure previously described as knob-like appendages by O'Flaherty et al. [26], extending from their base plates (likely "clumped/aggregated" base plate appendices) and clearly visible in Figure 1. Estimations were made on the dimensions of these phages (Table 1). Capsid heights were estimated as 92.9 ± 4.0 nm (B1), 87.0 ± 2.1 nm (JA1) and 92.9 ± 3.8 nm (K). Tail dimension were also estimated as $233.0 \pm 4.4 \times 23.4 \pm 1.2$ nm (B1), $231.5 \pm 4.7 \times 22.7 \pm 0.9$ nm (JA1), and $227.5 \pm 5.5 \times 23.8 \pm 1.0$ nm (K), and base plates/knobs complexes were estimated as $30.1 \pm 1.8 \times 47.2 \pm 3.7$ nm (B1), $32.5 \pm 7.9 \times 45.8 \pm 1.4$ nm (JA1), and $36.6 \pm 5.1 \times 41.7 \pm 2.6$ nm (K). Owing to the similar morphology of all three phages, a host range study was conducted to explore possible differences in host spectra across a number of hospital isolates. Twenty-one of these isolates represented the entire collection of MRSA sequence-types identified in Ireland by the National MRSA Reference Laboratory (Dublin, Ireland), and includes the commonly encountered ST22-MRSA-IV, which has been predominant in Irish hospitals since the late 1990s [29]. The other two *S. aureus* strains used in this study were included as additional phage propagation strains. Host range was assessed by plaque assay technique on lawns of various MRSA strains listed in Table 2. The efficiency of plaquing (EOP) was used to represent the degree to which each of the phages studied infected all 23 staphylococcal strains. Phage JA1 had the broadest host range, forming plaques on 18 out of the 23 staphylococcal strains examined. B1 also had a broad host range and was capable of forming plaques on 17 isolates (with some in common with the 18 lysed by phage JA1). Phage K had the narrowest host range, forming plaques on only 10 of the isolates (including its propagating strain DPC5246). All 23 staphylococcal strains were effectively lysed by at least one of the three phages, with the exception of E1139 (IV) ST45 and E1185 (IV) ST12, whose EOP were significantly low at 3.88×10^{-6} and 1.16×10^{-6} respectively; as well as 3488 (VV) ST8, which was resistant to all three phages. Plaque size ranged from 0.5 mm to 1.5 mm, with a halo occurring in some instances (Table 3 and Supplementary Materials, Figure S1). The wide host range encountered in this study is common among K-like phages and has been reported for other staphylococcal K-like phages, such as JD007, which infected 95% of *S. aureus* isolates obtained from several hospitals in Shanghai, China [30].

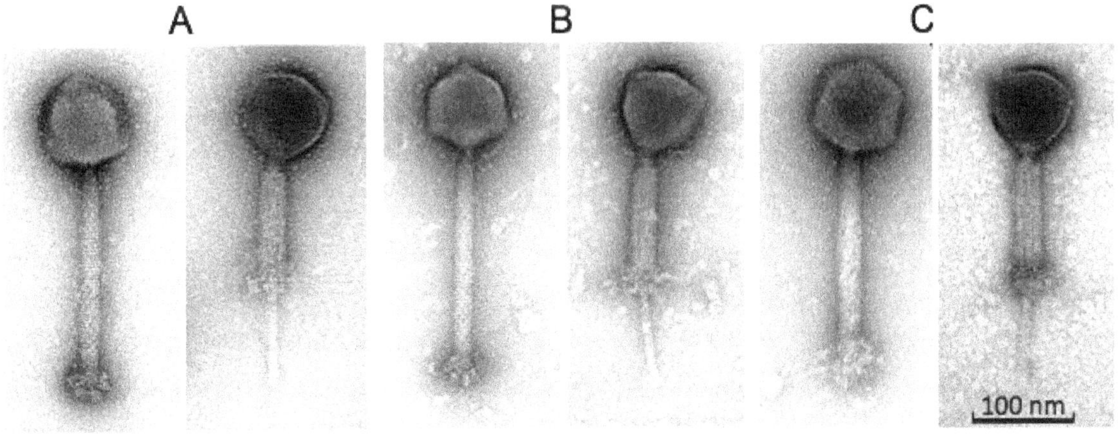

Figure 1. Transmission electron micrographs of phages B1 (**A**), JA1 (**B**), and K (**C**) showing their icosahedral capsid and their long contractile tail (both extended and contracted)

Table 1. Dimensions of staphylococcal phages B1, JA1, and K derived from micrographs obtained from transmission electron microscopy.

Phages	Head (nm)	Tail Length (nm) (incl. "knob")	Tail Width (nm)	Baseplate "knob" Length (nm)	Baseplate "knob" Width (nm)
B1	92.9 ± 4.0 (n = 11)	233.0 ± 4.4 (n = 12)	23.4 ± 1.2 (n = 12)	30.1 ± 1.8 (n = 12)	47.2 ± 3.7 (n = 10)
JA1	87.0 ± 2.1 (n = 9)	231.5 ± 4.7 (n = 9)	22.7 ± 0.9 (n = 9)	32.5 ± 7.9 (n = 9)	45.8 ± 1.4 (n = 9)
K	92.9 ± 3.8 (n = 16)	227.5 ± 5.5 (n = 16)	23.8 ± 1.0 (n = 16)	36.6 ± 5.1 (n = 16)	41.7 ± 2.6 (n = 16)

Table 2. Host ranges of staphylococcal phages B1, JA1, and K against methicillin-resistant *Staphylococcus aureus* (MRSA) strains from the Irish National Reference Laboratory (St. James's Hospital Dublin, Ireland) including the efficiency of plaquing (EOP) of these strains.

S. aureus Strain	Phage K	Phage B1	Phage JA1
DPC5246*	1.00 ± 0.0	1.00 ± 0.0	8.98×10^{-1} ± 0.8
CIT281189*	No infection	No infection	1.00 ± 0.0
0.0066 (IIIV) ST239	No infection	No infection	2.59 ± 2.5
0.1206 (IV) ST250	No infection	3.89×10^{-1} ± 0.3	1.35 ± 1.2
0.1239 (III) ST239	No infection	1.46×10^{-1} ± 0.1	4.17×10^{-2} ± 0.0
0.1345 (II) ST5	No infection	No infection	2.08×10^{-1} ± 0.1
0073 (III) ST239	No infection	3.21×10^{-1} ± 0.2	No infection
0104 (III) ST239	No infection	3.95×10^{-1} ± 0.2	1.82 ± 1.6
0220 (II) ST5	3.03×10^{-1} ± 0.1	2.17×10^{-1} ± 0.2	2.38×10^{-1} ± 0.2
0242 (IV) ST30	4.43×10^{-1} ± 0.1	5.23×10^{-1} ± 0.5	4.90×10^{-1} ± 0.3
0308 (IA) ST247	1.40 ± 0.2	1.36 ± 1.3	1.71 ± 1.6
3045 (IIV) ST8	No infection	4.93×10^{-2} ± 0.0	1.69 ± 0.7
3144 (IIV) ST8	No infection	1.21 ± 1.0	2.17 ± 1.2
3488 (VV) ST8	No infection	No infection	No infection
3581 (IA) ST247	No infection	No infection	9.26×10^{-1} ± 0.7
3594 (II) ST36	4.38×10^{-1} ± 0.1	8.67×10^{-1} ± 0.4	1.06 ± 0.7
3596 (IIV) ST8	2.49×10^{-4} ± 0.0	1.29 ± 0.9	3.59 ± 2.7
E1038 (IIV) ST8	1.27×10^{-4} ± 0.0	2.02×10^{-1} ± 0.2	1.89 ± 1.4
E1139 (IV) ST45	No infection	3.88×10^{-6} ± 0.0	No infection
E1174 (IV) ST22	7.03×10^{-1} ± 0.7	3.11×10^{-1} ± 0.2	No infection
E1185 (IV) ST12	1.16×10^{-6} ± 0.0	No infection	No infection
E1202 (II) ST496	No infection	4.79×10^{-1} ± 0.2	9.49×10^{-1} ± 0.8
M03/0073 (III) ST239	1.76 ± 0.5	1.51 ± 0.8	2.30 ± 0.7

* *S. aureus* strains for phage propagation; data is represented as means ± standard deviations based on triplicate measurements.

Table 3. Zone sizes and morphologies of B1, JA1, and K plaques formed on MRSA strains collected from the Irish National MRSA Reference Laboratory (St. James's Hospital Dublin, Ireland).

S. aureus Strain	Phage K	Phage B1	Phage JA1
DPC5246	2 mm	1 mm with halo to 2 mm	1 mm with halo to 2 mm
CIT281189	No plaques	No plaques	1.5 mm
0.0066 (IIV) ST239	No plaques	No plaques	1 mm
0.1206 (IV) ST250	No plaques	2 mm	0.5 mm with halo to 1 mm
0.1239 (III) ST239	No plaques	0.5 mm, faint plaques	1 mm
0.1345 (II) ST5	No plaques	No plaques	1 mm
0073 (III) ST239	No plaques	0.5 mm	No plaques
0104 (III) ST239	No plaques	0.5 mm	1 mm
0220 (II) ST5	0.5 mm	1 mm	1 mm
0242 (IV) ST30	1 mm	1.5 mm	1.5 mm
0308 (IA) ST247	1 mm	1 mm	0.5 mm, faint plaques
3045 (IIV) ST8	No plaques	1 mm	1 mm

Table 3. *Cont.*

S. aureus Strain	Phage K	Phage B1	Phage JA1
3144 (IIV) ST8	No plaques	1.5 mm, faint plaques	1 mm
3488 (VV) ST8	No plaques	0.5 mm, faint plaques	0.5 mm with halo to 1 mm
3581 (IA) ST247	No plaques	No plaques	1 mm
3594 (II) ST36	1.5 mm	1 mm	1.5 mm
3596 (IIV) ST8	0.5 mm	0.5 mm with halo to 1.5 mm	0.5 mm with halo to 1.5 mm
E1038 (IIV) ST8	0.5 mm, faint plaques	0.5 mm, faint plaques	1.5 mm
E1139 (IV) ST45	No plaques	0.5 mm, faint plaques	No plaques
E1174 (IV) ST22	0.5 mm, faint plaques	0.5 mm	No plaques
E1185 (IV) ST12	0.5 mm, faint plaques	No plaques	No plaques
E1202 (II) ST496	No plaques	1 mm	0.5 mm
M03/0073 (III) ST239	2 mm	0.5 mm with halo to 1.5 mm	0.5 mm with halo to 1.5 mm

2.3. Phage Adsorption on Phage Resistant Isolates

While some level of phage insensitivity was encountered against all three phages, phage K was the frequently insensitive virion to the *S. aureus* strains tested, and thus, was chosen to evaluate whether or not adsorption inhibition played a role in its insensitivity. Phage K was able to adsorb to all phage-insensitive strains to approximately the same extent as the propagating strain DPC5246. This rules out the possibility of adsorption inhibition playing a role in the narrow host range encountered with phage K in comparison to both phages B1 and JA1 (Supplementary Materials, Figure S2). Additionally, adsorption studies with phages B1 and JA1 indicated that adsorption did not play a role in the differences observed.

2.4. Genome Comparison between Phages B1, JA1, and K

The genome of phage K is 139,831 bp in size with long terminal repeats (LTRs) of 8486 bp [31]. Genomes of similar sizes were obtained for phages B1 and JA1, these being 140,808 bp and 139,484 bp, respectively. Examination of sequence reads allowed the identification of LTRs for these phages, due to the identification of a region within their genomes with roughly double the average number of reads, these regions being 8076 bp and 7651 bp in size for phages B1 and JA1, respectively. This approach to the determination of terminal repeats has been utilized for a number of phages [32–34]. The sequences of all three phages, when analyzed, contained the 12 bp inverted repeat sequences 5′-TAAGTACCTGGG-3′ and 5′-CCCAGGTACTTA-3′, which separates the LTRs from the non-redundant part of the phage DNA, and are characteristic of K-like phages [22,35]. Thus, the entire packaged genome sizes are 148,884 bp (B1), 147,135 bp (JA1), and 148,317 bp (K). Phage K possessed 212 ORFs in its genome [31,36], whereas phages B1 and JA1 possessed 219 (Supplementary Materials, Table S1) and 215 ORFs (Supplementary Materials, Table S2) respectively.

Nucleotide pairwise sequence alignment based on BLASTN revealed phages B1 and JA1 (including their LTRs) to be 99% identical to each other, thus can be considered different isolates of the same phage species [37]. On the other hand, phages B1 and JA1 (including their LTRs) showed 95% and 94% identity (respectively) to phage K, placing these phages on the boundary of speciation.

The examination of 100 bp sequences upstream of each ORFs on the non-redundant genome of these phages, using MEME [38], identified 44 and 43 RpoD-like promoters for phages B1 and JA1, respectively. It was observed that these promoters where heavily concentrated in regions with ORFs encoding short hypothetical proteins and those with functions associated with nucleotide metabolism and DNA replication, rather than those associated with virion structure (Supplementary Materials, Tables S3 and S4). A similar finding was also reported with K-like phage vB_SauM-fRuSau02 [21]. Additionally, 30 Rho-independent terminators were identified on the non-redundant genomes for both B1 and JA1 (Supplementary Materials, Tables S5 and S6).

Four ORFs present in phage B1 were observed to be absent in JA1 (Table 4). These ORFs encoded two putative terminal repeat-encoded proteins (PhageB1_009, 016) and two proteins of unknown function (phageB1_202, 203). Although both B1 and JA1 had similar content of ORFs with 1% difference between their genomes, both phages varied in their host range on the *S. aureus* strains they infected. This variation is likely attributed to the difference encountered in their genome. Additionally, multiple ORFs present in phage K but absent in both B1 and JA1 were encountered (Figure 2, Table 5). Furthermore, ORFs present in both phages B1 and JA1 but absent in K were also encountered (Figure 2, Table 6). These ORFs are discussed below.

Table 4. List of missing ORFs present in phage B1 but absent in phage JA1.

ORFs	Amino Acid Numbers	Protein Size (kDa)	Predicted Function
PhageB1_009	112	13.5	Terminal repeat encoded protein
PhageB1_016	107	12.4	Terminal repeat encoded protein
PhageB1_202	32	3.5	Unknown
PhageB1_203	104	11.6	Unknown

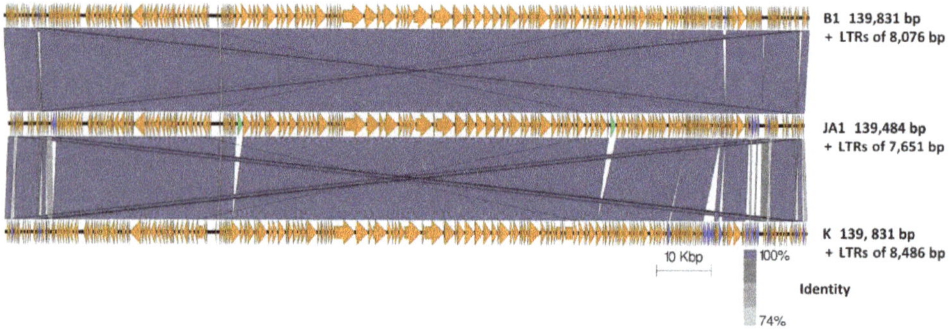

Figure 2. Genome comparison of phages B1, JA1, and K (including their long terminal repeats) using currently available annotations employing BLASTN and visualized with Easyfig. Regions of sequence similarity are connected by the shaded area, using a grey scale; genome maps consisting of orange arrows indicating the location of ORFs along the phage genomes, with unshared ORFs highlighted in blue with those indicating unshared homing endonuclease highlighted in green.

Table 5. List of missing ORFs and their predicted putative functions absent in both phages B1 and JA1 but present in phage K.

ORFs	Amino Acid Number	Protein Size (kDa)	Predicted Function
PhageK_004	108	12.7	Unknown
PhageK_016*	107	12.4	Unknown
PhageK_019	57	4.7	Unknown
PhageK_020	89	10.2	Unknown
PhageK_168	185	21.7	Predicted to contain a transmembrane region based on InterProScan
PhageK_187	101	11.7	Unknown
PhageK_188	123	13.8	Predicted to contain a transmembrane region based on InterProScan
PhageK_189	78	9.2	Unknown
PhageK_190	175	20.6	Predicted as a putative metallophoshatase
PhageK_191	106	12.9	Unknown
PhageK_192	76	8.9	Predicted to contain a transmembrane region based on InterProScan
PhageK_196	226	25.8	Unknown
PhageK_205	83	9.7	Unknown
PhageK_206	98	11.2	Unknown
PhageK_208	99	11.6	Unknown
PhageK_209	75	8.9	Unknown
PhageK_211	117	13.9	Predicted to possess a transmembrane region based on InterProScan
PhageK_212	128	15.6	Unknown

* ORF that phage JA1 does not share with phage K.

Table 6. List of missing ORFs and their predicted function absent in phage K but present in phages B1 and JA1.

ORFs	Amino Acid Number	Protein Size (kDa)	Predicted Function
PhageJA1_003 (PhageB1_003)	96	11.3	Unknown
PhageJA1_020 (PhageB1_022)	161	19.1	Unknown
PhageJA1_021 (PhageB1_023)	135	16.5	Unknown
PhageJA1_084 (PhageB1_087)	323	39.6	Predicted as a putative endonuclease interrupting the terminase large subunit [PhageJA1_083 (PhageB1_086) and PhageJA1_085 (PhageB1_088)]
PhageJA1_152 (PhageB1_155)	322	38.3	Predicted as a putative endonuclease containing a LAGLIDADG-like domain and an Intein splicing domain and interrupts the DNA repair protein [PhageJA1_151 (PhageB1_154) and PhageJA1_153 (PhageB1_156)]
PhageJA1_206 (PhageB1_212)	73	8.9	Unknown
PhageJA1_208 (PhageB1_214)	169	20.3	HHpred indicates homology to cell wall hydrolases
PhageJA1_209 (PhageB1_215)	109	12.6	Unknown
PhageJA1_211 (PhageB1_217)	104	12.0	Unknown
PhageJA1_212 (PhageB1_218)	55	6.5	Unknown
PhageJA1_213 (PhageB1_219)	33	3.7	Predicted to possess a transmembrane region based on InterProScan

2.4.1. Characteristic Features of Phage K ORFs Absent in Both JA1 and B1

Seventeen ORFs present in phage K were absent in both phages B1 and JA1, with one additional ORF found not to be shared between JA1 and K. These ORFs are listed in Table 5. No function could be assigned to these with the exception of phageK_190, which based on NCBI conserved domain search possessed a metallophosphatase-like domain (cd07390; E value; 3.94×10^{-30}) and is a member of the metallophosphatase (MPP) superfamily. Families within this superfamily of enzymes are functionally diverse, involved in the cleavage of phosphoester bonds, and include Mre11/SbcD-like exonucleases, Dbr1-like RNA lariat debranching enzymes, YfcE-like phosphodiesterases, purple acid phosphatases (PAPs), YbbF-like UDP-2,3-diacylglucosamine hydrolases, and acid sphingomyelinases (ASMases) [39].

2.4.2. Characteristic Features of Phages B1 and JA1 ORFs Absent in Phage K

Eleven ORFs present in both phages B1 and JA1 were absent in phage K (Table 6). No putative function could be assigned to the majority of these ORFs based on BLASTP, InterProScan or HHpred analysis, with the exception of phageJA1_084 (phageB1_087) and phageJA1_152 (phageB1_155), which encoded homing endonucleases interrupting both the terminase large subunit and the DNA repair protein, respectively. These homing endonucleases are site-specific DNA endonucleases capable of initiating DNA breaks leading to repair and recombination event that results in the integration of this endonuclease ORF into a gene that was previously lacking it [40]. The presence of these mobile genetic elements is common among known staphylococcal phages of the subfamily *Spounavirinae*, and these endonucleases ORFs are known to insert themselves into essential phage genes [21,41]. Additionally, HHpred analysis indicated ORFs PhageJA1_208 and PhageB1_214 to possess remote homology to cell-degrading proteins. The majority of these ORFs were found to be located next to the genome termini of JA1 and B1, with genes located in this region having been previously reported in similar phages to be expressed early in phage development [35]. Such proteins are usually involved in subversion of the host's machinery to aid phage takeover [42,43].

2.4.3. Comparison of Phages K, B1, and JA1 with other Similar Therapeutic Phages (Team1, vB_SauM-fRuSau02, Sb-1 and ISP)

Four additional staphylococcal phages that originate in commercial phage therapeutic mixtures are Team1, vB_SauM-fRuSau02, Sb-1 and ISP, as discussed earlier [19–24]. These phages were also reported to possess wide host ranges towards a number of clinically relevant *S. aureus* strains. Although similar, these phages have several feature differences from each other and from phages B1 and JA1. Comparison of nucleotide identities (BLASTN) with phage K shows that they belong to the genus *Kayvirus* (Supplementary Materials, Table S7) possessing genomes of similar sizes, apart from Sb-1, being smaller than would be expected, suggesting the genome submission may have been incomplete (Figure 3). Additionally, the arrangement of ORFs is quite similar. Furthermore, tRNA genes of these phages were also examined. All seven phages were found to possess the same four tRNA genes for methionine, tryptophan, phenylalanine, and aspartic acid (Supplementary Materials, Table S8). The eleven ORFs which were present in B1 and JA1 but absent in K (Table 6, Supplementary Materials, Figure S3) were similarly present in Team 1, vB_SauM-fRuSau02, Sb-1 and ISP. And likewise, the ORFs present in K, but absent in both B1 and JA1, were also missing in these phages. However, vB_SauM-fRuSau02 possesses a much shorter putative tail protein (RS_159) of 73 amino acids compared to the phage K counterpart (PhageK_151) of 170 amino acids. Non-hypothetical proteins that differed between these phages were a membrane protein (Phage B1_180, PhageJA1_177, and Phage_170) and an ATPase-like protein (Protein id: CCA65911.1 for phage ISP). Other ORFs that differed among these phages were mostly hypothetical proteins.

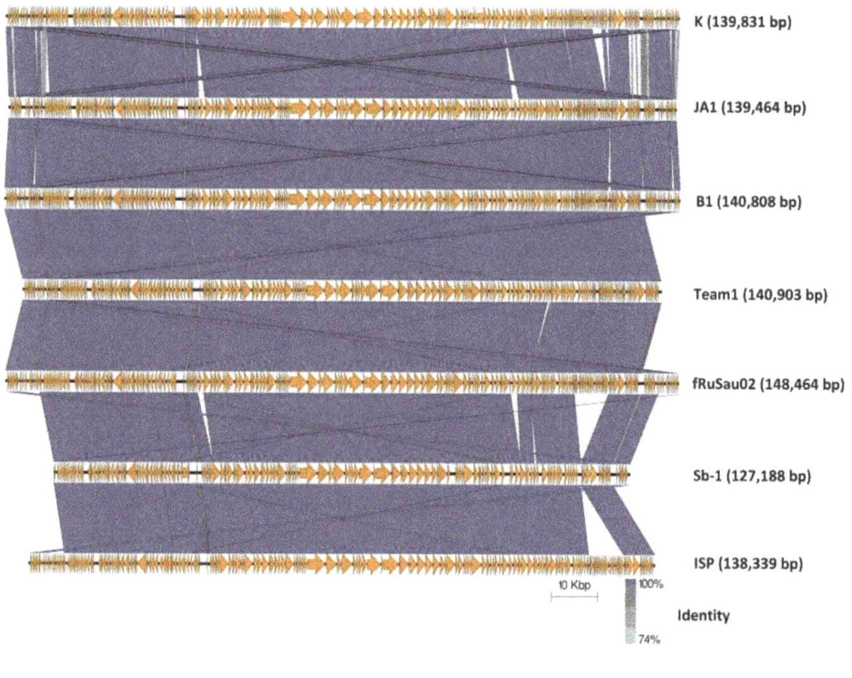

Figure 3. Genome comparison of phage K with the six staphylococcal phages employed in commercial phages mixture (B1, JA1, Team 1 [22–24], vB_SauM-fRuSau02 [21], Sb-1 [19] and ISP [20]) using currently available annotations employing BLASTN and visualized with Easyfig.

S. aureus employ several defense strategies against viral attack [10,44] and these, such as restriction modification systems [45] and CRISPR-Cas systems [46], may vary from strain to strain. These defenses along with several variations encountered at the genetic level across phages B1, JA1, and K may explain the differences in host ranges observed in this study.

3. Materials and Methods

3.1. Bacterial Strains, Phage and Growth Requirement

Phages B1 and JA1 were isolated from a commercial phage cocktail purchased from the George Eliava Institute of Bacteriophage, Microbiology and Virology, Tbilisi, Georgia. The MRSA strains utilized in this study were all acquired from the Irish National MRSA Reference Laboratory, Dublin, Ireland [2] with the exception of DPC5246 and CIT281189, which are routine propagation strains utilized in our laboratory [26,36]. These strains were routinely cultured in Brain Heart Infusion broth (BHI; Sigma, St. Louis, MO, USA) at 37 °C with shaking or on BHI plates containing 1.5% (*w/v*) bacteriological agar (Sigma). All strains were stocked in BHI containing 40% glycerol and stored at −80 °C.

3.2. CsCl Gradient Purification

Isopycnic centrifugation through CsCl gradients was performed as previously described [47], with a number of modifications. A high titer phage lysate (>1 × 10^9 plaque forming units [PFU] mL^{-1}), was precipitated using polyethylene glycol (15% *w/v* PEG8000, 1 M NaCl) at 4 °C overnight and centrifuged, after which the pellet was resuspended in TMN buffer (10 mM Tris-HCl pH 7.4, 10 mM $MgSO_4{\cdot}7H_2O$, 0.5 M NaCl). The resulting phage preparation was placed onto a CsCl step gradient composed of 1.3, 1.5, and 1.7 g/mL layers and spun in a 100 Ti rotor (Beckman Coulter, Brea, CA, USA) at 200,480 *g* for 3 h at 4 °C. The resulting phage preparations were dialyzed in Tris-HCl buffer (10 mM, pH 7.5) at 4 °C.

3.3. Phage Host Range and Adsorption Study

Host range assay was performed for phages B1, JA1, and K using the plaque assay plating technique (Tables 2 and 3). This was done in triplicate for three independent experiments. The efficiency of plaquing (EOP) was determined by dividing the phage titer on each test strain by the phage titer of the reference strain (*S. aureus* DPC5246, in the case of phages B1 and K, and *S. aureus* CIT281189 for phage JA1) [48]. An adsorption assay was performed according to the protocol previously described elsewhere with some modification [49]. Briefly, MRSA strains were grown to an optical density (OD) of 0.2 at 600 nm (estimated cell count at 10^8 colony forming unit (cfu) mL^{-1}) and 100 µL of cells were mixed with 100 µL of respective phage titered at approximately 1 × 10^7 PFU/mL for a multiplicity of infection (MOI) of 0.1. The resulting mixtures were incubated at room temperature for 5 min to allow for phage adsorption. The bound phages were separated from the free phages by centrifugation at 14,000 rpm for 5 min. Adsorption of the phage on each strain was determined by subtracting the number of unbound phage (per mL) from the total input PFU/mL. Adsorption efficiency was expressed as a percentage relative to the propagating strain DPC5246.

3.4. Transmission Electron Microscopy

Electron microscopic analysis was performed following negative staining of the CsCl gradient prepared phages on freshly prepared carbon films with 2% (*w/v*) uranyl acetate. Electron micrographs were taken using a Tecnai 10 transmission electron microscope (FEI Thermo Fisher, Eindhoven, the Netherlands) at an acceleration voltage of 80 kV with a MegaView G2 CDD camera (EMSIS, Muenster, Germany).

3.5. Phage DNA Isolation

Phage DNA extraction was performed on CsCl purified high titer phages. These were initially treated with $MgCl_2$ followed by pre-treatment with DNase and RNase for 60 min at 37 °C. Following that subsequent treatment with SDS, EDTA and proteinase K with further incubation for 60 min at 55 °C. DNA extractions were then performed on the pre-treated samples with phenol/chloroform/isoamyl alcohol (25:24:1 *v/v/v*) and chloroform/isoamyl alcohol (24:1 *v/v*). DNA precipitation was achieved using sodium acetate and 95% ethanol. DNA quality and quantity were estimated using a Nanodrop (ND-1000) and visualized following agarose gel electrophoresis

3.6. *Phage DNA Sequencing*

DNA sequencing was performed with a high throughput Illumina HiSeq system sequencing (GATC Biotech, Konstanz, Germany). Library preparation was performed by DNA fragmentation together with adapter ligation. The libraries were then measured and quantified on a Fragment Analyzer and then sequenced to generate 2 × 300 bp paired-end reads. *De novo* assembly was performed using CLC Bio Genomics Workbench v8.0 (Aarhus, Denmark).

3.7. *Bioinformatic Analysis*

Open reading frames (ORFs) for the sequenced phages were predicted with Glimmer [50] and GenemarkS [51]. Putative functions were assigned to these ORFs using BLASTP (https://blast.ncbi.nlm.nih.gov/Blast.cgi?PAGE=Proteins), HHpred (https://toolkit.tuebingen.mpg.de/#/tools/hhpred; [52]) and InterProscan (http://www.ebi.ac.uk/interpro/search/sequence-search; [53]). Transfer RNA was predicted using tRNAscan-SE (http://lowelab.ucsc.edu/tRNAscan-SE/; [54]) and ARAGORN (http://130.235.46.10/ARAGORN/; [55]). Potential promoters were predicted using MEME (Multiple Em for Motif Elicitation) (http://meme-suite.org/tools/meme; [38]), followed by manual curation. Potential Rho-independent terminators were identified using ARNold (http://rna.igmors.u-psud.fr/toolbox/arnold; [56]) with Mfold QuikFold (http://unafold.rna.albany.edu/?q=DINAMelt/Quickfold; [57]) using RNA energy rules 3.0 to verify predictions. Artemis Comparison Tool (ACT) was used for the identification of feature variations between the genomes of phages, with homology being assessed with BLASTN [58] Genome comparison maps between phages were visualized using the Easyfig visualization tool [59]. K-like *Staphylococcus* phages used in comparative studies were K (KF766114), Team 1 (KC012913), vB_SauM-fRuSau02 (MF398190), Sb-1 (HQ163896) and ISP (FR852584).

3.8. *Nucleotide Sequence Accession Number*

The genome sequence for phages B1 and JA1 were deposited into GenBank under the accession numbers MG656408 and MF405094, respectively.

4. Conclusions

Host range of three highly similar phages was performed in this study, and it was identified that phages B1 and JA1 from the Fersisi commercial phage mix had a much broader host range in comparison to phage K on a representative Irish bank of clinical MRSA sequence type isolates. Comparisons of their genomes lead to the identification of several ORFs absent in phage K, but present in both phages B1 and JA1. These ORFs were also identified in several other staphylococcal phages sourced from commercial phage mixtures (B1, JA1, Team 1 [22–24], vB_SauM-fRuSau02 [21], Sb-1 [19] and ISP [20]), also with a reported wide host range. The exact role of these ORFs is currently unknown. However, these ORFs along with several variations encountered at the genetic level between these phages may, in part, explain their different host range. Unfortunately, information is lacking on the influences of various phage resistance systems, which may be active in *Staphylococcus aureus*. Phage research also needs to focus more on elucidation of the functions of hypothetical proteins to allow greater understanding of how phages overcome such systems.

Supplementary Materials: The following are available online at http://www.mdpi.com/2079-6382/7/2/37/s1, Figure S1: Plaque morphologies of phages B1, JA1 and K with common morphology types encountered in their host range study to include plaques sizes of 2mm (A), 0.5mm (B) and 1.0mm (C), Figure S2: *Staphylococcus* phage K adsorption to strains of *Staphylococcus aureus* resistant to infection by, in comparison host strain DPC5246, Figure S3: Comparison of regions within the genome of phage K to closely related staphylococcal phages, Table S1: Annotation of the staphylococcal phage vB_SauM_B1, Table S2: Annotation of the staphylococcal phage vB_SauM_JA1, Table S3: Predicted Rho-like promoters of *Staphylococcus* phage B1 genome found using MEME, Table S4: Predicted Rho-like promoters of *Staphylococcus* phage JA1 genome found using MEME, Table S5: High ΔG rho-independent terminators predicted in the genome *Staphylococcus* phage B1 identified using ARNold and QuikFold, Table S6: High ΔG rho-independent terminators predicted in the genome *Staphylococcus* phage JA1 identified using ARNold and QuikFold, Table S7: Percentage similarity based on BLASTN of broad host range *Staphylococcus* phages that form commercial phage cocktails to that of *Staphylococcus* phage K, Table S8: tRNA genes of phages B1, JA1, K, vB_SauM-fRuSau02, ISP, Sb-1, Team 1.

Author Contributions: J.A. conducted the majority of lab work and wrote the manuscript, C.B. assisted with bioinformatics, writing, and critically read the manuscript; S.A.M. assisted with the phage host-range work; N.C. provided the Fersisi therapeutic phages and their information, and critically read the manuscript, E.M.G. isolated and helped characterize phage B1, J.OM and O.M. were co-supervisors of J.A. and both critically read the manuscript, H.N. and C.F. were responsible for electron microscopy and phage measurements, and A.C. conceived, funded, guided the study and critically read the manuscript.

Acknowledgments: This work was supported by Science Foundation Ireland, project reference 12/R1/2335. We thank undergraduate students Aoife Keating, Ceile Berkery and Adonai Djankah for their technical assistance with the host range studies and Angela Back for assistance with the electron microscope preparations.

References

1. Tong, S.Y.C.; Davis, J.S.; Eichenberger, E.; Holland, T.L.; Fowler, V.G. *Staphylococcus aureus* infections: Epidemiology, pathophysiology, clinical manifestations, and management. *Clin. Microbiol. Rev.* **2015**, *28*, 603–661. [CrossRef] [PubMed]
2. Shore, A.C.; Rossney, A.S.; O'Connell, B.; Herra, C.M.; Sullivan, D.J.; Humphreys, H.; Coleman, D.C. Detection of staphylococcal cassette chromosome mec-associated DNA segments in multiresistant methicillin-susceptible *Staphylococcus aureus* (MSSA) and identification of *Staphylococcus epidermidis* ccrAB4 in both methicillin-resistant *S. aureus* and MSSA. *Antimicrob. Agents Chemother.* **2008**, *52*, 4407–4419. [CrossRef] [PubMed]
3. Hiramatsu, K.; Cui, L.; Kuroda, M.; Ito, T. The emergence and evolution of methicillin-resistant *Staphylococcus aureus*. *Trends Microbiol.* **2001**, *9*, 486–493. [CrossRef]
4. Jevons, M.P. "Celbenin"—Resistant Staphylococci. *BMJ* **1961**, *1*, 124–125. [CrossRef]
5. Klein, E.; Smith, D.L.; Laxminarayan, R. Hospitalizations and Deaths Caused by Methicillin-Resistant *Staphylococcus aureus*, United States, 1999–2005. *Emerg. Infect. Dis.* **2007**, *13*, 1840–1846. [CrossRef] [PubMed]
6. O'Flaherty, S.; Ross, R.P.; Coffey, A. Bacteriophage and their lysins for elimination of infectious bacteria. *FEMS Microbiol. Rev.* **2009**, *33*, 801–819. [CrossRef] [PubMed]
7. Schmelcher, M.; Loessner, M.J. Application of bacteriophages for detection of foodborne pathogens. *Bacteriophage* **2014**, *4*, e28137. [CrossRef] [PubMed]
8. Wittebole, X.; De Roock, S.; Opal, S.M. A historical overview of bacteriophage therapy as an alternative to antibiotics for the treatment of bacterial pathogens. *Virulence* **2014**, *5*, 226–235. [CrossRef] [PubMed]
9. Bertozzi Silva, J.; Storms, Z.; Sauvageau, D. Host receptors for bacteriophage adsorption. *FEMS Microbiol. Lett.* **2016**, *363*, 1–11. [CrossRef] [PubMed]
10. Hyman, P.; Abedon, S.T. Bacteriophage Host Range and Bacterial Resistance. In *Advances in Applied Microbiology*, 1st ed.; Laskin, A.I., Sarislani, S., Gadd, G.M., Eds.; Elsevier Inc.: Cambridge, MA, USA, 2010; Volume 70, pp. 217–248, ISBN 9780123809919.
11. Labrie, S.J.; Samson, J.E.; Moineau, S. Bacteriophage resistance mechanisms. *Nat. Rev. Microbiol.* **2010**, *8*, 317–327. [CrossRef] [PubMed]
12. Hall, A.R.; Scanlan, P.D.; Buckling, A. Bacteria-Phage Coevolution and the Emergence of Generalist Pathogens. *Am. Nat.* **2011**, *177*, 44–53. [CrossRef] [PubMed]
13. Hall, J.P.J.; Harrison, E.; Brockhurst, M.A. Viral host-adaptation: Insights from evolution experiments with phages. *Curr. Opin. Virol.* **2013**, *3*, 572–577. [CrossRef] [PubMed]

14. Samson, J.E.; Magadán, A.H.; Sabri, M.; Moineau, S. Revenge of the phages: Defeating bacterial defences. *Nat. Rev. Microbiol.* **2013**, *11*, 675–687. [CrossRef] [PubMed]
15. Sulakvelidze, A.; Alavidze, Z.; Morris, J.G. Bacteriophage therapy. *Antimicrob. Agents Chemother.* **2001**, *45*, 649–659. [CrossRef] [PubMed]
16. Abedon, S.T.; Kuhl, S.J.; Blasdel, B.G.; Kutter, E.M. Phage treatment of human infections. *Bacteriophage* **2011**, *1*, 66–85. [CrossRef] [PubMed]
17. Villarroel, J.; Larsen, M.V.; Kilstrup, M.; Nielsen, M. Metagenomic analysis of therapeutic PYO phage cocktails from 1997 to 2014. *Viruses* **2017**, *9*. [CrossRef] [PubMed]
18. Zschach, H.; Joensen, K.G.; Lindhard, B.; Lund, O.; Goderdzishvili, M.; Chkonia, I.; Jgenti, G.; Kvatadze, N.; Alavidze, Z.; Kutter, E.M.; et al. What can we learn from a metagenomic analysis of a georgian bacteriophage cocktail? *Viruses* **2015**, *7*, 6570–6589. [CrossRef] [PubMed]
19. Kvachadze, L.; Balarjishvili, N.; Meskhi, T.; Tevdoradze, E.; Skhirtladze, N.; Pataridze, T.; Adamia, R.; Topuria, T.; Kutter, E.; Rohde, C.; et al. Evaluation of lytic activity of staphylococcal bacteriophage Sb-1 against freshly isolated clinical pathogens. *Microb. Biotechnol.* **2011**, *4*, 643–650. [CrossRef] [PubMed]
20. Vandersteegen, K.; Mattheus, W.; Ceyssens, P.J.; Bilocq, F.; de Vos, D.; Pirnay, J.P.; Noben, J.P.; Merabishvili, M.; Lipinska, U.; Hermans, K.; et al. Microbiological and molecular assessment of bacteriophage ISP for the control of *Staphylococcus aureus*. *PLoS ONE* **2011**, *6*, e24418. [CrossRef] [PubMed]
21. Leskinen, K.; Tuomala, H.; Wicklund, A.; Horsma-Heikkinen, J.; Kuusela, P.; Skurnik, M.; Kiljunen, S. Characterization of vB_SauM-fRuSau02, a Twort-Like Bacteriophage Isolated from a Therapeutic Phage Cocktail. *Viruses* **2017**, *9*, 258. [CrossRef] [PubMed]
22. El Haddad, L.; Abdallah, N.B.; Plante, P.L.; Dumaresq, J.; Katsarava, R.; Labrie, S.; Corbeil, J.; St-Gelais, D.; Moineau, S. Improving the safety of *Staphylococcus aureus* polyvalent phages by their production on a *Staphylococcus xylosus* strain. *PLoS ONE* **2014**, *9*, e102600. [CrossRef] [PubMed]
23. Markoishvili, K.; Tsitlanadze, G.; Katsarava, R.; Morris, J.G.; Sulakvelidze, A. A novel sustained-release matrix based on biodegradable poly(ester amide)s and impregnated with bacteriophages and an antibiotic shows promise in management of infected venous stasis ulcers and other poorly healing wounds. *Int. J. Dermatol.* **2002**, *41*, 453–458. [CrossRef] [PubMed]
24. Jikia, D.; Chkhaidze, N.; Imedashvili, E.; Mgaloblishvili, I.; Tsitlanadze, G.; Katsarava, R.; Morris, J.G.; Sulakvelidze, A. The use of a novel biodegradable preparation capable of the sustained release of bacteriophages and ciprofloxacin, in the complex treatment of multidrug-resistant *Staphylococcus aureus*-infected local radiation injuries caused by exposure to Sr90. *Clin. Exp. Dermatol.* **2005**, *30*, 23–26. [CrossRef] [PubMed]
25. Adriaenssens, E.M.; Clokie, C.M.R.; Sullivan, M.B.; Gillis, A.; Jens Kuhn, B.H.; Kropinski, A.M. Taxonomy of prokaryotic viruses: 2016 update from the ICTV bacterial and archaeal viruses subcommittee. *Arch. Virol.* **2017**, *162*, 1153–1157. [CrossRef] [PubMed]
26. O'Flaherty, S.; Ross, R.P.; Meaney, W.; Fitzgerald, G.F.; Elbreki, M.F.; Coffey, A. Potential of the Polyvalent Anti-Staphylococcus Bacteriophage K for Control of Antibiotic-Resistant Staphylococci from Hospitals. *Appl. Environ. Microbiol.* **2005**, *71*, 1836–1842. [CrossRef] [PubMed]
27. Rountree, P.M. The serological differentiation of staphylococcal bacteriophages. *J. Gen. Microbiol.* **1949**, *3*, 164–173. [CrossRef] [PubMed]
28. Ackermann, H.W. Frequency of morphological phage descriptions in the year 2000. *Arch. Virol.* **2001**, *146*, 843–857. [CrossRef] [PubMed]
29. Rossney, A.S.; Lawrence, M.J.; Morgan, P.M.; Fitzgibbon, M.M.; Shore, A.; Coleman, D.C.; Keane, C.T.; O'Connell, B. Epidemiological typing of MRSA isolates from blood cultures taken in Irish hospitals participating in the European Antimicrobial Resistance Surveillance System (1999–2003). *Eur. J. Clin. Microbiol. Infect. Dis.* **2006**, *25*, 79–89. [CrossRef] [PubMed]
30. Cui, Z.; Feng, T.; Gu, F.; Li, Q.; Dong, K.; Zhang, Y.; Zhu, Y.; Han, L.; Qin, J.; Guo, X. Characterization and complete genome of the virulent Myoviridae phage JD007 active against a variety of *Staphylococcus aureus* isolates from different hospitals in Shanghai, China. *Virol. J.* **2017**, *14*, 26. [CrossRef] [PubMed]
31. Gill, J.J. Revised Genome Sequence of *Staphylococcus aureus* Bacteriophage K. *Genome Announc.* **2014**, *2*, 12–13. [CrossRef] [PubMed]
32. Buttimer, C.; Hendrix, H.; Oliveira, H.; Casey, A.; Neve, H.; McAuliffe, O.; Paul Ross, R.; Hill, C.; Noben, J.P.; O'Mahony, J.; et al. Things are getting hairy: Enterobacteria bacteriophage vB_PcaM_CBB. *Front. Microbiol.* **2017**, *8*, 1–16. [CrossRef] [PubMed]

33. Li, S.; Fan, H.; An, X.; Fan, H.; Jiang, H.; Chen, Y.; Tong, Y. Scrutinizing virus genome termini by high-throughput sequencing. *PLoS ONE* **2014**, *9*, e85806. [CrossRef] [PubMed]
34. Fouts, D.E.; Klumpp, J.; Bishop-Lilly, K.A.; Rajavel, M.; Willner, K.M.; Butani, A.; Henry, M.; Biswas, B.; Li, M.; Albert, M.J.; et al. Whole genome sequencing and comparative genomic analyses of two *Vibrio cholerae* O139 Bengal-specific Podoviruses to other N4-like phages reveal extensive genetic diversity. *Virol. J.* **2013**, *10*, 165. [CrossRef] [PubMed]
35. Łobocka, M.; Hejnowicz, M.S.; Dąbrowski, K.; Gozdek, A.; Kosakowski, J.; Witkowska, M.; Ulatowska, M.I.; Weber-Dąbrowska, B.; Kwiatek, M.; Parasion, S.; et al. Genomics of staphylococcal Twort-like phages—Potential therapeutics of the post-antibiotic era. *Adv. Virus Res.* **2012**, *83*, 143–216. [CrossRef] [PubMed]
36. O'Flaherty, S.; Coffey, A.; Edwards, R.; Meaney, W.; Fitzgerald, G.F.; Ross, R.P. Genome of Staphylococcal Phage K: A New Lineage of Myoviridae Infecting Gram-Positive Bacteria with a Low G+C Content. *J. Bacteriol.* **2004**, *186*, 2862–2871. [CrossRef] [PubMed]
37. Adriaenssens, E.M.; Rodney Brister, J. How to name and classify your phage: An informal guide. *Viruses* **2017**, *9*, 70. [CrossRef] [PubMed]
38. Bailey, T.L.; Boden, M.; Buske, F.A.; Frith, M.; Grant, C.E.; Clementi, L.; Ren, J.; Li, W.W.; Noble, W.S. MEME SUITE: Tools for motif discovery and searching. *Nucleic Acids Res.* **2009**, *37*, W202–W208. [CrossRef] [PubMed]
39. Matange, N.; Podobnik, M.; Visweswariah, S.S. Metallophosphoesterases: structural fidelity with functional promiscuity. *Biochem. J.* **2015**, *467*, 201–216. [CrossRef] [PubMed]
40. Gogarten, J.P.; Hilario, E. Inteins, introns, and homing endonucleases: recent revelations about the life cycle of parasitic genetic elements. *BMC Evol. Biol.* **2006**, *6*, 94. [CrossRef] [PubMed]
41. Vandersteegen, K.; Kropinski, A.M.; Nash, J.H.E.; Noben, J.-P.; Hermans, K.; Lavigne, R. Romulus and Remus, two phage isolates representing a distinct clade within the Twortlikevirus genus, display suitable properties for phage therapy applications. *J. Virol.* **2013**, *87*, 3237–3247. [CrossRef] [PubMed]
42. Wei, P.; Stewart, C.R. A Cytotoxic Early Gene of *Bacillus subtilis* Bacteriophage SPOl. *J. Bacteriol.* **1993**, *175*, 7887–7900. [CrossRef] [PubMed]
43. Stewart, C.R.; Gaslightwala, I.; Hinata, K.; Krolikowski, K.A.; Needleman, D.S.; Peng, A.S.Y.; Peterman, M.A.; Tobias, A.; Wei, P. Genes and regulatory sites of the "host-takeover module" in the terminal redundancy of *Bacillus subtilis* bacteriophage SPO1. *Virology* **1998**, *246*, 329–340. [CrossRef] [PubMed]
44. Seed, K.D. Battling Phages: How Bacteria Defend against Viral Attack. *PLoS Pathog.* **2015**, *11*, e1004847. [CrossRef] [PubMed]
45. Roberts, G.A.; Houston, P.J.; White, J.H.; Chen, K.; Stephanou, A.S.; Cooper, L.P.; Dryden, D.T.F.; Lindsay, J.A. Impact of target site distribution for Type i restriction enzymes on the evolution of methicillin-resistant *Staphylococcus aureus* (MRSA) populations. *Nucleic Acids Res.* **2013**, *41*, 7472–7484. [CrossRef] [PubMed]
46. Cao, L.; Gao, C.H.; Zhu, J.; Zhao, L.; Wu, Q.; Li, M.; Sun, B. Identification and functional study of type III—A CRISPR-Cas systems in clinical isolates of *Staphylococcus aureus*. *Int. J. Med. Microbiol.* **2016**, *306*, 686–696. [CrossRef] [PubMed]
47. Sambrook, J.; Russell, D.W. Purification of bacteriophage lamda particles by isopycnic centrifugation through CsCl gradients. In *Molecular Cloning: A Laboratory Manual*; Cold Spring Harbor Laboratory Press: New York, NY, USA, 2001; Volume 1, p. 247, ISBN 0879695773.
48. Gutiérrez, D.; Vandenheuvel, D.; Martínez, B.; Rodríguez, A.; Lavigne, R.; García, P. Two Phages, philPLA-RODI and philPLA-C1C, Lyse Mono- and Dual-Species Staphylococcal Biofilms. *Appl. Environ. Microbiol.* **2015**, *81*, 3336–3348. [CrossRef] [PubMed]
49. Li, X.; Koç, C.; Kühner, P.; Stierhof, Y.-D.; Krismer, B.; Enright, M.C.; Penadés, J.R.; Wolz, C.; Stehle, T.; Cambillau, C.; et al. An essential role for the baseplate protein Gp45 in phage adsorption to *Staphylococcus aureus*. *Sci. Rep.* **2016**, *6*, 26455. [CrossRef] [PubMed]
50. Delcher, A. Improved microbial gene identification with GLIMMER. *Nucleic Acids Res.* **1999**, *27*, 4636–4641. [CrossRef] [PubMed]
51. Besemer, J.; Lomsadze, A.; Borodovsky, M. GeneMarkS: A self-training method for prediction of gene starts in microbial genomes. Implications for finding sequence motifs in regulatory regions. *Nucleic Acids Res.* **2001**, *29*, 2607–2618. [CrossRef] [PubMed]
52. Söding, J.; Biegert, A.; Lupas, A.N. The HHpred interactive server for protein homology detection and structure prediction. *Nucleic Acids Res.* **2005**, *33*, W244–W248. [CrossRef] [PubMed]

53. Mitchell, A.; Chang, H.-Y.; Daugherty, L.; Fraser, M.; Hunter, S.; Lopez, R.; McAnulla, C.; McMenamin, C.; Nuka, G.; Pesseat, S.; et al. The InterPro protein families database: The classification resource after 15 years. *Nucleic Acids Res.* **2015**, *43*, D213–D221. [CrossRef] [PubMed]
54. Lowe, T.M.; Eddy, S.R. tRNAscan-SE: A program for improved detection of transfer RNA genes in genomic sequence. *Nucleic Acids Res.* **1997**, *25*, 955–964. [CrossRef] [PubMed]
55. Laslett, D.; Canback, B. ARAGORN, a program to detect tRNA genes and tmRNA genes in nucleotide sequences. *Nucleic Acids Res.* **2004**, *32*, 11–16. [CrossRef] [PubMed]
56. Naville, M.; Ghuillot-Gaudeffroy, A.; Marchais, A.; Gautheret, D. ARNold: A web tool for the prediction of rho-independent transcription terminators. *RNA Biol.* **2011**, *8*, 11–13. [CrossRef] [PubMed]
57. Zuker, M. Mfold web server for nucleic acid folding and hybridization prediction. *Nucleic Acids Res.* **2003**, *31*, 3406–3415. [CrossRef] [PubMed]
58. Carver, T.J.; Rutherford, K.M.; Berriman, M.; Rajandream, M.-A.; Barrell, B.G.; Parkhill, J. ACT: The Artemis comparison tool. *Bioinformatics* **2005**, *21*, 3422–3423. [CrossRef] [PubMed]
59. Sullivan, M.J.; Petty, N.K.; Beatson, S.A. Easyfig: A genome comparison visualizer. *Bioinformatics* **2011**, *27*, 1009–1010. [CrossRef] [PubMed]

3

Nisin in Combination with Cinnamaldehyde and EDTA to Control Growth of *Escherichia coli* Strains of Swine Origin

Des Field [1,*,†], Inès Baghou [1,†], Mary C. Rea [2,3], Gillian E. Gardiner [4], R. Paul Ross [1,3] and Colin Hill [1,3,*]

1 School of Microbiology, University College Cork, Cork T12 YT20, Ireland; ines.baghou@mycit.ie (I.B.); p.ross@ucc.ie (R.P.R.)
2 Teagasc Food Research Centre, Moorepark, Fermoy, Co., Cork P61 C996, Ireland; mary.rea@teagasc.ie
3 APC Microbiome Institute, University College Cork, Cork T12 YT20, Ireland
4 Department of Science, Waterford Institute of Technology, Waterford X91 K0EK, Ireland; ggardiner@wit.ie
* Correspondence: des.field@ucc.ie (D.F.); c.hill@ucc.ie (C.H.)

† These authors contributed equally.

Academic Editor: Leonard Amaral

Abstract: Post-weaning diarrhoea (PWD) due to enterotoxigenic *Escherichia coli* (ETEC) is an economically important disease in pig production worldwide. Although antibiotics have contributed significantly to mitigate the economic losses caused by PWD, there is major concern over the increased incidence of antimicrobial resistance among bacteria isolated from pigs. Consequently, suitable alternatives that are safe and effective are urgently required. Many naturally occurring compounds, including the antimicrobial peptide nisin and a number of plant essential oils, have been widely studied and are reported to be effective as antimicrobial agents against pathogenic microorganisms. Here, we evaluate the potential of nisin in combination with the essential oil cinnamaldehyde and ethylenediaminetetraacetic acid (EDTA) to control the growth of *E. coli* strains of swine origin including two characterized as ETEC. The results reveal that the use of nisin (10 μM) with low concentrations of trans-cinnamaldehyde (125 μg/mL) and EDTA (0.25–2%) resulted in extended lag phases of growth compared to when either antimicrobial is used alone. Further analysis through kill curves revealed that an approximate 1-log reduction in *E. coli* cell counts was observed against the majority of targets tested following 3 h incubation. These results highlight the potential benefits of combining the natural antimicrobial nisin with trans-cinnamaldehyde and EDTA as a new approach for the inhibition of *E. coli* strains of swine origin.

Keywords: antimicrobial resistance; antibiotics; antimicrobial peptide; enterotoxigenic *E. coli*; nisin; bacteriocin; essential oil; cinnamaldehyde; EDTA

---

1. Introduction

Post-weaning diarrhea (PWD) is one of the most life-threatening diseases in the swine industry worldwide. It is commonly associated with the proliferation of enterotoxigenic *Escherichia coli* (ETEC) in the pig intestine resulting in mortality, dehydration, weight loss and retarded growth [1]. Current control strategies frequently involve polymyxins, macrolides and fluoroquinolones, antibiotics that are also critically important in human medicine [2]. However, the routine use of in-feed antibiotics was banned in the European Union (EU) in 2006 (Regulation EC/1831/2003), although their use is still permitted under veterinary prescription as the need arises. Moreover, in recent times the use of antimicrobials in food production animals has come under considerable scrutiny, given that recent genomic and metagenomic studies in humans, animals and in the environment have brought to light the existence of a reservoir of antibiotic resistance genes that could be mobilized and transferred from these sources to human pathogens [3–5]. In addition, the use of zinc oxide (ZnO) at pharmacological concentrations (i.e., concentrations in excess of normal dietary requirements) will no longer be a therapeutic option for the prevention and control of PWD and bowel oedema in young pigs in the EU. This follows the recent ruling by the Committee for Medicinal Products for Veterinary Use (CVMP) to ban its use. Consequently, there is increasing emphasis on practices to reduce antibiotic usage in animal husbandry by promoting prudent use initiatives, as well as exploring the implementation of potential alternatives for the use of antibiotics and zinc oxide in livestock production.

One group of antimicrobials that have been at the forefront of alternative antibiotic research for decades are the lantibiotic class of bacteriocins (bacterially produced, small, heat-stable peptides that are active against other bacteria). The best known lantibiotic is nisin A, a 34-amino acid polycyclic peptide that exhibits antibacterial activity against a wide range of clinical and food-borne pathogens and is widely used as a natural food biopreservative [6]. Although nisin is not currently used for medical applications, it has realized commercial applications in the veterinary industry for the prevention/treatment of bovine mastitis [7,8]. It functions by a distinctive dual mode of action involving binding to lipid II, an essential precursor of the bacterial cell wall, followed by insertion into the membrane of the target cell to form a pore [9–11]. As a consequence of these two distinct and cooperative mechanisms, no significant resistance to nisin A has been observed despite its widespread use over several decades by the food industry [12]. Consequently, lantibiotics such as nisin A possess enormous potential for therapeutic applications, not only as alternatives but also as synergists with other antimicrobials. For example, aromatic plant oils have been widely investigated due to their antimicrobial activities and numerous studies have demonstrated the synergistic activities of nisin and essential oil combinations including thymol [13], carvacrol [14,15] and cinnamaldehyde [16], amongst others. Similarly, the activity of nisin can be enhanced through the addition of chelating agents such as ethylenediaminetetraacetic acid (EDTA) [17,18]. Recently, Al Atya and coworkers demonstrated the effectiveness of nisin in combination with colistin towards *E. coli* strains of swine origin [19]. Importantly, the combination proved effective against both planktonic and biofilm cultures of *E. coli* strains exhibiting a colistin-resistance phenotype, validating the potential of such strategies to reduce the effective dose required for these antibiotics to help prevent or delay the further spread of resistance. Indeed, such approaches are all the more urgent given the directive that all EU Member States are required to achieve a reduction of approximately 65% in the current sales of colistin for veterinary use at an EU level by 2020 (https://www.cdc.gov/drugresistance/tatfar/tatfar-recomendations.html). However, if the use of colistin and other critical antibiotics is to be diminished or replaced in animal husbandry, suitable alternatives that are safe and efficient must be found.

Here we assess the efficacy of nisin in combination with a variety of essential oils and EDTA, and establish that a nisin + EDTA + cinnamaldehyde combination exhibits significantly greater anti-*E coli* activity compared to the use of either antimicrobial alone.

2. Results

2.1. Bacterial Susceptibility to Antimicrobial Compounds

Minimum inhibitory concentration assays (MICs) with purified nisin A peptide and the essential oils thymol, carvacrol and trans-cinnamaldehyde were determined against *E. coli* targets of pig origin, including two characterized as ETEC (K88F4 and F18ab) in order to ascertain appropriate concentrations for combinatorial assays. Additionally, MIC assays were also carried out to establish the relative sensitivity or resistance to a range of antibiotics including penicillin, erythromycin, chloramphenicol, tetracycline, cefuroxime, ceftazidime, colistin and polymyxin B. Activity against the target strains required a relatively high concentration of nisin (200 μg/mL). This value was in agreement with data obtained by Naghmouchi and co-workers against a panel of Gram-negative strains [20] and, yet again, highlights the relative resistance of Gram-negative bacteria to nisin compared to Gram-positive strains which can have MICs in the nanomolar (nM) range. The majority of the *E. coli* targets were resistant to erythromycin, tetracycline and penicillin, with the exception of *E. coli* F2S2, which remained sensitive to chloramphenicol and tetracycline (Table 1) and were overall in agreement with previous studies with *E. coli* strains of swine origin [19,21]. Colistin and polymyxin B exhibited almost identical activity against 4 of 5 of the target strains and were in close agreement with previously established figures against sensitive strains of *E. coli* [19,22]. The exception was the ETEC F18ab strain which exhibited an MIC of 25 μg/mL for both polymyxin and colistin (Table 1), indicative of resistance to these antimicrobials. Furthermore, all of the target strains remained sensitive to the cephalosporin antibiotics ceftazidime, cefuroxime and cefradine, while resistance to cefoxitin was observed for all strains. The susceptibility of the bacterial strains to the essential oils thymol, carvacrol and trans-cinnamaldehyde was also assessed in order to ascertain appropriate concentrations for combinatorial assays. Cinnamaldehyde proved to be the most active of the essential oils with an inhibitory concentration of 1250 μg mL^{-1} which was within the 400–1322 μg mL^{-1} range established by previous studies [23].

Table 1. Minimum inhibitory concentration determinations of nisin A, and the essential oils thymol, carvacrol and trans-cinnamaldehyde against *E. coli* strains of swine origin. ‡ denotes enterotoxigenic *Escherichia coli* (ETEC) strains. Results are expressed as the mean of triplicate assays.

Antibiotic	*E. coli* Strain				
	F150F3	F2S2	K88F4 ‡	F3P3	F18ab ‡
Chloramphenicol	>50	12.5	>50	>50	12.5
Tetracycline	>50	1.56	50	25	50
Penicillin G	>50	25	25	25	12.5
Streptomycin	>50	25	>50	12.5	1.56
Cefoxitin	>50	>50	>50	>50	>50
Erythromycin	>50	>50	>50	>50	50
Lincomycin	>50	>50	>50	>50	>50
Ceftazidine	<0.4	<0.4	<0.4	<0.4	<0.4
Cefuroxime	6.25	3.12	6.25	6.25	6.25
Cefradine	25	12.5	25	25	12.5
Cefsulodin	>50	50	50	50	50
Colistin	0.39	0.39	<0.2	<0.2	25
Polymyxin B	0.39	0.39	<0.2	<0.2	25
Carvacrol	>1250	>1250	>1250	>1250	>1250
Cinnamaldehyde	1250	1250	1250	>1250	1250
Thymol	>1250	>1250	>1250	>1250	>1250
Nisin	200	200	200	200	200

2.2. Growth Curve-Based Comparisons of the Activity of Nisin A and Natural Antimicrobial Combinations

Having established the MIC values for nisin A and a range of essential oils against the panel of *E. coli* strains, growth curves were performed in order to reveal the impact of sub-lethal concentrations of nisin A, cinnamaldehyde and EDTA (alone and in combination) on bacterial growth. The final concentration of nisin or cinnamaldehyde used for each organism was a fraction of the previously determined MIC value (i.e., 1/10×, 1/6×, 1/4×, etc.) and combinations thereof. Initial growth curves were carried out with EDTA to establish levels that were marginally inhibitory compared to a control strain in the absence of EDTA for each of the strains. Nisin at 1/6× MIC (33 μg/mL) had little or no impact on the growth of the targets *E. coli* K88F4 (Figure 1A), *E. coli* F3P3 (Figure 1B) or *E. coli* F2S2 (Figure 1C), affirming the relatively poor activity of nisin against Gram-negative bacteria. Similarly, a slight lag in growth was observed for both EDTA and cinnamaldehyde (at 1/10× MIC; 125 μg/mL) when compared to the untreated control (Figure 1). However, pronounced inhibitory effects were recorded when nisin was used in combination with cinnamaldehyde and EDTA against *E. coli* K88F4 (Figure 1A), *E. coli* F3P3 (Figure 1B), *E. coli* F2S2 (Figure 1C), as observed by the exceptionally extended lag phase in all cases compared to the untreated control. Notably, the combination also proved effective against the colistin and polymyxin B-resistant ETEC F18ab strain (Figure 1D).

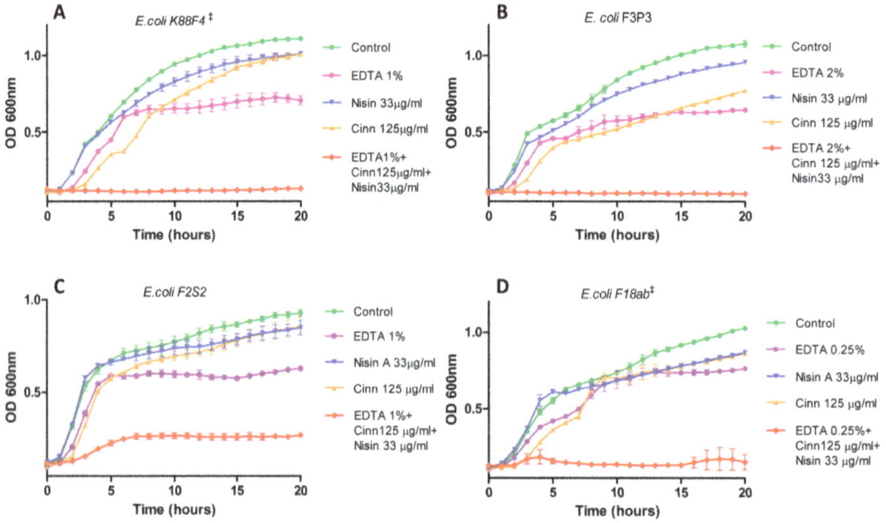

Figure 1. Growth curve analysis of (**A**) *E. coli* K88F4 in the presence of 1/6× minimum inhibitory concentration (MIC; 33 μg/mL) nisin A (blue inverted triangle), 1/10× MIC (125 μg/mL) cinnamaldehyde (orange triangle), ethylenediaminetetraacetic acid (EDTA) 1.0% (purple circle) in combination (red diamond) and untreated control (green circle), (**B**) *E. coli* F3P3 in the presence of 1/6× MIC (33 μg/mL) nisin A (blue inverted triangle), 1/10× MIC (125 μg/mL) cinnamaldehyde (orange triangle), EDTA 2% (purple circle), in combination (red diamond) and untreated control (green circle), (**C**) *E. coli* F2S2 in the presence of 1/6× MIC (33 μg/mL) nisin A (blue inverted triangle), 1/10× MIC (125 μg/mL) cinnamaldehyde (orange triangle), EDTA 1% (purple circle), in combination (red diamond) and untreated control (green circle) and (**D**) *E. coli* F18ab in the presence of 1/6× MIC (33 μg/mL) nisin A (blue inverted triangle), 1/10× MIC (125 μg/mL) cinnamaldehyde (orange triangle), EDTA 0.25% (purple circle), in combination (red diamond) and untreated control (green circle). ‡ denotes ETEC strains.

2.3. Kill Assay Determination of the Activity of Nisin A and Natural Antimicrobial Combinations

Following on from the data established by growth curves, the bactericidal activity of nisin in combination with cinnamaldehyde and EDTA against the target *E. coli* was investigated utilising kill assays within a defined period of time (3 h). *E. coli* F2S2, *E. coli* K88F4, *E. coli* F3P3 and *E. coli* F18ab at a concentration of 1×10^7 cfu were exposed to nisin (33 μg/mL), cinnamaldehyde (125 μg/mL) and EDTA (1%, 2%, 2%, 0.25%, respectively) at 37 °C for 3 h.

In general, an approximate 1-log reduction in *E. coli* counts was observed for the antimicrobial combination compared to the initial inoculum (Figure 2). When compared to the untreated control, a 2-log differential in cell numbers was observed between the antimicrobial combination and the control in each case for *E. coli* K88F4, ($p < 0.046$), *E. coli* F3P3 ($p < 0.043$) and *E. coli* F2S2 ($p < 0.005$). The exception was *E. coli* F18ab whereby cell numbers remained static (2.9×10^7 cfu/mL; Figure 2) following 3 h of incubation. In contrast, the untreated control had increased to 2.3×10^8 cfu/mL.

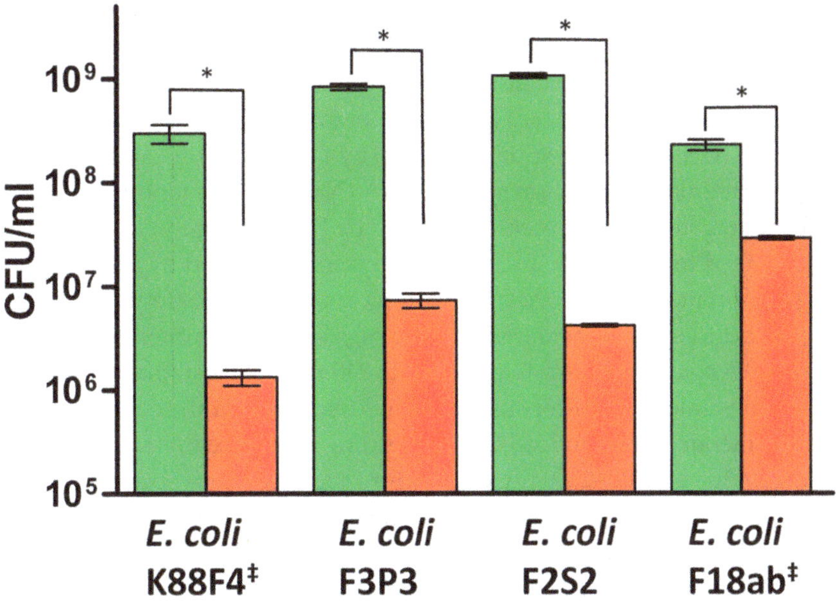

Figure 2. Kill effect of nisin in combination with cinnamaldehyde and EDTA against *E. coli* strains of swine origin. Kill assay performed over a defined 3 h period with *E. coli* K88F4 in the presence of nisin (33 μg/mL) + cinnamaldehyde (125 μg/mL) + EDTA (1%) and untreated control (Green), *E. coli* F3P3 in the presence of nisin (33 μg/mL) + cinnamaldehyde (125 μg/mL) + EDTA (2%) (Red) and untreated control (Green), *E. coli* F2S2 in the presence of nisin (33 μg/mL) + cinnamaldehyde (125 μg/mL) + EDTA (1%) EDTA 2% (Red) and untreated control (Green), *E. coli* F18ab in the presence of nisin (33 μg/mL) + cinnamaldehyde (125 μg/mL) + EDTA (0.25%) (Red) and untreated control (Green). Asterisks rating of * indicates statistically significant differences between groups ($p \leq 0.05$). ‡ denotes ETEC strains.

3. Discussion

Post-weaning diarrhea is an economically important enteric disease in pigs resulting in significant financial losses. It is commonly associated with the proliferation of ETEC, a pathotype characterized by the production of enterotoxins and adhesins, both essential for disease development [24] that act on the intestinal epithelium of pigs. Alarmingly, critically important antibiotics such as fluoroquinolones, aminoglycosides and polymyxins are sold in vast quantities for use in pigs during the post-weaning period in many countries worldwide [25]. However, the emergence of bacterial resistance to these antibiotics has dictated that effective and sustainable alternative approaches to tackling microbial disease in both humans and livestock must be identified. Here, we set out to examine for the first time the ability of nisin, when used in conjunction with a selection of natural antimicrobials including essential oils, to control several *E. coli* strains of swine origin, including two characterized as ETEC, with the ultimate aim of identifying superior antimicrobial combinations. Following MIC determinations and growth curve analysis in the presence of nisin + cinnamaldehyde + EDTA combinations, substantial enhanced inhibitory relationships were observed. The results reveal that sub-inhibitory levels of nisin (1/6× MIC) and cinnamaldehyde (1/10× MIC) supplemented with EDTA (0.25–2%) can effectively control the growth of *E. coli* numbers in laboratory media. In contrast, nisin was ineffective against the *E. coli* targets when used independently. Indeed, considerable work has been conducted to enhance the poor antibacterial activity of nisin toward Gram-negative bacteria (due to the outer membrane of the Gram-negative cell wall that acts as a physical barrier, obstructing access of the peptides to the cytoplasmic membrane). Such strategies have included destabilization of the outer membrane by combining with essential oils that contain aldehydes, terpenes and phenolic compounds [26,27]. Other strategies have involved nisin and chelating agents such as EDTA, which acts by removing Mg^{2+} and Ca^{2+} ions essential for stabilizing the lipopolysaccharide

(LPS) outer membrane of Gram-negative bacteria [18,28]. Our investigations also highlight the enhanced potency of nisin when combined with trans-cinnamaldehyde and EDTA, implying that combinations of two or more antimicrobials, which affect different targets, exhibit great potential as a new approach against pathogenic-resistant bacteria. Moreover, all the aforementioned antimicrobials are classified as GRAS (Generally Recognized as Safe) by the FDA (Food and Drug Administration). Notably, a product containing the sodium salt of EDTA (Na_2EDTA), a tannin-rich extract of *Castanea sativa*, thyme oil and oregano oil was recently assessed by EFSA for use with pigs at a recommended dose of 1000 mg/kg feed to reduce the incidence of dysentery caused by *Brachyspira hyodysenteriae* and so improve performance [29]. Furthermore, the European Food Safety Authority (EFSA) panel concluded that the additive was considered safe for pigs at the recommended dose of 1000 mg/kg feed of which Na_2EDTA constituted 24% (equivalent to 240 mg). None of the active constituents raised safety concerns for consumers when considered individually and at the concentrations delivered to feed using the recommended dose. Indeed, animal feeding studies to investigate EDTA toxicity have established an LD_{50} value of 2000–2200 mg/kg bw for rats, while a no observed adverse effect level (NOAEL) of 500 mg/kg bw per day for Na_2EDTA and Na_3EDTA was determined from a 90-day study in rats and in a long-term (2-year) study in rats and mice [30]. However, rats fed 1%, 5% or 10% disodium salt of EDTA for 90 days had significantly lower food consumption and weight gain than controls [31]. Although the concentrations of EDTA used in this study (0.25–2%) exceed the maximum permitted dose (by 10–100 fold), reductions in EDTA concentration may be achieved through Response Surface Methodology which has been used very effectively to analyze, predict and model systems that require optimization of multiple factors and has been used previously for nisin, EDTA and pH combinations [32]. Alternatively, other chelators could be investigated as well as the use of other natural antimicrobial compounds such as organic acids, which have been shown to control PWD and enhance growth performance in pigs [33–35] and have been shown to act synergistically with nisin [36].

Several studies have investigated the ability of essential oil compounds to control the proliferation of pathogenic bacteria, as well as contribute to better gut health in pigs and potentially replace the use of antibiotic growth promoters which have been prohibited in the European Union since 2006 [37]. For example, Li and co-workers demonstrated that the addition of encapsulated essential oils (thymol and cinnamaldehyde) improved feed intake and growth rate, reduced the incidence of diarrhoea and resulted in a positive modulation of microbial populations measured in the faeces, with a reduction of *E. coli* and an increase of *Lactobacillus* counts [38]. Similarly, addition of an essential oil to weaner pig diets showed evidence of a reduction in *Salmonella* faecal shedding and numbers of coliforms and *Salmonella* in cecal digesta [39], and administration of an encapsulated blend of formic acid, citric acid and essential oils [40] to finishing pigs for 28 days prior to slaughter reduced *Salmonella* seroprevalence and demonstrated potential for the prevention of *Salmonella* shedding. In addition, the inclusion of cinnamaldehyde with blended organic acids and a permeabilising agent in the diets of weaned pigs experimentally infected with ETEC was found to decrease faecal *E. coli* concentrations, with no effect on the concentration of faecal lactobacilli [41]. While there is a paucity of studies involving nisin and pigs, the benefits of incorporating nisin into the diets of poultry [42] and rabbits [43] have been established.

In this study, we have provided proof of concept that the natural antimicrobial peptide nisin in combination with natural plant extracts such as trans-cinnamaldehyde could expand the spectrum of useful therapeutics and form a novel strategy in the control of ETEC infection in post-weaning pigs. However, in vivo studies along with genomic characterization and transcriptomic and proteomic profiling of the gut microbiota will be necessary to validate the antimicrobial efficacy and safety of these antimicrobial combinations for use in pigs.

4. Materials and Methods

4.1. Bacterial Strains and Growth Conditions

Lactococcus lactis NZ9700 (a nisin A producing strain used for peptide purification) was grown in M17 broth supplemented with 0.5% glucose (GM17) or GM17 agar at 30 °C. *E. coli* strains F150F3, F2S2, F3P3, K88F4 and F18ab were grown in Luria–Bertani (LB) broth (5 g/L yeast extract [Oxoid, Hampshire, UK], 10 g/L tryptone [Oxoid] and 10 g/L NaCl [Merck, Nottingham UK]), incubated overnight at 37 °C and shaken at 170 rpm. *E. coli* strains F150F3, F2S2 and F3P3 were isolates from pooled faecal samples from across different pig production stages and the designation F refers to Farm. Enterotoxigenic *E. coli* (ETEC) strains K88F4 and F18ab were PCR-positive for F4 and F18 adhesins, respectively. *E. coli* K88F4 was determined to be serotype O147 and positive for STb, LT and EAST1 toxins but negative for STa. *E. coli* F18ab was determined to be serotype O141 and negative for STa, STb, EAST1 and LT toxins.

4.2. Minimum Inhibitory Concentration Assays

Minimum inhibitory concentration (MIC) determinations were carried out in triplicate in 96-well microtitre plates (Sarstedt, Rheinbach, Germany) as described previously [36,37]. Briefly, target strains were grown overnight in the appropriate conditions and medium, subcultured into fresh broth and allowed to grow to an OD_{600} of ~0.5 and diluted to a final concentration of 10^5 cfu mL^{-1} in a volume of 0.2 mL. Chloramphenicol, penicillin G, erythromycin, tetracycline, colistin and polymyxin B (Sigma, Steinheim, Germany) were resuspended in LB broth to a stock concentration of 128 or 256 µg/mL. The antibiotics were adjusted to 16, 32, 64 or 128 µg/mL starting concentration and 2-fold serial dilutions of each compound were made in 96-well plates for a total of 12 dilutions. The MIC assays of essential oils were carried out as above but were diluted to a starting concentration of 2 mg/mL for serial dilution of thymol, carvacrol and trans-cinnamaldehyde. Purified nisin was adjusted to a 120 µM (400 µg/mL) starting concentration and 2-fold serial dilutions were carried out. The target strain was then added and after incubation for 16 h at 37 °C, the MIC was read as the lowest concentration causing inhibition of visible growth.

4.3. Nisin Purification

Nisin was purified according to previously described protocols [44–46]. The purified nisin peptide was subjected to MALDI-ToF Mass Spectrometric analysis to confirm purity before use.

4.4. Growth Curve Experiments

For growth experiments, overnight cultures were transferred (10^7 cfu mL^{-1} in a volume of 1.0 mL) into LB supplemented with the relevant concentration of nisin A and antibiotic/peptide or essential oil/peptide/EDTA combinations, and subsequently 0.2 mL was transferred to 96-well microtitre plates (Sarstedt). Cell growth was measured spectrophotometrically over 24 h or 48 h periods by using a SpectraMax M3 spectrophotometer (Molecular Devices, Sunnyvale, CA, USA).

4.5. Kill Assay Analysis

For kill assays, overnight cultures of target strains were transferred into LB broth (1 mL) containing nisin-purified peptide in combination with cinnamaldehyde and EDTA at the appropriate concentration. Samples were incubated for 3 h at 37 °C before serial dilution in Ringers solution followed by enumeration on LB agar plates. All experiments were carried out in triplicate.

4.6. Statistical Analysis

E. coli data were checked for normality and homogeneity of variances using the Shapiro–Wilk test and Levene's test, respectively. All comparisons were based on the mean ± standard deviation. Parametric data were analyzed using independent *t*-tests. Non-parametric data were analyzed by the Mann–Whitney U-test. All tests were performed using a 5% level of significance. All statistically significant results are complimented with the corresponding effect size using Cohen's d classification.

5. Conclusions

The increasing pressure on the livestock industry to halt the use of in-feed antibiotics has initiated new research to find safe and efficient alternatives. The combination of nisin peptides, essential oils such as cinnamaldehyde, and EDTA could pave the way for new treatment concepts when it comes to PWD, in particular towards Gram-negative bacteria including drug-resistant ETEC.

Acknowledgments: D.F., M.C.R., C.H. and R.R. are supported by the Irish Government under the National Development Plan, through SFI Investigator awards to C.H. and R.R. (10/IN.1/B3027), and the APC Microbiome Institute under Grant Number SFI/12/RC/2273. We thank Paula O'Connor for mass spectrometry analysis. We also thank Prof. Nola Leonard at the University College Dublin for providing *E. coli* isolates and the Agri-Food and BioSciences Institute (AFBI), Stormont, Northern Ireland, for providing ETEC strains.

Author Contributions: D.F. and I.B. contributed equally to the manuscript. Conceived and designed the experiments: D.F., C.H. and R.R. Performed the experiments: I.B., D.F. Analyzed the data: D.F., I.B., M.C.R., G.E.G. and C.H. Contributed reagents/materials/analysis tools: D.F., G.E.G., C.H. and R.P.R. Wrote the paper: D.F., I.B., R.P.R. and C.H.

References

1. Rhouma, M.; Letellier, A.; Beaudry, F.; Fairbrother, J.M. Post weaning diarrhea in pigs: Risk factors and non-colistin-based control strategies. *Acta Vet. Scand.* **2017**, *59*. [CrossRef] [PubMed]
2. De Briyne, N.; Atkinson, J.; Pokludová, L.; Borriello, S.P. Antibiotics used most commonly to treat animals in Europe. *Vet. Rec.* **2014**, *175*. [CrossRef] [PubMed]
3. Rolain, J.-M. Food and human gut as reservoirs of transferable antibiotic resistance encoding genes. *Front. Microbiol.* **2013**, *4*. [CrossRef] [PubMed]
4. Liu, Y.-Y.; Wang, Y.; Walsh, T.R.; Yi, L.X.; Zhang, R.; Spencer, J.; Yu, L.F. Emergence of plasmid-mediated colistin resistance mechanism MCR-1 in animals and human beings in China: A microbiological and molecular biological study. *Lancet Infect. Dis.* **2016**, *16*, 161–168. [CrossRef]
5. Haenni, M.; Poirel, L.; Kieffer, N.; Châtre, P.; Saras, E.; Métayer, V.; Madec, J.Y. Co-occurrence of extended spectrum β lactamase and MCR-1 encoding genes on plasmids. *Lancet Infect. Dis.* **2016**, *16*, 281–282. [CrossRef]
6. Delves-Broughton, J.; Blackburn, P.; Evans, R.J.; Hugenholtz, J. Applications of the bacteriocin, nisin. *Antonie Van Leeuwenhoek* **1996**, *69*, 193–202. [CrossRef] [PubMed]
7. Cao, L.T.; Wu, J.Q.; Xie, F.; Hu, S.H.; Mo, Y. Efficacy of nisin in treatment of clinical mastitis in lactating dairy cows. *J. Dairy Sci.* **2007**, *90*, 3980–3985. [CrossRef] [PubMed]
8. Wu, J.; Hu, S.; Cao, L. Therapeutic effect of nisin Z on subclinical mastitis in lactating cows. *Antimicrob. Agents Chemother.* **2007**, *51*, 3131–3135. [CrossRef] [PubMed]
9. Breukink, E.; de Kruijff, B. Lipid II as a target for antibiotics. *Nat. Rev. Drug Discov.* **2006**, *5*, 321–332. [CrossRef] [PubMed]
10. Wiedemann, I.; Breukink, E.; van Kraaij, C.; Kuipers, O.P.; Bierbaum, G.; de Kruijff, B.; Sahl, H.G. Specific binding of nisin to the peptidoglycan precursor lipid II combines pore formation and inhibition of cell wall biosynthesis for potent antibiotic activity. *J. Biol. Chem.* **2001**, *276*, 1772–1779. [CrossRef] [PubMed]
11. Bonelli, R.R.; Schneider, T.; Sahl, H.G.; Wiedemann, I. Insights into in vivo activities of lantibiotics from gallidermin and epidermin mode-of-action studies. *Antimicrob. Agents Chemother.* **2006**, *50*, 1449–1457. [CrossRef] [PubMed]
12. Breukink, E.; de Kruijff, B. The lantibiotic nisin, a special case or not? *Biochim. Biophys. Acta* **1999**, *1462*, 223–234. [CrossRef]
13. Ettayebi, K.; El Yamani, J.; Rossi-Hassani, B. Synergistic effects of nisin and thymol on antimicrobial activities in *Listeria monocytogenes* and *Bacillus subtilis*. *FEMS Microbiol. Lett.* **2000**, *183*, 191–195. [CrossRef] [PubMed]

14. Pol, I.E.; Smid, E.J. Combined action of nisin and carvacrol on *Bacillus cereus* and *Listeria monocytogenes*. *Lett. Appl. Microbiol.* **1999**, *29*, 166–170. [CrossRef] [PubMed]
15. Periago, P.M.; Moezelaar, R. Combined effect of nisin and carvacrol at different pH and temperature levels on the viability of different strains of *Bacillus cereus*. *Int. J. Food Microbiol.* **2001**, *68*, 141–148. [CrossRef]
16. Field, D.; Daly, K.; O'Connor, P.M.; Cotter, P.D.; Hill, C.; Ross, R.P. Efficacies of nisin A and nisin V semipurified preparations alone and in combination with plant essential oils for controlling *Listeria monocytogenes*. *Appl. Environ. Microbiol.* **2015**, *81*, 2762–2769. [CrossRef] [PubMed]
17. Branen, J.K.; Davidson, P.M. Enhancement of nisin, lysozyme, and monolaurin antimicrobial activities by ethylenediaminetetraacetic acid and lactoferrin. *Int. J. Food Microbiol.* **2004**, *90*, 63–74. [CrossRef]
18. Boziaris, I.S.; Adams, M.R. Effect of chelators and nisin produced in situ on inhibition and inactivation of gram negatives. *Int. J. Food Microbiol.* **1999**, *53*, 105–113. [CrossRef]
19. Al Atya, A.K.; Abriouel, H.; Kempf, I.; Jouy, E.; Auclair, E.; Vachée, A.; Drider, D. Effects of colistin and bacteriocins combinations on the in vitro growth of *Escherichia coli* strains from swine origin. *Probiot. Antimicrob. Proteins* **2016**, *8*, 183–190. [CrossRef] [PubMed]
20. Naghmouchi, K.; Baah, J.; Hober, D.; Jouy, E.; Rubrecht, C.; Sané, F.; Drider, D. Synergistic effect between colistin and bacteriocins in controlling gram-negative pathogens and their potential to reduce antibiotic toxicity in mammalian epithelial cells. *Antimicrob. Agents Chemother.* **2013**, *57*, 2719–2725. [CrossRef] [PubMed]
21. Meng, Q.; Bai, X.; Zhao, A.; Lan, R.; Du, H.; Wang, T.; Jin, D. Characterization of Shiga toxin-producing *Escherichia coli* isolated from healthy pigs in China. *BMC Microbiol.* **2014**, *14*. [CrossRef] [PubMed]
22. Corvec, S.; Tafin, U.F.; Betrisey, B.; Borens, O.; Trampuz, A. Activities of fosfomycin, tigecycline, colistin, and gentamicin against extended-spectrum-β-lactamase-producing *Escherichia coli* in a foreign-body infection model. *Antimicrob. Agents Chemother.* **2013**, *57*, 1421–1427. [CrossRef] [PubMed]
23. Hyldgaard, M.; Mygind, T.; Meyer, R.L. Essential oils in food preservation: Mode of action, synergies, and interactions with food matrix components. *Front. Microbiol.* **2012**, *3*. [CrossRef] [PubMed]
24. Nagy, B.; Fekete, P.Z. Enterotoxigenic *Escherichia coli* in veterinary medicine. *Int. J. Med. Microbiol.* **2005**, *295*, 443–454. [CrossRef] [PubMed]
25. Peng, M.; Salaheen, S.; Biswas, D. Animal health: Global antibiotic issues A2. In *Encyclopedia of Agriculture and Food Systems*; Van Alfen, N.K., Ed.; Academic Press: Oxford, UK, 2014; pp. 346–357.
26. Alves, F.C.; Barbosa, L.N.; Andrade, B.F.; Albano, M.; Furtado, F.B.; Pereira, A.F.M.; Júnior, A.F. Short communication: Inhibitory activities of the lantibiotic nisin combined with phenolic compounds against *Staphylococcus aureus* and *Listeria monocytogenes* in cow milk. *J. Dairy Sci.* **2016**, *99*, 1831–1836. [CrossRef] [PubMed]
27. Campion, A.; Morrissey, R.; Field, D.; Cotter, P.D.; Hill, C.; Ross, R.P. Use of enhanced nisin derivatives in combination with food-grade oils or citric acid to control *Cronobacter sakazakii* and *Escherichia coli* O157:H7. *Food Microbiol.* **2017**, *65*, 254–263. [CrossRef] [PubMed]
28. Zhou, L.; van Heel, A.J.; Montalban-Lopez, M.; Kuipers, O.P. Potentiating the activity of nisin against *Escherichia coli*. *Front. Cell Dev. Biol.* **2016**, *4*. [CrossRef] [PubMed]
29. Aquilina, G.; Azimonti, G.; Bampidis, V.; Bastos, M.D.L.; Bories, G.; Chesson, A.; Kouba, M. Products or Substances used in Animal, Safety and efficacy of Diarr-Stop S Plus® (Na2EDTA, tannin-rich extract of *Castanea sativa*, thyme oil and oregano oil) as a feed additive for pigs for fattening. *EFSA J.* **2016**, *14*. [CrossRef]
30. Wynn, J.E.; Riet, B.V.; Borzelleca, J.F. The toxicity and pharmacodynamics of EGTA: Oral administration to rats and comparisons with EDTA. *Toxicol. Appl. Pharmacol.* **1970**, *16*, 807–817. [CrossRef]
31. Yang, F.Y.; Lin, Z.H.; Li, S.G. Reversal of mitochondrial swelling by ethylenediaminetetraacetate. *Sci. Sin.* **1964**, *13*, 1518–1522. [PubMed]
32. Khan, A.; Vu, K.D.; Riedl, B.; Lacroix, M. Optimization of the antimicrobial activity of nisin, Na-EDTA and pH against gram-negative and gram-positive bacteria. *LWT Food Sci. Technol.* **2015**, *61*, 124–129. [CrossRef]
33. Partanen, K.H.; Mroz, Z. Organic acids for performance enhancement in pig diets. *Nutr. Res. Rev.* **1999**, *12*, 117–145. [CrossRef] [PubMed]
34. Tsiloyiannis, V.K.; Kyriakis, S.C.; Vlemmas, J.; Sarris, K. The effect of organic acids on the control of post-weaning oedema disease of piglets. *Res. Vet. Sci.* **2001**, *70*, 281–285. [CrossRef] [PubMed]

35. Suiryanrayna, M.; Ramana, J.V. A review of the effects of dietary organic acids fed to swine. *J. Anim. Sci. Biotechnol.* **2015**, *6*. [CrossRef] [PubMed]
36. Zhao, X.; Zhen, Z.; Wang, X.; Guo, N. Synergy of a combination of nisin and citric acid against *Staphylococcus aureus* and *Listeria monocytogenes*. *Food Addit. Contam. Part A* **2017**, *34*, 2058–2068. [CrossRef] [PubMed]
37. Zeng, Z.; Zhang, S.; Wang, H.; Piao, X. Essential oil and aromatic plants as feed additives in non-ruminant nutrition: A review. *J. Anim. Sci. Biotechnol.* **2015**, *6*. [CrossRef] [PubMed]
38. Li, S.Y.; Ru, Y.J.; Liu, M.; Xu, B.; Péron, A.; Shi, X.G. The effect of essential oils on performance, immunity and gut microbial population in weaner pigs. *Livest. Sci.* **2012**, *145*, 119–123. [CrossRef]
39. Michiels, J.; Missotten, J.; Rasschaert, G.; Dierick, N.; Heyndrickx, M.; De Smet, S. Effect of organic acids on Salmonella colonization and shedding in weaned piglets in a seeder model. *J. Food Prot.* **2012**, *75*, 1974–1983. [CrossRef] [PubMed]
40. Walia, K.; Argüello, H.; Lynch, H.; Leonard, F.C.; Grant, J.; Yearsley, D.; Lawlor, P.G. Effect of strategic administration of an encapsulated blend of formic acid, citric acid, and essential oils on Salmonella carriage, seroprevalence, and growth of finishing pigs. *Prev. Vet. Med.* **2017**, *137*, 28–35. [CrossRef] [PubMed]
41. Stensland, I.; Kim, J.C.; Bowring, B.; Collins, A.M.; Mansfield, J.P.; Pluske, J.R.A. Comparison of diets supplemented with a feed additive containing organic acids, cinnamaldehyde and a permeabilizing complex, or zinc oxide, on post-weaning diarrhoea, selected bacterial populations, blood measures and performance in weaned pigs experimentally infected with enterotoxigenic *E. coli*. *Animals* **2015**, *5*, 1147–1168. [CrossRef]
42. Józefiak, D.; Kierończyk, B.; Juśkiewicz, J.; Zduńczyk, Z.; Rawski, M.; Długosz, J.; Højberg, O. Dietary nisin modulates the gastrointestinal microbial ecology and enhances growth performance of the broiler chickens. *PLoS ONE* **2013**, *8*, e85347. [CrossRef] [PubMed]
43. Laukova, A.; Chrastinová, L'.; Plachá, I.; Kandričáková, A.; Szabóová, R.; Strompfová, V.; Žitňan, R. Beneficial effect of lantibiotic nisin in rabbit husbandry. *Probiot. Antimicrob. Proteins* **2014**, *6*, 41–46. [CrossRef] [PubMed]
44. Field, D.; Quigley, L.; O'Connor, P.M.; Rea, M.C.; Daly, K.; Cotter, P.D.; Ross, R.P. Studies with bioengineered nisin peptides highlight the broad-spectrum potency of nisin V. *Microb. Biotechnol.* **2010**, *3*, 473–486. [CrossRef] [PubMed]
45. Field, D.; Begley, M.; O'Connor, P.M.; Daly, K.M.; Hugenholtz, F.; Cotter, P.D.; Ross, R.P. Bioengineered nisin A derivatives with enhanced activity against both gram positive and gram negative pathogens. *PLoS ONE* **2012**, *7*, e46884. [CrossRef] [PubMed]
46. Healy, B.; Field, D.; O'Connor, P.M.; Hill, C.; Cotter, P.D.; Ross, R.P. Intensive mutagenesis of the nisin hinge leads to the rational design of enhanced derivatives. *PLoS ONE* **2013**, *8*, e79563. [CrossRef] [PubMed]

4

Efficacy of an Optimised Bacteriophage Cocktail to Clear *Clostridium difficile* in a Batch Fermentation Model

Janet Y. Nale [1], Tamsin A. Redgwell [2], Andrew Millard [1] and Martha R. J. Clokie [1,*]

1 Department of Infection, Immunity and Inflammation, University of Leicester, Leicester LE1 9HN, UK; jn142@le.ac.uk (J.Y.N.); adm39@leicester.ac.uk (A.M.)

2 School of Life Sciences, University of Warwick, Coventry CV4 7AL, UK; T.Redgwell@warwick.ac.uk

* Correspondence: mrjc1@le.ac.uk

Abstract: *Clostridium difficile* infection (CDI) is a major cause of infectious diarrhea. Conventional antibiotics are not universally effective for all ribotypes, and can trigger dysbiosis, resistance and recurrent infection. Thus, novel therapeutics are needed to replace and/or supplement the current antibiotics. Here, we describe the activity of an optimised 4-phage cocktail to clear cultures of a clinical ribotype 014/020 strain in fermentation vessels spiked with combined fecal slurries from four healthy volunteers. After 5 h, we observed ~6-log reductions in *C. difficile* abundance in the prophylaxis regimen and complete *C. difficile* eradication after 24 h following prophylactic or remedial regimens. Viability assays revealed that commensal enterococci, bifidobacteria, lactobacilli, total anaerobes, and enterobacteria were not affected by either regimens, but a ~2-log increase in the enterobacteria, lactobacilli, and total anaerobe abundance was seen in the phage-only-treated vessel compared to other treatments. The impact of the phage treatments on components of the microbiota was further assayed using metagenomic analysis. Together, our data supports the therapeutic application of our optimised phage cocktail to treat CDI. Also, the increase in specific commensals observed in the phage-treated control could prevent further colonisation of *C. difficile*, and thus provide protection from infection being able to establish.

Keywords: *Clostridium difficile*; *Clostridium difficile* infection; bacteriophages; phage therapy; microbiome; in vitro fermentation model

---

1. Introduction

Antimicrobial resistance is a global health threat to clinical practice and public health [1–4]. It is estimated that the continued rise in multidrug resistance (MDR) will cause 10 million people to die worldwide by 2050 and cost 100 trillion USD [5]. To effectively control bacterial infections, novel effective antimicrobials with target specificity and high efficiency are urgently needed [6–8]. Although bacteriophages or phages (viruses which specifically lyse bacteria) were first isolated over 100 years ago, for a long period they were mainly the focus of fundamental research. However, particularly over the last decade, there has been an increasing interest in the isolation, characterisation and development of phages for therapeutic use in humans, animals, and plants [9–13]. This revived interest is mainly driven by problems associated with ineffective antibiotics. These natural bacterial predators have the potential to provide a safe and suitable supplement, or replacement for antibiotics because of their specificity and amplification at the site of infection [14–17]. Indeed, phage products have been developed for medical use, and some can be found as over-the-counter medicines and are used as decontamination agents in food industries [10,18–20].

Clostridium difficile is a notorious nosocomial bacterium that remains a major cause of infectious diarrhea, with high morbidity and mortality in the elderly and in immunocompromised patients worldwide [21–25]. *C. difficile* surveillance for the United Kingdom showed that there were 19,269 reported cases of *C. difficile* infection (CDI) and 488 (~3%) fatalities in 2015. In the US, ~500,000 CDI cases are reported annually, with approximate 30,000 deaths, 20% recurrent rates, and an estimated treatment cost of ~$10,000 per case [21,22,26]. CDI is becoming increasingly difficult to treat because of the emergence of severe and antibiotic-resistant ribotypes, and very limited treatment options [6,27,28]. Currently, only three antibiotics are available on the market for CDI treatment. Metronidazole is cheap, largely effective, and is recommended for initial use in moderate or non-severe episodes [29–31]. However, there are problems associated with its efficacy to treat some important prevalent and clinically relevant ribotypes, resistance has also been seen towards this antibiotic, and it is associated with health-related complications such as low birth weight [30,32,33]. Vancomycin is the antibiotic of choice for moderate to severe CDI but its use, particularly if long-term, can promote the emergence of vancomycin-resistant enterococci [34,35]. Also reduced susceptibility have been reported in *C. difficile* leading to recurrent infection, thus it is suboptimal [36,37]. Fidaxomicin is a highly specific antibiotic that has been shown to be effective when vancomycin treatment has failed [38] but it is expensive ($3360 compared to $1273 for vancomycin or $21.90 for metronidazole—all per course) and may not be cost-effective for some strain-specific CDIs [39–41]. This complex relationship between *C. difficile* and antibiotics is compounded by the fact that they generally have a detrimental impact on the gut microbiota, which leads to dysbiosis that then enables *C. difficile* to colonise the gut and cause disease. Therefore, there is a clear need to develop additional antimicrobials with increased target specificity in order to efficiently remove this pathogen but leave other components of the gut microbiota intact [6,10].

Previous reports have described the isolation of phages that specifically target *C. difficile* and demonstrated the use of different in vivo and in vitro models to test the specificity and efficacy of the phages to selectively eradicate this bacterium [42–46]. The commonly used in vivo model for CDI and *C. difficile* phage therapy is the hamster model, which is useful as hamsters demonstrate the classical CDI clinical symptoms seen in humans [47,48]. However, the model is difficult to use because of the exquisite sensitivity of hamsters to *C. difficile* toxins, high costs, and inherent technical issues associated with working with these animals [49,50]. Therefore, alternative models such as the wax moth *Galleria mellonella* larva have been developed as suitable replacement models to probe many aspects of CDI phage therapy [46]. Other models that have been used to study *C. difficile* phage therapy are the in vitro gut and batch fermentation models [44,51]. Although these models have been developed to study the gut microbiome and pharmokinetics of antibiotics, very few studies have applied them to study *C. difficile* phage therapy [38,50,52].

The four myoviruses CDHM1, 2, 5, and 6 used in this study were isolated from the environment and were well characterised in our laboratory [45,53]. This optimised phage cocktail was the first phage mix shown to completely clear *C. difficile* in pure cultures and it was also shown to prevent biofilm formation in vitro. In addition, the phages reduced colonisation in vivo in both hamster and wax moth larva CDI models [45,46]. The data obtained from these models provided novel insights into the therapeutic applications of these phages to treat CDI. However, more information is needed in order to determine the specificity of this phage set to *C. difficile*, and to establish their ability to clear the target pathogen in the presence of competitive pressure from other components of the human gut microbiota. Indeed, no previous publications have examined the potential impact of the application of *C. difficile* phages on the human microbiome. Therefore, we developed and present results from an in vitro phage therapy assay using a batch fermentation model. To do this, we obtained human feces from a specific age profile of healthy volunteers (with full ethical consent) in order to examine the impacts of our phage set on a wide range of human microbiota. The work was designed to: (i) determine the efficacy of our optimised phage cocktail to clear a clinically relevant ribotype 014/020 strain in the presence of the gut microbiota, (ii) test the efficiency of the phages using prophylactic or remedial regimens in the targeted eradication of the bacterium in the batch fermentation model, and (iii) ascertain the potential synergistic or antagonistic effect of phage application on culturable and unculturable components of the human gut microbiome.

2. Results

2.1. Individual Donors Have a Unique Microbiome Composition

To determine the specificity and efficacy of the phages to clear *C. difficile* in the presence of competitive pressure from representative human gut microbiota, we spiked five fermentation vessels containing a minimal medium with combined fecal slurries obtained from four healthy volunteers [54–56]. The donors were comprised of individuals from diverse ethnic and age groups (a 70-year-old white British woman, 44-year-old black woman, 17-year-old black girl, and 7-year-old white British boy) to capture a wide range of human gut microbial diversity. Prior to mixing the fecal slurries together, we determined the microbiome composition from the individual donors by resuspending the fecal matter in the minimal medium and enumerating the bacteria present on selective agar media targeting five commonly occurring gut commensals [44,51]. We observed that approximately 10^5–10^6 CFU/mL (colony-forming unit per milliliter) of enterococci counts were detected from all the four donors. Similar counts were observed with the lactobacilli group, except that the abundance of this bacterium was very low, hence it was undetectable in the teenager. Relatively higher counts were observed in the total anaerobes and enterobacteria, which ranged from 10^6 to 10^7 CFU/mL in all the donors. The bifidobacterial counts were quite variable, from very low counts of ~10^3 CFU/mL in the teenager, to 10^5 and 10^6 CFU/mL in the infant and adult, respectively, and 10^7 CFU/mL in the elderly donor lady. Interestingly, but not unexpectedly, we did not recover *C. difficile* from any of the donors. When the fecal matter was mixed together and assayed, it was observed that the total anaerobes and enterobacterial numbers were the highest with ~10^6 CFU/mL, but ~10^5 CFU/mL was being contributed by the enterococci, lactobacilli, and bifidobacteria (Figure 1).

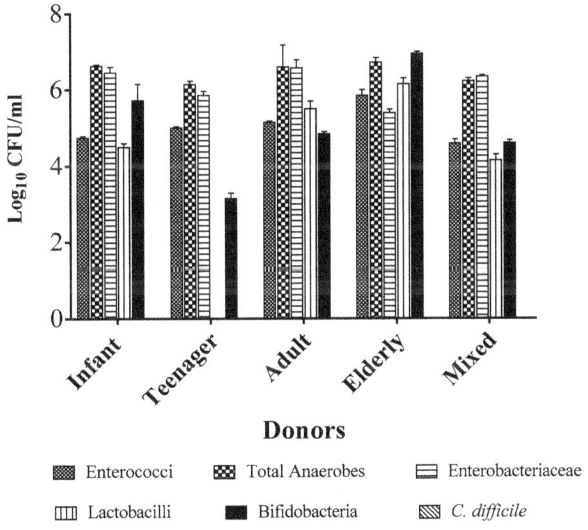

Figure 1. Contributory culturable bacterial counts from each of the individual donors and final cumulative counts of each bacterium added to the fermentation vessels. The bacteria present in the fecal sample of each donor were determined by recovery on selective medium for each bacterial grouping, after which, the samples were mixed together in relatively equal amounts and used to prime the fermentation vessels. The data was analysed using GraphPad Prism 7. Error bars are SEMs of three biological replicates.

2.2. Phages Cleared *C. difficile* in the Batch Fermentation Model

We determined the ability of the phage cocktail to clear CD105LC2 (ribotype 014/020 clinical strain) in the batch fermentation model using two treatments. In the prophylactic regimen, the fecal slurries were exposed to a dose of the phage cocktail followed by a mixture of the phages and bacteria, and subsequently by two doses of the phage cocktail (Table 1). In the first 5 h following bacteria and phage exposure, we observed a ~6-log reduction of CFU/mL of *C. difficile* counts in the prophylactic regimen compared to the bacterial control. When the fermentation vessels were treated remedially, the phage cocktail was added after culturing the bacteria for 5 h. At the 24 h time point (19 h post-phage treatment in the remedial regimen), *C. difficile* was eradicated in both the prophylactic and remedial treatment vessels, and this observation remained consistent from this time until the end of the experiment (72 h). As expected, *C. difficile* was not detected in the untreated (vessel 1) and the phage (vessel 3) controls. However, in the *C. difficile*-only control (vessel 2), we observed that after 5 h of incubation, *C. difficile* numbers began to drop from ~10^7 CFU/mL (at 5 h) to ~10^4 CFU/mL at 36, 48, and 72 h, respectively (Figure 2A).

Table 1. Bacteria and phage treatment regimens for the gut fermentation vessels.

Fermentation Vessels	Treatments	Time to Dose (h)						
		−2	0	5	24	36	48	72
1	Control untreated	-	M	M	M	M	M	-
2	*C. difficile* control	-	B	M	M	M	M	-
3	Control phage	-	P	P	P	P	M	-
4	Prophylaxis	P	P+B	P	P	M	M	-
5	Remedial	-	B	P	P	P	P	-

Five vessels containing combined fecal slurries from four healthy volunteers were treated with 2 mL each of 6–8 × 10^8 CFU/mL of *C. difficile* culture (B), 2–6 × 10^9 PFU/mL (plaque-forming units per milliliter) of phage cocktail (P), and/or minimal medium (M) at the time points shown above [51]. At each time point, 2 mL of samples from the vessels were removed and replaced with an equal volume of the bacteria, phage or medium. The time points were selected based on our prior in vitro data on the phages, which showed that the phages maintained clearance of CD105LC2 cultures at the first 5 and 24 h time points [45]. The additional 36 and 48 h time points were based on previous fermentation studies [51].

2.3. *Impact of Phage Treatmens on the Viability of other Components of the Culturable Gut Microbiota*

After establishing the efficacy of the phage cocktail to clear *C. difficile* in the batch fermentation model, we investigated their impact on five common major bacterial groups in the human gut. We did this by conducting viability assays on selective media for bifidobacteria, enterococci, enterobacteria, lactobacilli, and total anaerobes in the five fermentation vessels at all the time points examined [44,51].

Bifidobacterial numbers were relatively constant in both the treatment regimens and the three controls throughout the experiment. The ~10^5 CFU/mL of bacteria observed at 0 h decreased to ~10^4 CFU/mL in all the treatment regimens as well as in the controls at 5 h. The bacterial numbers remained relatively stable at this level until the end of the experiment (72 h). There was no significant difference in the number of bacteria left in all the treatment vessels at the end of the 72 h time period of the experiment ($p = 0.05$) (Figure 2B).

The enterococci abundance showed distinct changes depending on the treatment. Relatively equal numbers, ~10^5 CFU/mL of bacteria, were observed at the beginning of the experiment (0 h) in all the treatment vessels, and this number remained consistent until 24 h. After this time, the bacterial numbers dropped to ~10^4 CFU/mL in vessels 1 and 2, which corresponded to the untreated and *C. difficile* controls, respectively, both not treated with the phages. The numbers for this group of bacteria continued to drop in vessels 1 and 2, and after 72 h, only ~10^3 CFU/mL of bacteria were recovered. However, in all the phage-treated vessels comprising the phage control (vessel 3), the prophylactic (vessel 4), and the remedial regimens (vessel 5), the enterococci detected remained relatively stable at ~10^5 CFU/mL from 5 h to 72 h (Figure 2C).

For the enterobacteria, the numbers increased from ~10^6 to 10^8 CFU/mL within the first 5 h of the experiment in all the fermentation vessels. After 24 h, the bacterial numbers remained stable in the phage-only treated control, but lower numbers (10^7 CFU/mL) were observed in the untreated vessel

(vessel 1) and the prophylaxis vessel (vessel 3). The remedial and the bacterial control vessels had even lower numbers (10^6 CFU/mL). After 24 h, higher enterobacterial numbers (~10^8 CFU/mL) were seen in the phage-only treated vessel (vessel 3), which remained stable throughout the experiment. In the other vessels (vessels 1, 2, 4, and 5), however, the bacterial counts remained lower (at ~10^6 CFU/mL) than in the phage-treated vessel at 24 h until the experiment was terminated. At the end of the experiment, ~2-log CFU/mL higher numbers of enterobacteria were observed in the phage-only treated vessel (vessel 3), compared to the other vessels (Figure 2D).

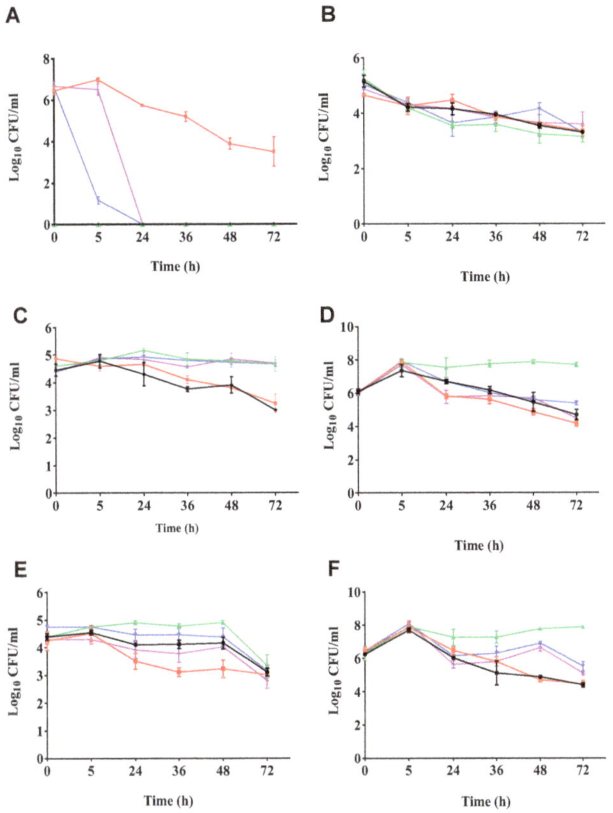

Figure 2. Impact of phage treatment on *C. difficile* and other components of the gut microbiota. The impact of phage treatment was ascertained by recovering the bacteria on selective media for (**A**) *C. difficile*; (**B**) bifidobacteria; (**C**) enterococci; (**D**) enterobacteria; (**E**) lactobacilli; (**F**) total anaerobes. The bacterial counts of the different treatment vessels and time points are presented. Black lines, vessel 1, untreated slurries; red lines, vessel 2, *C. difficile* control; green lines, vessel 3, phage-only-treated control; blue lines, vessel 4, prophylaxis regimen, and purple lines, vessel 5, remedial regimen. The data was analysed using GraphPad Prism 7. Error bars are SEMs of 3 biological replicates.

We also assayed for lactobacilli counts in all the treatment vessels over the time points. We observed that equal numbers (~10^5 CFU/mL) of the bacteria were detected in the beginning of the experiment at 5 h in all the vessels. At the 24 h time point, the phage-only treated and the prophylactic-treated vessels had higher bacterial numbers than the remedial regimen, the *C. difficile*, and the untreated control vessels. In all the vessels, the bacterial numbers remained stable at this level and at the subsequent three time points of 24, 36, and 48 h, but steadily declined to ~10^3 CFU/mL at 72 h (Figure 2E).

The final bacterial group assayed on selective media was the total anaerobes. As observed for the enterococci, the total number of anaerobes increased markedly from ~10^6 CFU/mL at 0 h to 10^8 CFU/mL at 5 h in all the vessels. However, the total number of anaerobes (~10^7 CFU/mL) in the phage-only treated control vessel (vessel 3) was ~1-log CFU/mL higher than in the other four treatment vessels (vessels 1, 2, 4, and 5) at 24 and 36 h. At 48 h however, the total anaerobe count was higher in the phage-only treatment (vessel 3), with ~10^8 CFU/mL recovered, followed by the prophylaxis and remedial regimen vessels with ~10^6 CFU/mL of bacteria detected. The control untreated slurries (vessel 1) and the *C. difficile* control (vessel 2) had relatively lower numbers (~10^5 CFU/mL) at 72 h (Figure 2F).

2.4. Metagenomics Analysis of the Impact of Phage Treatment on the Total Microbiome within the Gut Fermentation Vessels

The viability assays confirmed a complete eradication of *C. difficile* at the 24 h after phage treatment in both the prophylactic and remedial fermentation vessels. The beginning of an effect on five other bacterial groups was also observed. To probe these observations more deeply and to determine the impact on the components of the microbiota, including those that cannot be cultured, the total DNA from the five treatment vessels at the 24 h time point was extracted and used as a template for whole metagenomics analysis. The total reads per vessel at 24 h were mapped to relevant sequences representing all three domains of life (Table 2). The percentage of reads for each domain was normalised against the total number of reads found in each vessel. The highest percentage of reads for bacteria was found in vessel 5, with 99.11%, whereas the lowest percentage of reads was found in vessel 1, with 97.76% reads. We observed that Firmicutes, Bacteroidetes, Proteobacteria, Actinobacteria, Cyanobacteria, Euryarchaeota, Verrucomicrobia, Deinococcus-Thermus, Spirochaetes and Synergistetes abundances were consistently the most abundant among the bacterial phyla examined, irrespective of the treatment vessel (Table S1, Figure 3A–D,Fi). Although the individual groups of bacteria remained consistent in all treatments, their abundances varied considerably in the vessels. We observed that percent reads mapped to Actinobacteria were higher in the none-phage-treated vessels (vessel 1, 26.2% and vessel 2, 26.9%) compared to vessels 3 (22.4%), 4 (23.8%), and 5 (25.3), which corresponded to phage-treated vessels (Table S1, Figure 3A–E). This pattern in all the vessels was also observed for the Bacteroidetes, for which the reads found in non-phage-treated vessels were higher compared to those in phage-treated vessels (Table S1). In contrast, the Deinococcus levels were higher in vessels 3, 4, and 5, which contained the phages, but reduced in non-phage-treated vessels (vessels 1 and 2). The Firmicutes and Verrucomicrobia had reduced abundance in the phage-only-treated slurries compared to the other four vessels (Table S1). Conversely, the Cyanobacteria, Enterobacteriaceae, and Proteobacteria abundance was elevated at 24 h in the phage-only-treated control vessel compared to the other four vessels. The abundance of the Spirochaetes in the prophylaxis treatment regimens was comparable to the level found in the untreated slurries (vessel 1). Consistent with our viability assays, we observed that Bifidobacteriaceae, Enterobacteriaceae, Lactobacillales as well as the Coriobacteriaceae, Bacteroidaceae, Porphyromonadaceae, Rikenellaceae, Eubacteriaceae, Lachnospiraceae, Rhizobiales, Desulfovibrionales and Ruminococcacea abundances were considerably high in vessel 3 from the metagenomics data (Figure 3A–D,Fi).

Table 2. Reads mapped to the three domains of life.

Domain	Clade Reads in Each Vessel (%)				
	V1	V2	V3	V4	V5
Bacteria	89,526 (97.76)	74,116 (99.05)	23,061 (98.89)	96,888 (98.77)	103,406 (99.11)
Archaea	2030 (2.217)	646 (0.8633)	19 (0.08148)	926 (0.944)	764 (0.7323)
Viruses	18 (0.01966)	64 (0.08553)	240 (1.029)	284 (0.2895)	165 (0.1581)
Total	91,574	74,826	23,320	98,098	104,335

Whole genome sequencing was conducted on DNA samples extracted at the 24 h time point. The data was analysed using Pavian.

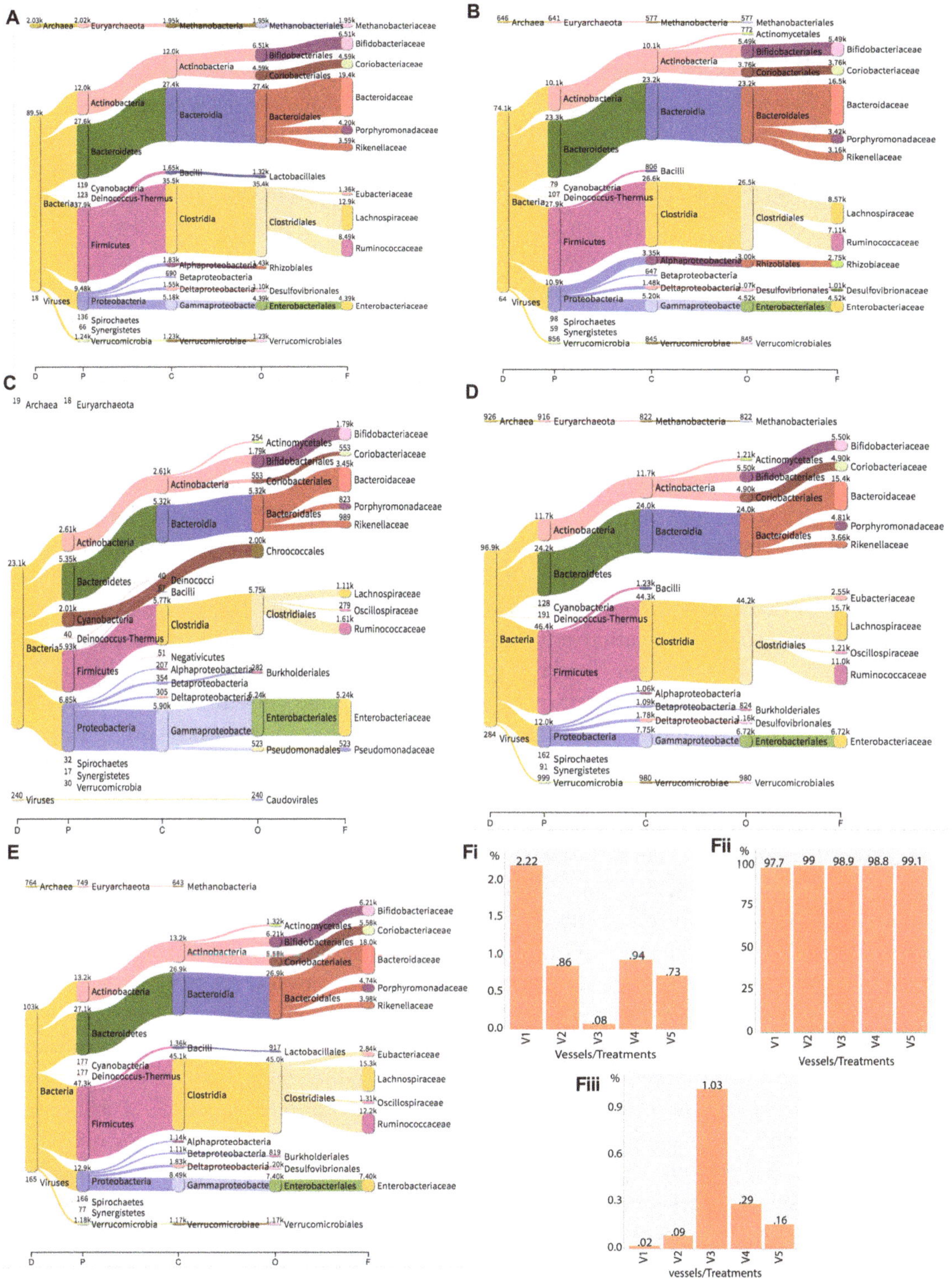

Figure 3. Analysis of the 10 most abundant taxa from Archea, Bacteria, and Viruses as ascertained by the metagenomics data. Total genomic DNA was extracted at 24 h time point from (**A**) vessel 1, untreated slurries; (**B**) vessel 2, *C. difficile* control; (**C**) vessel 3, phage-only-treated control; (**D**) vessel 4, prophylaxis regimen; (**E**) vessel 5, remedial regimen. The samples were prepared using NexteraXT sample preparation kit and sequenced on MiSeq platform using V2 (2 × 250 bp) chemistry. The resulting fastq files were trimmed with Sickle, and the metagenomes were assembled using megahit. An overview of the 10 most abundant taxa: Phyla (P), Classes (C), order (O), and family (F) are shown for each treatment vessel, as visualised using Pavian. The percent reads mapped to Archaea, Bacteria, and Viruses in the vessels at 24 h are shown in (**Fi**), (**Fii**), and (**Fiii**), respectively.

The percentage of reads mapped to Archaea was found to be highest in the untreated vessel (vessel 1), with 2.2% reads mapped to this domain in this vessel at the 24 h time point. The remaining vessels, V2–5, had low percent reads (0.08–0.94) mapped to Archaea compared to the untreated vessel 1. The phylum Euryarchaeota, consisting of the family Methanobacteriaceae was consistently found in all the vessels, although its abundance was considerably lower in the phage-only-treated vessel (vessel 3) (Figure 3Fii).

Consistent with the other two phyla, we found reads corresponding to viruses to be represented in all the treatment vessels. For the percentages of reads which mapped to the viruses, we found the highest level in vessel 3 (phage-only-treated vessel) with 1.029% of the total reads, and lower levels in all other treatment vessels (vessel 1, 2, 4, and 5). Vessel 1 had the lowest percent viral reads (0.0196) compared to vessels 2, 3, 4, and 5, which had 0.08553, 1.029, 0.2895, and 0.1581%, respectively (Figure 3Fiii).

3. Discussion

The need for alternative therapeutics to combat antibiotic resistance is clear [5,57]. The challenges posed by MDR are current and serious and so cannot be ignored. Consequently, significant resources are being channeled towards understanding the root causes of MDR and developing effective approaches to tackle the associated health threats [8,58,59]. There is an urgent clinical unmet need for novel treatments for *C. difficile*, the causal agent of CDI [6,60]. Recent reviews on past, current, and future options for CDI treatment concluded that phage therapy has significant potential as a treatment because of its specificity, amplification at infection sites, and minimal deleterious impact to the gut microbiome [6,16,43]. The development of phage treatments for this pathogen has been hampered by the lack of strictly virulent phages. Furthermore, although past data has demonstrated the efficacy of *C. difficile* phages to clear the bacterium in vitro and in vivo, there is the lack of preclinical data to ascertain the impact of these phages on the human gut microbiome [45,46]. Previously, we developed the first effective *C. difficile* phage cocktail, which consists of four well-characterised, broad host range myoviruses [45,46]. In this study, we showed as a proof of concept that the cocktail can effectively clear a clinically prevalent *C. difficile* ribotype isolate in a batch fermentation model, and that their application promotes the growth of other human gut commensals.

The two previous reports on *C. difficile* phage therapy using in vitro gut models used a batch fermentation model over a 48 h time period [51] or a three-component continuous colon model over a 35 day period [44]. In both assays, the effect of one phage, ΦCD27, to clear NCTC11204, a ribotype 001 strain, was investigated. The two reports are consistent with our observation that the prophylactic regimen is more effective at clearing *C. difficile* than the remedial regimen. Although both previous data sets showed a significant reduction (~6-log CFU/mL) in the prophylaxis treatment, *C. difficile* (~1-log CFU/mL) was still detected in the 48 h report [51], and up to 10^8 CFU/mL of cells or spores were detected in the 35 day report at the end of the assays [44]. Whilst ΦCD27 was shown to be active in the prophylactic regimen, the regrowth observed could be attributed either to resistance-developing, an inherent insensitivity of the bacterium to the phages, or the generation of resistant lysogenic clones, as shown when the bacterium was treated with the phage at a multiplicity of infection (MOI) of 7 [51]. Since all published *C. difficile* phages are temperate and encode an integrase gene, which mediates their integration into host genomes, the development of lysogenic mutants using a single phage for therapy occurs, as shown in previous reports [45,47,51]. In our previous work and in work presented here, we have demonstrated that the impacts of lysogeny and/or phage or antibiotic resistance are mitigated by the application of an optimised diverse phage cocktail [45,46]. *C. difficile* was fully lysed regardless of whether a prophylactic or remedial regimen was applied, and remained undetectable till the end of the experiment (72 h), as shown in this study (Figure 2A) and in our previous in vitro models [45,46]. The phages used here exhibit a complementary effect, whereby resistant or lysogenic clones produced by one phage or antibiotic treatment become susceptible to infection by another phage in the mix, leading to complete eradication of *C. difficile* in vitro and significant reduction of colonisation in vivo [45,46].

The advantages of using a phage cocktail was also demonstrated in our remedial regimen, where we observed a ~7-log CFU/mL reduction in *C. difficile* counts, and the bacterium was completely eliminated from vessel 5 (remedial regimen) within 24 h of the post-phage treatment without any detectable regrowth (Figure 2A). In contrast, there was only a >1-log CFU/mL reduction when the single phage ΦCD27 was applied remedially at an MOI of 10 at this time and at subsequent time points, and no observable impact was reported when the phage was applied at an MOI of 7 [51]. The lower remedial impact of *C. difficile* phages was also observed in other in vitro assays [45–48]. Obviously, these data further support the fact that phage therapy for CDI will require the application of optimised phage combinations, as previously reported for treating other bacterial species [13,61]. Although our phage cocktail was optimised for the ribotype 014/020, work is currently ongoing in our laboratory to determine suitable phage combinations for other prevalent and severe ribotypes.

In our fermentation model, we have for the first time studied the impact of phages on microbiomes derived from fecal samples from four healthy volunteers from different age groups and ethnicities to prime the fermentation vessels. Although we used fecal matter from healthy live volunteers from different age groups, other work used human fecal matter of deceased individuals [62] or healthy elderly individuals [44,51,52,56]. Whilst the elderly group reflects the majority of people commonly predisposed to CDI because of their weak immune system, other age groups are also susceptible to the pathogen, though to a lesser extent [63,64]. In addition, human gut microbiomes have been shown to vary greatly and be shaped by individual lifestyles, age groups, and geographical regions, and have been studied in combined emulsions (Figure 1) [54,55,65].

Although *C. difficile* is often a natural human commensal, we did not recover it from the fecal samples of our donors using our viability assays. *C. difficile* is generally considered to be an opportunistic bacterium and could remain in the gut of a healthy individual without causing disease until there is a disruption of the microbial balance (dysbiosis) through antibiotic use, triggering *C. difficile* to colonise the gut and causing disease [6,66,67]. *C. difficile* could possibly be present in the guts of our donors but in low abundance, hence it could not be detected in the feces [67]. In addition, the decline in *C. difficile* counts, as observed in the bacterial control after 24 h, has been reported previously and could reflect the response of the bacterium outside the natural gut environment or the depletion of nutrients in the medium used [44,51].

Our observations from the viability assays and metagenomic analysis show that both the prophylactic or remedial phage regimens did not have a significant detrimental impact on the five bacterial groups examined and concur with other previous phage therapy assays [44,51]. Similarly, we did not observe a huge difference in the abundance of bacteria in the phage-treated vessels and controls in the metagenomics data, and this clearly supports the advantages of phage therapy over antibiotics [68]. Because of their specificity, phages are able to infect the targeted bacteria, preserving the commensal niche as opposed to chemical antibiotics, which have a broader activity and may induce superinfection by some species such as *C. difficile* [15,69].

Prior to our work, no data had examined the impact of just *C. difficile* phages on other components of the microbiota during therapy. The two previously published fermentation model reports examined the impact of phages on *C. difficile* clearance and the corresponding impact on other commensals but did not examine the effect of phages alone on the gut microbiota [44,51]. Here, we showed that the abundances of certain gut commensals were elevated and restored to the initial levels of the donor samples during phage administration, and this clearly links to the high viral abundance found in vessel 3 (Table 2). This observation strongly suggests that the phages could promote the growth of natural human bacteria, providing health benefits, and thus could protect the gut from *C. difficile* colonisation [69]. The possible roles of phages in the restoration of the gut microbiomes of CDI patients have previously been reported and may provide biological insights into the mechanisms of fecal transplantation. For example, previous data showed that fecal matter containing higher diversity of Caudovirales led to increased richness, diversity, and evenness of these viral particles when transplanted to CDI patients. A concomitant increase in the abundance of other gut commensals (such as Proteobacteria and Actinobacteria) and the resultant resolution of CDI were also observed in the majority of the recipient patients [70]. Similarly, the administration of fecal filtrates from healthy humans via nasojejunal tubes restored the normal stool habits and eliminated CDI symptoms in five symptomatic chronic relapsing CDI patients in another study [71].

4. Materials and Methods

4.1. Bacterial Isolates and Phage Cocktail Used in This Study

In this study, two *C. difficile* isolates were examined. The first, CD105HE1, is an environmental isolate of ribotype 076 and was used as the propagating host for the phages [53]. The second bacterial isolate, CD105LC2, was the test strain for the gut fermentation model and belonged to the clinically prevalent ribotype 014/020 [45]. The bacterial isolates were routinely cultured on brain heart infusion (BHI) agar (Oxoid, Hampshire, UK) supplemented with 7% defibrinated horse blood (Thermo Scientific, Hampshire, UK) for 48 h prior to use, or stored in cryogenic storage tubes (Abtek Biologicals Ltd., Liverpool, UK) at −80 °C. The bacterial culture used for the gut fermentation experiments was produced by inoculating a single colony of the test bacterium in 5 mL of pre-reduced fastidious anaerobic broth (BioConnections, Knypersley, UK) and incubating anaerobically (10% H_2, 5% CO_2 and 85% N_2, Don Whitley Scientific, West Yorkshire, UK) at 37 °C for 18–24 h. A 1:100 dilution of the overnight culture was prepared in 10 mL BHI broth, incubated until OD_{550}~0.25–0.3 (~10^8 CFU/mL) was attained, and used to inoculate the fermentation vessels. All liquid culture media were pre-reduced anaerobically at 37 °C for at least 1 h prior to use.

An optimised phage cocktail containing four *C. difficile* myoviruses, CDHM1, 2, 5, and 6 was used for phage therapy in this study. The individual phages were isolated from the environment and characterised previously in our laboratory [45,46], and propagated individually in liquid cultures of the environmental isolate CD105HE1 to produce 10^{10} PFU/mL of infective phage particles [45,53]. Prior to use, the phages were diluted to 10^9 PFU/mL in BHI and mixed in equal proportions to constitute the cocktail, which was kept at 4 °C for short-term storage or in 25% glycerol for long-term storage at −80 °C.

4.2. Gut Fermentation Model Set-Up

The gut fermentation model examined here was adapted from previous *C. difficile* phage studies [51] with slight modifications. The fermentation vessels were comprised of five 250 mL capacity Duran bottles containing 135 mL of a minimal medium containing 0.2% peptone, yeast extract, $NaHCO_2$, and Tween 80, 0.01% NaCl, 0.004% each of K_2HPO_4 and $KHPO_4$, 0.001% of $MgSO_4{\cdot}7H_2O$, $CaCl{\cdot}2H_2O$, and vitamin K (in 5% aqueous solution), 0.005% each of Cysteine HCl and bile salts, and 0.0002% haemin (dissolved in 400 μL of 1 M NaOH). The pH of the medium was adjusted to and maintained at ~6.8 throughout the experiment, using filter sterilised NaOH and HCl. The medium was pre-reduced anaerobically at 37 °C for 24 h before use.

Freshly voided fecal samples were collected from four donors comprising a heathy White infant British boy (7 years old), a Black African teenage girl (17 years old), a Black African adult lady (44 years old) and a White British Elderly lady (70 years old). All donors were healthy at the time of sample collection and had not had antibiotics for 6 months prior to the time of sampling [56]. The fecal matter was passed at will into sterile plastic bowls before being transferred to Elkay 30 mL polystyrene transport tubes fortified with spoons. The samples were immediately stored under ice, and analysed within 2 h of collection. Under anaerobic conditions, approximately 5 g (approximately one spoonful within the Elkay tube) of each stool sample was diluted in 20 mL of the minimal media and mixed by inversion until all fecal materials were completely suspended to form a fecal emulsion or slurry.

One milliliter of each sample slurry was taken to determine the donors' contributory microbiota. To do this, the culturable bacteria present in each fecal sample were ascertained by a viability assay on selective media for *C. difficile* (Brazier's CCEY medium, BioConnections, Knypersley, UK), bifidobacteria (BSM medium, Sigma, Steinheim, Germany), total anaerobe (Wilkins-Chalgren anaerobic agar, Oxoid, Hampshire UK), lactobaccilli (Rogosa agar, Oxoid, Hampshire, UK), enterobacteria (MacConkey agar, Sigma, Steinheim, Germany), and Gram-positive cocci (Slanetz-Bartley agar, Oxoid, Hampshire, UK), prepared according to the manufactures' recommendations. Afterwards, equal volumes of the fecal slurries were thoroughly mixed together, and 15 mL of the combined slurries was added to each of the fermentation vessels and further pre-reduced (anaerobically at 37 °C) for 2 h (−2 h, Table 1). The fermentation vessels were continuously agitated throughout the duration of the experiment using a sterile magnetic stirrer set, at 100 rpm.

4.3. Bacteria and Phage Treatment of the Fermenation Vessels

The five fermentation vessels were treated with 2 mL each of 6–8 $\times$ 10^8 CFU/mL culture of the test strain CD105LC2 (B), 2–6 $\times$ 10^9 PFU/mL of phage cocktail (P), and/or the minimal medium (M) at the time points shown in Table 1. At each time point, a 2 mL sample was removed from each of the treatment vessels and replaced with an equal volume of either the phage, the bacteria, or the minimum media, as appropriate (Table 1). The 2 mL samples were used for bacterial enumeration and DNA extraction for that time point. Vessel 1 (control untreated) contained the minimal medium and the fecal slurry only, and, at time points 0, 5, 24, 36, and 48 h, 2 mL of the pre-reduced minimal medium was added. In vessel 2 (*C. difficile* control), the bacterial culture was added at time point 0 h, and subsequently at the 5, 24, and 36 h time points, and at 48 h 2 mL of the minimal medium was added. For vessel 3 (control phage), the phages were added at 0, 5, 24, and 36 h, and at 48 h 2 mL of the medium was added. In the prophylactic regimen (vessel 4), the phages were added during the pre-reduction time (−2 h, on the basis of our prior data on phage pre-treatment time during the prophylaxis regimen [46]) and followed by the mixture of the phage and bacterial inocula, added at the 0 h time point. Afterwards, the phages were added at 5 and 24 h, and the medium at 36 and 48 h in vessel 4. For the remedial regimen (vessel 5), the bacterial inoculum was added at the 0 h time point, followed by the phage cocktail at the 5, 24, 36, and 48 h time points. The experiment was terminated at 72 h, and at this time the bacterial numbers were enumerated as described above.

4.4. DNA Extraction, Metagenomics Sequencing, and Analysis

The DNA was extracted from 1 mL of the 2 mL aliquot taken from the treated vessels using FastDNA spin kit for feces (MP Biomedicals, Santa Ana, CA, USA). The DNA quality was ascertained using Nanodrop One (Thermo Fisher Scientific, Madison, WI, USA) and Qubit ds DNA HS Assay kit with Qubit 3 fluorometer (Invitrogen, Carlsbad, CA, USA). Total genomic DNA was prepared using the NexteraXT DNA sample preparation kit (Illumina, San Diego, CA, USA). Sequencing was performed on the MiSeq platform using V2 (2 $\times$ 250 bp) chemistry. The resulting fastq files were trimmed with Sickle using default parameters, and metagenomes were assembled using megahit. An overview of sample diversity for each metagenome was obtained using Kraken [72] and visualised using Pavian [73]. The reads were mapped against the genomes of interest using BWA-MEM [74]).

5. Conclusions

Taken together, our data showed that the phage cocktail examined specifically cleared *C. difficile* in both prophylactic and remedial regimens despite the competitive pressure imposed by the diverse human microbiota. Furthermore, a therapy using the optimised phages altered the human commensal bacteria such that specific bacterial groups associated with a healthy gut microbiota dominated. In summary, the use of phages removed the target pathogen and favorably modified the model gut microbiome. Both of these outcomes would be beneficial if the phages were to be used therapeutically, so our data supports their further development as therapeutic agents.

Acknowledgments: The project was funded by AmpliPhi Biosciences in collaboration with the University of Leicester to develop the phages for therapeutic purpose for CDI. The funders had no role in study design, data collection, and analysis or preparation of the manuscript.

Author Contributions: J.Y.N., M.R.J.C., and A.M. conceived and designed the experiments; J.Y.N. performed the gut fermentation assays; A.M. and T.A.R. conducted the metagenomics sequencing; J.Y.N., T.A.R., and A.M. analysed the data; J.Y.N. wrote the paper; J.Y.N., T.A.R., A.M., and M.R.J.C. edited the paper and approved the final version to be submitted.

Conflicts of Interest: Although this work was funded by AmpliPhi Biosciences and under the terms of a license agreement to the University of Leicester headed by MRJC, the license agreement has since been terminated, and thus there is no conflict of interest in terms of license revenue shares. Similarly, all the other authors declare that the research was conducted in the absence of any commercial or financial relationships that could be construed as a potential conflict of interest.

References

1. De Kraker, M.E.A.; Stewardson, A.J.; Harbarth, S. Will 10 million people die a year due to antimicrobial resistance by 2050? *PLoS Med.* **2016**, *13*, e1002184. [CrossRef] [PubMed]
2. De Kraker, M.E.A.; Davey, P.G.; Grundmann, H. Mortality and hospital stay associated with resistant *Staphylococcus aureus* and *Escherichia coli* bacteremia: Estimating the burden of antibiotic resistance in Europe. *PLoS Med.* **2011**, *8*, e1001104. [CrossRef] [PubMed]
3. Stewardson, A.J.; Allignol, A.; Beyersmann, J.; Graves, N.; Schumacher, M.; Meyer, R.; Tacconelli, E.; De Angelis, G.; Farina, C.; Pezzoli, F.; et al. The health and economic burden of bloodstream infections caused by antimicrobial-susceptible and non-susceptible Enterobacteriaceae and *Staphylococcus aureus* in European hospitals, 2010 and 2011: A multicentre retrospective cohort study. *Euro Surveill.* **2016**, *21*. [CrossRef] [PubMed]
4. Naylor, N.R.; Pouwels, K.B.; Hope, R.; Green, N.; Henderson, K.L.; Knight, G.M.; Atun, R.; Robotham, J.V.; Deeny, S. A national estimate of the health and cost burden of *Escherichia coli* bacteraemia in the hospital setting: The importance of antibiotic resistance. *bioRxiv* **2017**. [CrossRef]
5. O'Neil, J. Antimicrobial Resistance: Tackling a Crisis for the Health and Wealth of Nations. The Review on Antimicrobial Resistance 2014. Available online: https://amr-review.org/sites/default/files/AMR%20Review%20Paper%20-%20Tackling%20a%20crisis%20for%20the%20health%20and%20wealth%20of%20nations_1.pdf (accessed on 31 December 2017).
6. Zucca, M.; Scutera, S.; Savoia, D. Novel avenues for *Clostridium difficile* infection drug discovery. *Expert Opin. Drug Discov.* **2013**, *8*, 459–477. [CrossRef] [PubMed]
7. Wise, R.; Blaser, M.J.; Carrs, O.; Cassell, G.; Fishman, N.; Guidos, R.; Levy, S.; Powers, J.; Norrby, R.; Tillotson, G.; et al. The urgent need for new antibacterial agents. *J. Antimicrob. Chemother.* **2011**, *66*, 1939–1940. [CrossRef] [PubMed]
8. Rai, J.; Randhawa, G.K.; Kaur, M. Recent advances in antibacterial drugs. *Int. J. Appl. Med. Res.* **2013**, *3*, 3–10.
9. Kutter, E.M.; Kuhl, S.J.; Abedon, S.T. Re-establishing a place for phage therapy in Western medicine. *Future Microbiol.* **2015**, *10*, 685–688. [CrossRef] [PubMed]
10. Abedon, S.T.; Kuhl, S.J.; Blasdel, B.G.; Kutter, E.M. Phage treatment of human infections. *Bacteriophage* **2011**, *1*, 66–85. [CrossRef] [PubMed]
11. Buttimer, C.; McAuliffe, O.; Ross, R.P.; Hill, C.; O'Mahony, J.; Coffey, A. Bacteriophages and bacterial plant diseases. *Front. Microbiol.* **2017**, *8*, 34. [CrossRef] [PubMed]
12. Cisek, A.A.; Dabrowska, I.; Gregorczyk, K.P.; Wyzewski, Z. Phage therapy in bacterial infections treatment: One hundred years after the discovery of bacteriophages. *Curr. Microbiol.* **2016**, *74*, 277–283. [CrossRef] [PubMed]

13. Regeimbal, J.M.; Jacobs, A.C.; Corey, B.W.; Henry, M.S.; Thompson, M.G.; Pavlicek, R.L.; Quinones, J.; Hannah, R.M.; Ghebremedhin, M.; Crane, N.J.; et al. Personalized therapeutic cocktail of wild environmental phages rescues mice from *Acinetobacter baumannii* wound infections. *Antimicrob. Agents Chemother.* **2016**, *60*, 5806–5816. [CrossRef] [PubMed]
14. Sulakvelidze, A.; Alavidze, Z.; Morris, J.G.J. Bacteriophage therapy. *Antimicrob. Agents Chemother.* **2001**, *45*, 649–659. [CrossRef] [PubMed]
15. Loc-Carrillo, C.; Abedon, S.T. Pros and cons of phage therapy. *Bacteriophage* **2011**, *1*, 111–114. [CrossRef] [PubMed]
16. Wittebole, X.; De Roock, S.; Opal, S.M. A historical overview of bacteriophage therapy as an alternative to antibiotics for the treatment of bacterial pathogens. *Virulence* **2014**, *5*, 226–235. [CrossRef] [PubMed]
17. Speck, P.; Smithyman, A. Safety and efficacy of phage therapy via the intravenous route. *FEMS Microbiol. Lett.* **2015**, *363*. [CrossRef] [PubMed]
18. Brüssow, H. What is needed for phage therapy to become a reality in Western medicine? *Virology* **2012**, *434*, 138–142. [CrossRef] [PubMed]
19. Slopek, S.; Weber-Dabrowska, B.; Dabrowski, M.; Kucharewicz-Krukowska, A. Results of bacteriophage treatment of suppurative bacterial infections in the years 1981–1986. *Arch. Immunol. Ther. Exp.* **1987**, *35*, 569–583.
20. EBI Food Safety. FDA and USDA Extend GRAS Approval for LISTEX for All Food Products. 2007. Available online: http://www.ebifoodsafety.com/en/news-2007.aspx (accessed on 31 December 2017).
21. Kwon, J.H.; Olsen, M.A.; Dubberke, E.R. The morbidity, mortality, and costs associated with *Clostridium difficile* infection. *Infect. Dis. Clin. N. Am.* **2015**, *29*, 123–134. [CrossRef] [PubMed]
22. Olsen, M.A.; Young-Xu, Y.; Stwalley, D.; Kelly, C.P.; Gerding, D.N.; Saeed, M.J.; Mahé, C.; Dubberke, E.R. The burden of *Clostridium difficile* infection: Estimates of the incidence of cdi from U.S. Administrative databases. *BMC Infect. Dis.* **2016**, *16*. [CrossRef] [PubMed]
23. Dubberke, E.R.; Olsen, M.A. Burden of *Clostridium difficile* on the healthcare system. *Clin. Infect. Dis.* **2012**, *55*, S88–S92. [CrossRef] [PubMed]
24. Bauer, M.P.; Notermans, D.W.; van Benthem, B.H.B.; Brazier, J.S.; Wilcox, M.H.; Rupnik, M.; Monnet, D.L.; van Dissel, J.T. *Clostridium difficile* infection in Europe: A hospital-based survey. *Lancet* **2011**, *377*, 63–73. [CrossRef]
25. Boyle, N.M.; Magaret, A.; Stednick, Z.; Morrison, A.; Butler-Wu, S.; Zerr, D.; Rogers, K.; Podczervinski, S.; Cheng, A.; Wald, A.; et al. Evaluating risk factors for *Clostridium difficile* infection in adult and pediatric hematopoietic cell transplant recipients. *Antimicrob. Resist. Infect. Control* **2015**, *4*. [CrossRef] [PubMed]
26. Lessa, F.C.; Mu, Y.; Bamberg, W.M.; Beldavs, Z.G.; Dumyati, G.K.; Dunn, J.R.; Farley, M.M.; Holzbauer, S.M.; Meek, J.I.; Phipps, E.C.; et al. Burden of *Clostridium difficile* infection in the United States. *N. Engl. J. Med.* **2015**, *372*, 825–834. [CrossRef] [PubMed]
27. Lessa, F.C.; Gould, C.V.; McDonald, L.C. Current status of *Clostridium difficile* infection epidemiology. *Clin. Infect. Dis.* **2012**, *55*, S65–S70. [CrossRef] [PubMed]
28. Kociolek, L.K.; Gerding, D.N. Breakthroughs in the treatment and prevention of *Clostridium difficile* infection. *Nat. Rev. Gastroenterol. Hepatol.* **2016**, *13*, 150–160. [CrossRef] [PubMed]
29. DuPont, H.L. Diagnosis and management of *Clostridium difficile* infection. *Clin. Gastroenterol. Hepatol.* **2013**, *11*, 1216–1223. [CrossRef] [PubMed]
30. Shah, D.; Dang, M.D.; Hasbun, R.; Koo, H.L.; Jiang, Z.D.; DuPont, H.L.; Garey, K.W. *Clostridium difficile infection*: Update on emerging antibiotic treatment options and antibiotic resistance. *Expert Rev. Anti-Infect. Ther.* **2010**, *8*, 555–564. [CrossRef] [PubMed]
31. Debast, S.B.; Bauer, M.P.; Kuijper, E.J. European society of clinical microbiology and infectious diseases: Update of the treatment guidance document for *Clostridium difficile* infection. *Clin. Microbiol. Infect.* **2014**, *20*, 1–26. [CrossRef] [PubMed]
32. Moura, I.; Spigaglia, P.; Barbanti, F.; Mastrantonio, P. Analysis of metronidazole susceptibility in different *Clostridium difficile* PCR ribotypes. *J. Antimicrob. Chemother.* **2013**, *68*, 362–365. [CrossRef] [PubMed]
33. Koss, C.A.; Baras, D.C.; Lane, S.D.; Aubry, R.; Marcus, M.; Markowitz, L.E.; Koumans, E.H. Investigation of metronidazole use during pregnancy and adverse birth outcomes. *Antimicrob. Agents Chemother.* **2012**, *56*, 4800–4805. [CrossRef] [PubMed]

34. Nelson, R.L.; Suda, K.J.; Evans, C.T. Antibiotic treatment for *Clostridium difficile*-associated diarrhoea in adults. *Cochrane Database Syst. Rev.* **2017**, *3*. [CrossRef] [PubMed]
35. Poduval, R.D.; Kamath, R.P.; Corpuz, M.; Norkus, E.P.; Pitchumoni, C.S. *Clostridium difficile* and vancomycin-resistant enterococcus: The new nosocomial alliance. *Am. J. Gastroenterol.* **2000**, *95*, 3513–3515. [CrossRef] [PubMed]
36. Bauer, M.P.; Kuijper, E.J.; van Dissel, J.T. European Society of Clinical Microbiology and Infectious Diseases (ESCMID): Treatment guidance document for *Clostridium difficile* infection (CDI). *Clin. Microbiol. Infect.* **2009**, *15*, 1067–1079. [CrossRef] [PubMed]
37. Baines, S.D.; Wilcox, M.H. Antimicrobial resistance and reduced susceptibility in *Clostridium difficile*: Potential consequences for induction, treatment, and recurrence of *C. difficile* infection. *Antibiotics* **2015**, *4*, 267–298. [CrossRef] [PubMed]
38. Chilton, C.H.; Crowther, G.S.; Freeman, J.; Todhunter, S.L.; Nicholson, S.; Longshaw, C.M.; Wilcox, M.H. Successful treatment of simulated *Clostridium difficile* infection in a human gut model by fidaxomicin first line and after vancomycin or metronidazole failure. *J. Antimicrob. Chemother.* **2014**, *69*, 451–462. [CrossRef] [PubMed]
39. Bartsch, S.M.; Umscheid, C.A.; Fishman, N.; Lee, B.Y. Is fidaxomicin worth the cost? An economic analysis. *Clin. Infect. Dis.* **2013**, *57*, 555–561. [CrossRef] [PubMed]
40. Stranges, P.M.; Hutton, D.W.; Collins, C.D. Cost-effectiveness analysis evaluating fidaxomicin versus oral vancomycin for the treatment of *Clostridium difficile* infection in the United States. *Value Health* **2013**, *16*, 297–304. [CrossRef] [PubMed]
41. Cruz, M.P. Fidaxomicin (Dificid), a novel oral macrocyclic antibacterial agent for the treatment of *Clostridium difficile*–associated diarrhea in adults. *Pharmacol. Ther.* **2012**, *37*, 278–281.
42. Hargreaves, K.R.; Clokie, M.R.J. *Clostridium difficile* phages: Still difficult? *Front. Microbiol.* **2014**, *5*. [CrossRef] [PubMed]
43. Sangster, W.; Hegarty, J.P.; Stewart, D.B. Phage therapy for *Clostridium difficile* infection: An alternative to antibiotics? *Semin. Colon Rectal Surg.* **2014**, *25*, 167–170. [CrossRef]
44. Meader, E.; Mayer, M.J.; Steverding, D.; Carding, S.R.; Narbad, A. Evaluation of bacteriophage therapy to control *Clostridium difficile* and toxin production in an in vitro human colon model system. *Anaerobe* **2013**, *22*, 25–30. [CrossRef] [PubMed]
45. Nale, J.Y.; Spencer, J.; Hargreaves, K.R.; Buckley, A.M.; Trzepiński, P.; Douce, G.R.; Clokie, M.R.J. Bacteriophage combinations significantly reduce *Clostridium difficile* growth in vitro and proliferation in vivo. *Antimicrob. Agents Chemother.* **2016**, *60*, 968–981. [CrossRef] [PubMed]
46. Nale, J.Y.; Chutia, M.; Carr, P.; Hickenbotham, P.; Clokie, M.R.J. 'Get in early'; biofilm and wax moth (*Galleria mellonella*) models reveal new insights into the therapeutic potential of *Clostridium difficile* bacteriophages. *Front. Microbiol.* **2016**, *7*. [CrossRef] [PubMed]
47. Ramesh, V.; Fralick, J.A.; Rolfe, R.D. Prevention of *Clostridium difficile*-induced ileocecitis with bacteriophage. *Anaerobe* **1999**, *5*, 69–78. [CrossRef]
48. Govind, R.; Fralick, J.A.; Rolfe, R.D. In vivo lysogenization of a *Clostridium difficile* bacteriophage ϕCD119. *Anaerobe* **2011**, *17*, 125–129.
49. Price, A.B.; Larson, H.E.; Crow, J. Morphology of experimental antibiotic-associated enterocolitis in the hamster: A model for human pseudomembranous colitis and antibiotic-associated diarrhoea. *Gut* **1979**, *20*, 467–475. [CrossRef] [PubMed]
50. Best, E.L.; Freeman, J.; Wilcox, M.H. Models for the study of *Clostridium difficile* infection. *Gut Microbes* **2012**, *3*, 145–167. [CrossRef] [PubMed]
51. Meader, E.; Mayer, M.J.; Gasson, M.J.; Steverding, D.; Carding, S.R.; Narbad, A. Bacteriophage treatment significantly reduces viable *Clostridium difficile* and prevents toxin production in an in vitro model system. *Anaerobe* **2010**, *16*, 549–554. [CrossRef] [PubMed]
52. Chilton, C.H.; Crowther, G.S.; Todhunter, S.L.; Nicholson, S.; Freeman, J.; Chesnel, L.; Wilcox, M.H. Efficacy of surotomycin in an in vitro gut model of *Clostridium difficile* infection. *J. Antimicrob. Chemother.* **2014**, *69*, 2426–2433. [CrossRef] [PubMed]
53. Hargreaves, K.R.; Kropinski, A.M.; Clokie, M.R.J. What does the talking?: Quorum sensing signalling genes discovered in a bacteriophage genome. *PLoS ONE* **2014**, *9*, e85131. [CrossRef] [PubMed]

54. Lloyd-Price, J.; Abu-Ali, G.; Huttenhower, C. The healthy human microbiome. *Genome Med.* **2016**, *8*. [CrossRef] [PubMed]
55. Browne, H.P.; Forster, S.C.; Anonye, B.O.; Kumar, N.; Neville, B.A.; Stares, M.D.; Goulding, D.; Lawley, T.D. Culturing of 'unculturable' human microbiota reveals novel taxa and extensive sporulation. *Nature* **2016**, *533*, 543–546. [CrossRef] [PubMed]
56. Baines, S.D.; Chilton, C.H.; Crowther, G.S.; Todhunter, S.L.; Freeman, J.; Wilcox, M.H. Evaluation of antimicrobial activity of ceftaroline against *Clostridium difficile* and propensity to induce *C. difficile* infection in an in vitro human gut model. *J. Antimicrob. Chemother.* **2013**, *68*, 1842–1849. [CrossRef] [PubMed]
57. Gould, I.M. The epidemiology of antibiotic resistance. *Int. J. Antimicrob. Agents* **2008**, *32*, S2–S9. [CrossRef] [PubMed]
58. Roberts, M.C.; McFarland, L.V.; Mullany, P.; Mulligan, M.E. Characterization of the genetic basis of antibiotic resistance in *Clostridium difficile*. *J. Antimicrob. Chemother.* **1994**, *33*, 419–429. [CrossRef] [PubMed]
59. Abhilash, M.; Vidya, A.G.; Jagadevi, T. Bacteriophage therapy: A war against antibiotic resistant bacteria. *Internet J. Altern. Med.* **2009**, *7*, 1.
60. Bauer, M.P.; van Dissel, J.T. Alternative strategies for *Clostridium difficile* infection. *Int. J. Antimicrob. Agents* **2009**, *33*, S51–S56. [CrossRef]
61. Wall, S.K.; Zhang, J.; Rostagno, M.H.; Ebner, P.D. Phage therapy to reduce preprocessing salmonella infections in market-weight swine. *Appl. Environ. Microbiol.* **2010**, *76*, 48–53. [CrossRef] [PubMed]
62. Macfarlane, G.T.; Macfarlane, S.; Gibson, G.R. Validation of a three-stage compound continuous culture system for investigating the effect of retention time on the ecology and metabolism of bacteria in the human colon. *Microb. Ecol.* **1998**, *35*, 180–187. [CrossRef] [PubMed]
63. Taslim, H. *Clostridium difficile* infection in the elderly. *Acta Medica Indonesiana* **2009**, *41*, 148–151. [PubMed]
64. McGowan, K.L.; Kader, H.A. *Clostridium difficile* infection in children. *Clin. Microbiol. Newsl.* **1999**, *21*, 49–53. [CrossRef]
65. Lagier, J.C.; Million, M.; Hugon, P.; Armougom, F.; Raoult, D. Human gut microbiota: Repertoire and variations. *Front. Cell. Infect. Microbiol.* **2012**, *2*. [CrossRef] [PubMed]
66. Antharam, V.C.; Li, E.C.; Ishmael, A.; Sharma, A.; Mai, V.; Rand, K.H. Intestinal dysbiosis and depletion of butyrogenic bacteria in *Clostridium difficile* infection and nosocomial diarrhea. *J. Clin. Microbiol.* **2013**, *51*, 2884–2892. [CrossRef] [PubMed]
67. Miyajima, F.; Roberts, P.; Swale, A.; Price, V.; Jones, M.; Horan, M.; Beeching, N.; Brazier, J.; Parry, C.; Pendleton, N.; et al. Characterisation and carriage ratio of *Clostridium difficile* strains isolated from a community-dwelling elderly population in the United Kingdom. *PLoS ONE* **2011**, *6*, e22804. [CrossRef] [PubMed]
68. Chan, B.K.; Abedon, S.T.; Loc-Carrillo, C. Phage cocktails and the future of phage therapy. *Future Microbiol.* **2013**, *8*, 769–783. [CrossRef] [PubMed]
69. Britton, R.A.; Young, V.B. Interaction between the intestinal microbiota and host in *Clostridium difficile* colonization resistance. *Trends Microbiol.* **2012**, *20*, 313–319. [CrossRef] [PubMed]
70. Zuo, T.; Wong, S.H.; Lam, K.; Lui, R.; Cheung, K.; Tang, W.; Ching, J.Y.L.; Chan, P.K.S.; Chan, M.C.W.; Wu, J.C.Y.; et al. Bacteriophage transfer during faecal microbiota transplantation in *Clostridium difficile* infection is associated with treatment outcome. *Gut* **2017**. [CrossRef] [PubMed]
71. Ott, S.J.; Waetzig, G.H.; Rehman, A.; Moltzau-Anderson, J.; Bharti, R.; Grasis, J.A.; Cassidy, L.; Tholey, A.; Fickenscher, H.; Seegert, D.; et al. Efficacy of sterile fecal filtrate transfer for treating patients with *Clostridium difficile* infection. *Gastroenterology* **2017**, *152*, 799–811. [CrossRef] [PubMed]
72. Wood, D.E.; Salzberg, S.L. Kraken: Ultrafast metagenomic sequence classification using exact alignments. *Genome Biol.* **2014**, *15*. [CrossRef] [PubMed]
73. Breitwieser, F.P.; Salzberg, S.L. Pavian: Interactive analysis of metagenomics data for microbiomics and pathogen identification. *bioRxiv* **2016**. [CrossRef]
74. Heng, L. Aligning Sequence Reads, Clone Sequences and Assembly Contigs with Bwa-Mem. Available online: https://arxiv.org/abs/1303.3997 (accessed on 31 December 2017).

5

Potentially Important Therapeutic Interactions between Antibiotics, and a Specially Engineered Emulsion Drug Vehicle Containing Krill-Oil-Based Phospholipids and Omega-3 Fatty Acids

David F. Driscoll

Stable Solutions LLC, Goleta, CA 93117, USA; d.driscoll@stablesolns.com

Abstract: The incidence of antimicrobial resistance (AMR) worldwide is increasing as the pipeline for the development of new chemotherapeutic entities is decreasing. Clearly, overexposure to antibiotics, including excessive dosing, is a key factor that fuels AMR. In fact, most of the new antibacterial agents under development are derivatives of existing classes of antibiotics. Novel approaches involving unique antimicrobial combinations, targets, and/or delivery systems are under intense investigation. An innovative combination of active pharmaceutical ingredients (APIs) consisting of antimicrobial drug(s), krill-oil-based phospholipids, and omega-3 fatty acid triglycerides, that may extend the therapeutic viability of currently effective antibiotics, at least until new chemical entities are introduced, is described.

Keywords: β-lactam antibiotics; β-lactamase inhibitors; krill oil phospholipids; omega-3 fatty acid triglycerides; antimicrobial resistance

---

1. Introduction

Antimicrobial resistance (AMR) is a worldwide concern. The United Nations, the WHO, and major pharmaceutical companies are committed to reducing AMR, with the latter providing a roadmap to achieve this goal by the year 2020 [1]. The roadmap includes four key commitments: (1) reduce the environmental impact of the production of antibiotics; (2) use antibiotics only in patients who need them; (3) improve access to existing and future antibiotics (including diagnostics and vaccines); (4) promote open collaborations between industry and public researchers. The fourth commitment broadly describes product development and the facilitation of the exchange of data on old antibiotics in efforts to fill specific gaps in the global pipeline.

Moreover, there has not been a successful pharmaceutical development of a newly discovered class of antibiotics in over 30 years. Therefore, all newer antibiotics that have reached the market since then have mostly been minor physicochemical modifications of existing drugs [2]. Consequently, if AMR exists to a certain class of antibiotics, it will eventually affect the modified congener that exhibits a similar structure–activity relationship. Therefore, alternative pharmaceutical strategies are being devised to optimize the delivery of particular antimicrobial agents or related APIs, or a combination of APIs. A more integrated approach that includes other pharmaceutical factors seems to be a reasonable additional consideration during drug development to reduce the incidence of AMR. Such factors include (a) precise dosing, (b) combination API therapy, (c) novel drug delivery systems, (d) shortened treatment intervals, and (e) restricted usage. The focus of this review will center on combination API therapy and novel drug delivery systems. In particular, an intravenous oil-in-water delivery system consisting of a combination of APIs will be described in the setting of bloodstream infections in the intensive care unit (ICU). Importantly, a major factor affecting the morbidity and mortality rates of septic ICU patients is the intensity of the accompanying systemic inflammatory response syndrome (SIRS).

A roadmap has recently (May 2016) been laid out by a multidisciplinary group of leading industry and academic experts "to identify the key scientific roadblocks to antibiotic discovery," supported by, and contained in, the Pew Charitable Trusts Report [2]. As of July 2016, of the 43 small molecule antibiotics under development, only 6 in the "pipeline" represent novel classes, and only one of which exhibits activity against Gram-negative bacteria [3]. A major emphasis in antibiotic research and development remains focused on the combination therapy of β-lactam antibiotics coupled with β-lactamase inhibitors (BLI), i.e., the application of two APIs. For example, the more recent antibiotic approvals for Gram-negative microorganisms, i.e., in 2014, US: ZERBAXA™ (ceftolozane–tazobactam) and, in 2015, US: AVACAZ™ (ceftazidime–avibactam), are BLI combination products consisting of a cephalosporin antibiotic (e.g., ceftazidime) and a BLI (e.g., avibactam). Although they provide better coverage against Gram-negative microorganisms vs. monotherapy, resistance has been observed [4]. Similarly, the first such combination therapy with penicillins, which are structurally related to cephalosporins and within the class of β-lactam antibiotics, was previously introduced 15 or more years ago, i.e., in 1997, US: UNASYN™ (ampicillin–sulbactam) and, in 2003, AUGMENTIN™ (amoxicillin–clavulanic acid), but the subsequent resistance to these therapies eventually led to the development of ZERBAXA™ and AVACAZ™.

Clearly, in the absence of a scientific breakthrough of new chemical classes of antimicrobial agents, alternative pharmaceutical strategies seem necessary. Over the last 30 years or so, pharmacokinetic (PK) techniques have been applied to support the optimal doses of antibiotics. Pharmacokinetics focuses on the time course of drug concentrations primarily in plasma, whereas pharmacodynamics (PD) relates the concentration of a drug in plasma to the observed pharmacological effect. Presently, combining PK/PD into a single statistical model is now routinely performed to assess the time course of the drug and the influence on its desired pharmacological effects, and this approach may be a more optimal way to dose BLI combinations [5]. Other proposed strategies in the search for viable antibiotic therapies for bloodstream infections include novel targeting agents and drug delivery systems [3]. Recent advancements in the analytical techniques applied to nanotechnology that allow more precise control of particle or droplet size distributions [6] have greatly added to the development of injectable dosage forms.

2. Bloodstream Infections in the ICU: SIRS, Sepsis, and Endotoxin—A Lethal Combination

Gram-negative sepsis is one of the most lethal bloodstreams infection in the ICU, and common pathogens include *Escherichia coli*, *Klebsiella pneumoniae*, and *Pseudomonas aeruginosa*. It is particularly lethal because the endotoxin or lipopolysaccharide produced accentuates the severity of the infection. Endotoxin, a component of the bacterial cell wall, is recognized by Toll-like receptors (TLRs) by the host, which binds this component and triggers activation of the nuclear factor kappa or the NFκB pathway, which in turn stimulates the synthesis and release of pro-inflammatory cytokines (e.g., tumor necrosis factor alpha (TNFα), interleukin-1 beta (IL-1β), and interleukin-6 (IL-6)) and stimulates other aspects of the immune system that increase the intensity of the metabolic response to infection. Thus, a vicious cycle ensues involving three main drivers that underlie the high mortality rate associated with Gram-negative sepsis: (1) SIRS, (2) sepsis, and (3) endotoxinemia. Consequently, using Gram-negative sepsis as a treatment model, a brief summary of these three variables (and later a sample intravenous combination-therapy regimen) is described.

2.1. *Systemic Inflammatory Response Syndrome (SIRS)*

In the intensive care unit (ICU) setting, all patients exhibit an acute inflammatory phase arising from high metabolic stresses affecting the function of vital organs (e.g., lungs, kidneys, heart, liver, and brain). If left unabated, the resulting multi-organ failure may produce a pronounced systemic inflammatory response syndrome (SIRS). As a key component of the metabolic response to injury, the increased endogenous production of eicosanoids (prostaglandins, thromboxanes, leukotrienes, and their downstream bioactive mediators, resolvins and protectins) is a vital part of the host response to SIRS. This heightened metabolic activity elicits an immune response that includes the production of other pro-inflammatory mediators (cytokines, chemokines, adhesion molecules, and reactive oxygen species) [7]. Hence, as inflammation increases, changes in selected (acute phase) proteins in plasma are also observed. Most notably, there is a reduction in the serum albumin level (resulting from extravascular pooling and heightened catabolism), as well as elevation of the C-reactive protein (CRP). As CRP is an acute phase protein, the magnitude of the increase in CRP is a reflection of the extent of metabolic and infectious-related stress, as well as tissue injury. When SIRS is accompanied by sepsis, the mortality rate progressively increases. There are numerous non-infectious causes as well, such as burn injury to >30% of body surface area, hemorrhagic shock, myocardial infarction, pancreatitis, and upper gastrointestinal bleeding. Similarly, there are numerous infectious causes of SIRS in the ICU, which include bacteremia, candidiasis, infectious endocarditis, pneumonia, and urinary tract infections. The clinical manifestations of SIRS in critically ill patients include the following four standard benchmarks (where diagnosis requires at least two of four to be present) in the diagnosis of this life-threatening illness [8]:

(1) a temperature of >38 °C or <36 °C;
(2) a heart rate of >90/minute;
(3) a respiratory rate of >20/minute (or $PaCO_2 < 32$ mmHg);
(4) a white blood cell count of >12,000/mm^3 or <4000/mm^3 (or 10% immature bands).

Once SIRS is diagnosed, additional pathological insults (i.e., co-morbid diseases) can lead to a deteriorating clinical state (i.e., known as the SIRS "cascade") that progressively increases the risk of mortality (%) that may start from a non-infectious source of SIRS (7%), progressing to an infectious SIRS insult: sepsis (16%) → severe sepsis (20%) → septic shock (46%) [9]. Current therapeutic approaches to SIRS include supportive medical therapies such as coronary vasodilation therapy, anti-ulcer regimens, appropriate antimicrobial therapy, blood product replacement, and even, for example, the strategic placement of surgical drains. Blocking the enhanced production of eicosanoids derived from omega-6 fatty acids by inhibiting the key enzymes that produce them (i.e., cyclooxygenases and/or lipoxygenases) is one way to reduce the intensity of SIRS. This has been achieved in critical care settings with injectable dosage forms of non-steroidal anti-inflammatory drugs (NSAIDs), such as ketorolac, which inhibits prostaglandin synthesis (i.e., selectively blocks cyclooxygenase-1 enzyme). However, in so doing, the drug increases the risk of damage to the gastrointestinal tract, the cardiovascular system, and the kidneys, and this is specifically detailed in the FDA's black-box warning (i.e., the strongest warning by the FDA for a drug with serious or fatal adverse reactions) that accompanies the package insert for ketorolac injection. Therefore, the NSAID therapy is currently viewed as potentially harmful in critically ill patients, and is not routinely applied in this setting. Additionally, metabolic therapies for SIRS include providing lipid substrates (essential fatty acids) that will modify the type of endogenous mediators that are produced, which fuel the inflammatory response—in particular, the production of prostaglandins (PGs), thromboxanes (TXAs), and leukotrienes (LKTs), i.e., the eicosanoids. Modifying the type of eicosanoids produced (e.g., from pro-inflammatory 2-series PGs and 4-series LKTs from omega-6 fatty acids to anti-inflammatory 3-series PGs and 5-series LKTs from omega-3 fatty acids) has been achieved by acutely altering the lipid substrate provided during the acute phase response. In this regard, the principal pro-inflammatory omega-6 fatty acids of interest are arachidonic acid (ARA) and linoleic acid (LA), while the key anti-inflammatory omega-3 fatty acids of interest are eicosapentaenoic acid (EPA) and docosahexaenoic acid (DHA). Modulating the intensity of the inflammatory response by altering the type of eicosanoids produced via intravenous infusion of omega-3 fatty acids seems to be an attractive alternative. For example, in a randomized controlled trial, 28 patients undergoing elective cardiopulmonary bypass surgery who received three perioperative intravenous lipid infusions containing omega-3 fatty acids had decreased biological and clinical signs of inflammation [10]. The acute provision of omega-3 fatty acids will be effectively incorporated into plasma cell membranes, and, as the preferred substrate over omega-6 fatty acids for the cyclooxygenase and lipoxygenase enzymes, such acids will ultimately produce anti-inflammatory eicosanoids. Importantly, providing omega-3 fatty acids intravenously greatly improves their bioavailability, i.e., changes in membrane composition (within 60 min of infusion [11]), over oral supplementation (requiring 6–8 weeks [12]). Thus, the anti-inflammatory effects can be achieved quickly—an absolute requirement in the clinical management of significant SIRS in the critical care setting.

2.2. Sepsis and Endotoxin

Blood infection or sepsis is a major cause of death in critically ill patients. Of those who survive, according to the Third International Consensus Definitions for Sepsis and Septic Shock (Sepsis-3) on 23 February 2016, they have "long-term physical, psychological, and cognitive disability with significant health care and social implications. [...] Sepsis is defined as the life-threatening organ dysfunction caused by a dysregulated host response to infection. [...] In lay terms, sepsis is a life-threatening condition that arises when the body's response to an infection injures its own tissues and organs" [13]. In the ICU, sepsis is a major form of metabolic stress, so it is associated with a heightened level of the systemic inflammatory response in ICU settings and often involves organ dysfunction.

In May 2016, a report from the Pew Charitable Trusts entitled "A Scientific Roadmap for Antibiotic Discovery" [2] acknowledges the fact that, for more than 30 years, there has been a "void" in the discovery of new classes of antibiotics. Not surprisingly, coinciding with this drought in pharmaceutical development (i.e., "no registered classes of antibiotics since 1984"), there has been a dramatic rise in antibiotic resistance (ABR), as noted in the declaration by the WHO that characterized this timespan as a "post-antibiotic era." A major priority is "understanding and overcoming barriers for drugs targeting Gram-negative bacteria," which is a leading cause of septic morbidity and mortality in ICU patients. In Gram-negative sepsis, endotoxins or lipopolysaccharides are the prime cause of increased morbidity and mortality because they trigger the immune response that includes the pronounced secretion of inflammatory mediators This is because the intensity of the metabolic response to injury and/or infection is a reflection of the patient's diet, and consumption of omega-6 rich soybean oil worldwide has been increasing. Consequently, if left unaddressed in the ICU patient, it can lead to septic shock with myocardial depression and renal impairment with mortality rates approaching 50% or higher. Although targeted API injectable therapies for bloodstream infections, such as those that antagonize or remove endotoxin from the bloodstream, seems to be a reasonable approach, there have been significant setbacks. For example, in 2009, an anti-endotoxin therapy was tried with a 10% phospholipid (PL-10) injectable emulsion (92.5 mg/mL of phosphatidyl choline, 7.75 mg/mL of sodium cholate, and 7.5 mg/mL of soybean oil) in two doses, compared to a placebo group in patients with confirmed or suspected Gram-negative severe sepsis [14]. The hypothesis was that the phospholipids would bind and neutralize endotoxin and lead to improved clinical outcomes. A total of 235 centers worldwide participated in the study, and the injectable emulsion was added to a pre-existing antibiotic regimen. Although the results were positive in previous large animal models of endotoxinemia (including one infection model) as well as during endotoxin challenge in normal human volunteers, the high phospholipid dose arm of the study (1350 mg or 13.5 mL of PL-10/kg; n = 182) was stopped on the recommendation of an Independent Safety Monitoring Committee due to an increase in life-threatening, serious adverse events detected in the fourth interim analysis. However, patient entry was completed in the lower dose arm (850 mg (or 8.5 mL of PL-10/kg; n = 598) and the placebo (n = 599) groups, but there were no differences in mortality, nor in the onset of new organ failure. More recently, there is another anti-endotoxin proposal that is being investigated, which involves coupling an antimicrobial drug effective against Gram-negative organisms with an extracorporeal blood purification technique [15]. Here, the antimicrobial drug polymyxin B is embedded in a polystyrene fiber and attached to a hemoperfusion device [16], but now, it appears to be no more effective than standard therapy [17]. In another novel approach, designed to mitigate the risk of mortality (based on an APACHE II score of $\geq$25) in adult ICU patients with severe sepsis, the intravenous administration of a recombinant form of human activated protein C (XIGRIS™) for 96 h was investigated and was reported to exert an anti-inflammatory effect by decreasing the leukocyte response to inflammatory cytokines (e.g., IL-6), resulting in reduced mortality [18]. However, in a follow-up study [19], the results could not be confirmed. Consequently, although there were no safety issues associated with the APIs in this study, the lack of clinical benefits prompted the manufacturer to withdraw the drug from the market on 25 October 2011.

3. New Therapeutic Combinations: Antibiotics + BLIs + Phospholipids + Omega-3 Fatty Acids

In addition to continuing to refine and, in some cases, develop more specific PK/PD models for a particular drug and/or dosage form, a novel drug delivery system has been developed, containing, for example, three or more APIs, as described below. What makes this dosage form unique is the use of ingredients that would normally be considered excipients (i.e., providing pharmaceutical stability and compatibility) but are used to exploit inherent pharmacological actions that exhibit API-related effects. The goal of course is to use them along with the primary API (antibiotic) in a synergistic manner that may reduce its dose (exposure), as well as favorably influence the clinical response to sepsis. That is, the excipient(s) to be included have an important dual function—a pharmaceutical role and a therapeutic role as an API. The pharmaceutical and pharmacological roles of the proposed intravenous formulation for Gram-negative sepsis is described below in Table 1.

Table 1. Sample composition of an API regimen in the treatment of Gram-negative Sepsis.

	Ingredient	Pharmaceutical Function	Therapeutic Function
1	Ceftolozane	—	β-lactam antibiotic
2	Tazobactam	—	β-lactamase inhibitor
3	krill oil phospholipids	Emulsifier	binds endotoxin; 2nd source of omega-3 fatty acids
4	enriched fish oil triglycerides	drug vehicle	major source of omega-3 fatty acids
5	medium chain triglyceride (MCT) oil	drug vehicle	improves lipid clearance
6	glycerol	tonicity agent	—
7	sodium oleate	co-emulsifier	binds endotoxin?
8	alpha-tocopherol	antioxidant	antioxidant delivery?
9	sterile water for injection	drug vehicle	—

Historically, the primary use of lipid injectable emulsions in the clinical setting have been for nutritional purposes, i.e., to deliver a dense source of fat calories and essential fatty acids. Subsequently, they were used as drug delivery vehicles for poorly water-soluble drugs such as propofol injectable emulsion. More recently, focus has been placed on the fatty acid composition of the oil phase with respect to the omega-3 and omega-6 fatty acid contents, and in particular, the effects on the systemic inflammatory response. Increasing the concentration of omega-3 fatty acids delivered during the acute phase of critical illness has an anti-inflammatory effect that may improve clinical outcomes [7]. Currently, a novel approach is to include polyfunctional components that have both pharmaceutical and pharmacological functions.

3.1. *Polyfunctional Ingredients*

3.1.1. Krill Oil Phospholipids

All phospholipids have the same unique character of possessing two hydrophobic nonpolar tail groups (sn-1 and sn-2 of the triglyceride structure) and a hydrophilic polar head group (sn-3 of the triacylglycerol structure) that imparts surface-active properties, i.e., a pharmaceutically effective emulsifier for the homogeneous dispersion of oil droplets in oil-in-water (o/w) injectable emulsions. This molecular arrangement allows the hydrophilic head groups and hydrophobic tail groups to align along the oil–water interface of the submicron droplets in a tight packing arrangement in order to electromechanically stabilize the emulsion. Krill oil phospholipids (KO-PLs) are unique compounds in that they are a marine-based PL and, as such, uniquely contain anti-inflammatory 20+ carbon, polyunsaturated omega-3 fatty acids EPA (20:5n3) and DHA (22:6n3). In contrast, the conventional PL from egg yolk phosphatides that come from hens that are fed vegetable grains high in pro-inflammatory 18-carbon omega-6 fatty acids and saturated fatty acids. In terms of the egg phospholipid fatty acid profile, it typically contains fatty acids—in decreasing order, palmitic (16:0), oleic (18:1n9), stearic (18:0), and linoleic (18:2n6) acids—that are attached to the available sn-1 and sn-2 positions, whereas 70–95% of the omega-3 fatty acids EPA (20:5n3) and DHA (22:6n3) are attached to the phospholipids in krill oil. This difference may have significant and unique implications for pharmaceutical actions of KO-PLs as emulsifying and/or solubilizing agents. For example, we know in living organisms that both EPA and DHA are not only the longest-chain fatty acids found in biological membranes, but they are also the most unsaturated (5 and 6 double bonds, respectively). They are highly flexible (having elastic compressibility) and can interconvert between multiple torsional states that can alter membrane order and fluidity. In pharmaceutical emulsions, these characteristics can uniquely alter the molecular packing arrangement that influences not only the shape of micelles, but also their surfactant properties. The "packing parameter P" is certainly influenced by the long hydrophobic tail, and this may be especially important with respect to the unique ability of omega-3 fatty acids to enhance their surfactant properties over shorter chain fatty acids with lower numbers of carbons, and degrees of unsaturation, or with saturated long-chain fatty acids, typically found in conventional egg phospholipids. These differences may be especially important for highly water-insoluble drugs intended for intravenous administration. Pharmaceutically, KO-PLs have potentially useful surfactant and drug-solubilizing activities.

Although krill oil is not a high source of omega-3 fatty acids (up to 35% of the fatty acid profile) compared to enriched fish oil (≥45%), it nonetheless makes an important contribution to the omega-3 fatty acids mainly provided by highly enriched fish oil triglycerides. This is a key consideration when EPA + DHA are provided in pharmacological doses in the treatment of SIRS that accompanies sepsis. In addition, as phospholipids, KO-PLs are capable of binding endotoxin produced during Gram-negative sepsis. In cell culture studies, KO-PL emulsions have been shown to protect against endotoxin-induced pro-inflammatory activation of macrophages [20]. As with any drug dose, and as described earlier, injectable phospholipids in high concentrations can be dangerous. In the Dellinger et al. study [14], however, the concentration of PL-10 emulsion that was infused was nearly an order of magnitude higher (10%) than the PL concentrations that have been safely given in injectable nutritional and drug emulsions (1.2%). Such differences (~log dose), as observed in typical dose-finding studies of any drug, often reveal the toxicity of many compounds. Pharmacologically, in safe and effective doses, KO-PLs have demonstrated potentially useful activity against SIRS and endotoxinemia. The safe and effective clinical dose of krill oil phospholipids will require future study, but for emulsion stability, concentrations between 0.6 and 1.8% have been safely given since the introduction of nutritional emulsions in 1961.

3.1.2. Fish Oil Triglycerides Enriched in Omega-3 Fatty Acids

According to the European Pharmacopoeia (EP), there are two pharmaceutical monographs for fish oil: EP Monograph 1352 entitled "Omega-3 Acid Triglycerides" and EP Monograph 1912 entitled "Fish Oil, Rich in Omega-3 Acids" [21]. EP 1912 is a natural fish oil that has been refined and made appropriate for human consumption. Of the total fatty acid profile, it contains about 30% (by weight) of the essential fatty acids EPA and DHA. Typically, this type of fish oil is contained in fish oil capsules used as oral supplements. In contrast, EP1352 is both refined and enriched (e.g., by molecular distillation) to increase the concentration of EPA and DHA to about 60% of the total fatty acid profile.

This type of fish oil is often used in injectable emulsions. The oil phase of conventional lipid injectable emulsions plays a key role as a carrier for poorly water-soluble drugs. An internal or dispersed phase consisting of mainly very long-chain (20–22 carbons) triglycerides of fish oil may assist in the solubilization of practically water-insoluble drugs, where conventional long-chain (16–18 carbons) triglycerides are not as effective. Pharmaceutically, fish oil triglycerides that are highly enriched with omega-3 fatty acids may result in improved delivery of the drug and/or pharmaceutical stability compared with conventional oils (soybean oil, medium chain triglyceride (MCT) oil, olive oil, etc.) used in intravenous lipid emulsions. Consequently, enriched fish oil triglycerides are the major source of omega-3 fatty acids in addition to those present in KO-PLs. When dosing, the effort should be focused on the absolute intakes of EPA + DHA and not on the omega-6/omega-3 ratio. The optimal intravenous dose that is effective in the treatment of SIRS, in the presence of sepsis, has not been determined. Based on an assessment of the literature on omega-3 fatty acids used to treat various inflammatory diseases, such as cardiovascular disease [22], a threshold dose of about 2 g of EPA + DHA per day appears to be necessary. It is worth noting that it may take several weeks of oral supplementation before clinical benefits are seen [7]. In contrast, the bioavailability of intravenous omega-3 fatty acids is fast (within 60 min of a bolus dose [11]). Therefore, close attention must be paid to identifying the ideal pharmacological dose range, ensuring that it is both safe and effective upon intravenous infusion in critically ill patients with SIRS + sepsis. The daily dose of omega-3 fatty acids necessary to favorably alter the clinical course of SIRS during sepsis will require future study, but intravenous doses of fish oil in the range of 1–6 g/day of EPA+DHA have been safely provided in ICU patients [23,24]. Furthermore, in patients with renal failure, the dose alterations for omega-3 fatty acids will likely parallel the modifications made for antibiotics, but this too will require future study.

3.1.3. Medium Chain Triglyceride Oil

MCTs consist of saturated fatty acids (no double bonds) containing between 6 and 12 carbon atoms. For use in lipid injectable emulsions, more than 95% of the fatty acids present are caprylic (8:0) and capric (10:0) acids (occupying the R′, R″, and R‴ below). Although triglyceride molecules are highly hydrophobic and therefore referred to as "neutral triglycerides," all of them possess three carbonyl groups that impart a slight polarity to the structure, as illustrated in Figure 1.

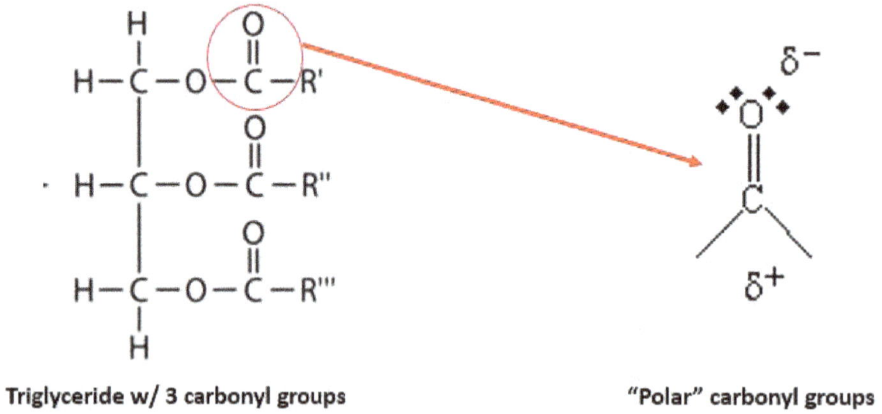

Figure 1. Triacylglycerol backbone and polar carbonyl groups.

These carbonyl structures allow triglycerides (to varying degrees) to be incorporated into the phospholipid bilayers of the egg lecithin surfactant at the oil–water interface. The shorter the hydrocarbon chain is, compared to the longer hydrocarbon chains that will orient to the oil phase, the closer the fatty acid will be to the aqueous phase. In a fish oil–MCT oil mixed emulsion, the unique MCT orientation has a significant impact on the physiochemical properties of the emulsion. It has been shown that MCTs displace Long Chain Triglycerides (LCTs) from the oil–water interface, and this behavior influences the intensity of the chemical stress imposed upon the emulsifier, which reduces the interfacial tension between the internal lipid phase and the external aqueous phase. For example, the interfacial tension of the 18-carbon oleic acid is 15.6 dyne/cm vs. 8.22 dyne/cm for the 8-carbon caprylic acid. Consequently, the stress upon the emulsifier at this oil–water interface is lower when MCTs are present. In fact, the pharmaceutical stability of lipid injectable emulsions is superior when MCTs are included with LCTs in mixed-oil emulsions [25]. Clinically speaking, these unique surface-active effects allow for the greater interaction with water-soluble proteins, such as the enzyme lipoprotein lipase, resulting in faster hydrolysis and clearance of mixed-oil lipid droplets upon infusion into the bloodstream [26]. That is, the longer the hydrocarbon chain length of the fatty acids present, the slower the clearance of lipid emulsions from the bloodstream, which may increase the risks of adverse events, especially in an ICU setting [21]. Therefore, from a pharmacological perspective, the presence of MCTs with fish oil triglycerides in lipid injectable emulsions improves the bioavailability and safety of the infusion.

3.1.4. Sodium Oleate

Of the five main free fatty acids present in the soybean oil-in-water injectable emulsion INTRALIPID™ (52% linoleic, 22% oleic, 13% palmitic, 8% linolenic, and 4% stearic), oleic acid is best known to exhibit surfactant properties. Whether or not this is related to its unique chemical structure (a single, *cis*-configured, double bond at the center of the hydrocarbon chain) is not known, but its increased presence in "aged" INTRALIPID emulsions improves its physical stability [27]. The fatty acids attached to the triglycerides in soybean oil-in-water emulsions will be hydrolyzed over time, and, because free fatty acids are potentially toxic upon intravenous administration (causing, for example, blood and liver abnormalities, pulmonary edema, ventilator defects, and kernicterus) [28], their formation must be limited during the shelf life of the product. Oleic acid's corresponding fatty acid salt (sodium oleate), however, is a safe excipient that retains the co-emulsifying properties and has been used for many years in commercially available lipid injectable emulsion products. Pharmaceutically speaking, along with the primary emulsifier, i.e., the surface-active phospholipids in krill oil, such products are the main stabilizers of the intravenous emulsion and allow sodium oleate to be safely infused. Anything that compromises the surfactant properties will promote the coalescence of submicron lipid droplets into large-diameter, and potentially embolic, fat globules that can occlude the pulmonary microvasculature (e.g., capillaries). As a consequence of its surface-active properties, sodium oleate may also play a complementary or synergistic role with phospholipids in the neutralization of endotoxin, but this has not been proven at this time. If true, this excipient also plays a therapeutic role in the formulation.

3.1.5. Alpha Tocopherol

From a pharmaceutical standpoint, alpha tocopherol or vitamin E is a critical stabilizing component routinely included in lipid injectable emulsions. This is particularly true if unsaturated fatty acids are present in the triglycerides that make up the oil phase of the emulsion. With the exception of MCT oil, all commonly used triglyceride oils contain unsaturated fatty acids. As the number of double bonds in the fatty acid increases, so too does the risk of oxidative degradation. For example, oleic acid is a monounsaturated fatty acid containing a single double bond; linoleic acid contains two double bonds; linolenic acid contains three; ARA has four, EPA has five, and DHA has six. Key measures in emulsions include the primary oxidation product (peroxide value) and the secondary oxidation product (anisidine), and these are routinely monitored over the course of the shelf life of the product. Importantly, given the highly polyunsaturated fatty acids present in fish oil used to treat SIRS, alpha tocopherol is a vital pharmaceutical excipient that preserves the quality and safety of the final injectable emulsion.

In addition, alpha tocopherol may have a systemic effect as an antioxidant. During severe critical illness and SIRS, oxidative stress is one of four hallmark events that need to be addressed (in addition to inflammation, ischemia, and immune dysfunction). Thus, the provision of alpha tocopherol may have a complementary therapeutic effect along with the omega-3 fatty acids in treating SIRS. However, this potential benefit, and the optimal dose needed to achieve both pharmaceutical and pharmacological benefits, has not yet been identified.

4. Conclusions

AMR is a clinically significant problem worldwide with lethal consequences, prompting numerous and diverse organizations in the search for therapeutic strategies in critically ill patients with bloodstream infections. Due to the lack of development of a new class of antibiotics in over 30 years, pharmaceutical methods may enhance pharmacological efficacy. For example, improvements in our understanding of PK/PD modeling, a novel dosage form design, and combination antimicrobial therapies may extend the activity against some of the most lethal microorganisms (e.g., Gram-negative bacteria) responsible for sepsis. In doing so, such pharmaceutical innovations may serve as a therapeutic bridge until new chemical entities to replace them are successfully developed. These pharmaceutical maneuvers can be applied to future antibiotics as well. It is clear that a multi-prong therapeutic approach, using a unique combination of pharmacological agents with potentially important antimicrobial and metabolic activities, is an important stratagem against AMR. The challenge ahead for this novel approach consists in identifying the effective concentrations of polyfunctional excipients, as well as "conventional" APIs, that safely achieve pharmaceutical and pharmacological functions.

Abbreviations

AMR	antimicrobial resistance
API	active pharmaceutical ingredient
PK/PD	pharmacokinetic/pharmacodynamics
ICU	intensive care unit
SIRS	systemic inflammatory response syndrome
CRP	C-reactive protein
PGs	prostaglandins
TXAs	thromboxanes
LKT	leukotrienes
FDA	Food and Drug Administration
NSAID	nonsteroidal anti-inflammatory drug
LA	linoleic acid
ARA	arachidonic acid
EPA	eicosapentaenoic acid
DHA	docosahexaenoic acid
KO	krill oil
PL	phospholipids
EP	European Pharmacopoeia
MCT	medium chain triglycerides
LCT	long chain triglycerides

References

1. Allergan; AstraZeneca; Cipla; DSM Sinochem Pharmaceuticals. *Industry Roadmap for Progress on Combating Antimicrobial Resistance*; F. Hoffman-La Roche Ltd.: Basel, Switzerland; GSK; Johnson & Johnson; Merck & Co., Inc.: Kenilworth, NJ, USA; Novartis: Basel, Switzerland; Pfizer: New York, NY, USA; Sanofi: Paris, France; Shionogi & Co., Ltd.: Osaka, Japan; Wockhardt: Mumbai, India, 2016.

2. Talkington, K.; Shore, C.; Kothari, P. *A Scientific Roadmap for Antibiotic Discovery*; The Pew Charitable Trust: Philadelphia, PA, USA, 2016.
3. Bush, K.; Page, M.G.P. What we may expect from novel antibacterial agents in the pipeline with respect to resistance and pharmacodynamic principles. *J. Pharmacokinet. Pharmacodyn.* **2017**, *44*, 113–132. [CrossRef] [PubMed]
4. Winkler, M.L.; Papp-Wallace, K.M.; Hujer, A.M.; Domitrovic, T.N.; Hujer, K.M.; Hurless, K.N.; Tuohy, M.; Hall, G.; Bonomo, R.A. Unexpected challenges in treating multidrug-resistant Gram-negative bacteria: Resistance to ceftazidime-avibactam in archived isolates of *Pseudomonas aeruginosa*. *Antimicrob. Agents Chemother.* **2015**, *59*, 1020–1029. [CrossRef] [PubMed]
5. Bush, K. A resurgence of β-lactamase inhibitor combinations effective against multidrug-resistant Gram-negative pathogens. *Int. J. Antimicrob. Agents* **2015**, *46*, 483–493. [CrossRef] [PubMed]
6. Driscoll, D.F.; Nicoli, D.F. Analytical methods for determining the size (distribution) in parenteral dispersions. In *Non-Biological Complex Drugs*; Crommelin, D.J.A., de Vlieger, J.S.B., Eds.; Springer: Cham, Switzerland, 2015; pp. 193–259.
7. Calder, P.J. Fatty acids and inflammation: The cutting edge between food and pharma. *Eur. J. Clin. Pharmacol.* **2011**, *668*, S50–S58. [CrossRef] [PubMed]
8. American College of Chest Physicians/Society of Critical Care Medicine Consensus Conference: Definitions for sepsis and organ failure and guidelines for the use of innovative therapies in sepsis. *Crit. Care Med.* **1992**, *20*, 864–874.
9. Rangel-Frausto, M.S.; Pittet, D.; Costigan, M.; Hwang, T.; Davis, C.S.; Wenzel, R.P. The natural history of the systemic inflammatory response syndrome (SIRS). A prospective study. *JAMA* **1995**, *273*, 117–123. [CrossRef] [PubMed]
10. Berger, M.M.; Delodder, F.; Liaudet, L.; Tozzi, P.; Schlaepfer, J.; Chiolero, R.L.; Tappy, L. Three short perioperative infusions of n-3 PUFAs reduce the systemic inflammation induced by cardiopulmonary bypass surgery: A randomized controlled trial. *Am. J. Clin. Nutr.* **2013**, *97*, 246–254. [CrossRef] [PubMed]
11. Carpentier, Y.A.; Hacquebard, M.; Portois, L.; Dupont, I.E.; Deckelbaum, R.J.; Malaisse, W.J. Rapid cellular enrichment of eicosapentaenoate after single intravenous injection of a novel medium-chain triacylglycerol:fish oil emulsion in humans. *Am. J. Clin. Nutr.* **2010**, *91*, 875–882. [CrossRef] [PubMed]
12. Endres, S.; Ghorbani, R.; Kelley, V.E.; Georgilis, K.; Lonnemann, G.; van der Meer, J.W.; Cannon, J.G.; Rogers, T.S.; Klempner, M.S.; Weber, P.C.; et al. The effect of dietary supplementation with n-3 polyunsaturated fatty acids on the synthesis of interleukin-1 and tumor necrosis factor by mononuclear cells. *N. Engl. J. Med.* **1989**, *320*, 265–271. [CrossRef] [PubMed]
13. Singer, M.; Deutschman, C.S.; Seymour, C.W.; Shankar-Hari, M.; Annane, D.; Bauer, M.; Bellomo, R.; Bernard, G.R.; Chiche, J.D.; Coopersmith, C.M.; et al. The Third International Consensus Definitions for Sepsis and Septic Shock (Sepsis-3). *JAMA* **2016**, *315*, 801–810. [CrossRef] [PubMed]
14. Dellenger, R.P.; Tomayko, J.F.; Angus, D.C.; Opal, S.; Cupo, M.A.; McDermott, S.; Ducher, A.; Calandra, T.; Cohen, J.; Lipid Infusion and Patient Outcomes in Sepsis (LIPOS) Investigators. Efficacy and safety of a phospholipid emulsion (GR270773) in Gram-negative severe sepsis: Results of a phase II multicenter, randomized, placebo-controlled, dose defining trial. *Crit. Care Med.* **2009**, *37*, 2929–2938. [CrossRef] [PubMed]
15. Virzi, G.M.; Clementi, A.; Brocca, A.; Ronco, C. Endotoxin effects on cardiac and renal functions and cardiorenal syndromes. *Blood Purif.* **2017**, *44*, 314–326. [CrossRef] [PubMed]
16. Klem, D.J.; Foster, D.; Schorr, C.A.; Kazempour, K.; Walker, P.M.; Dellinger, R.P. The EUPHRATES trial (Evaluating the Use of Polymyxin B. Hemoperfusion in a Randomized controlled trial of Adults Treated for Endotoxinemia and Septic shock): Study protocol for a randomized controlled trial. *Trials* **2014**, *15*, 218. [CrossRef]
17. Iba, T.; Fowler, L. Is polymyxin B-immobilized fiber column ineffective for septic shock? A discussion on the press release for EUPHRATES trial. *J. Intensive Care.* [CrossRef] [PubMed]
18. Bernard, G.R.; Vincent, J.L.; Laterre, P.F.; LaRosa, S.P.; Dhainaut, J.F.; Lopez-Rodriguez, A.; Steingrub, J.S.; Garber, G.E.; Helterbrand, J.D.; Ely, E.W.; et al. Efficacy and safety of recombinant human activated protein C for severe sepsis. *N. Engl. J. Med.* **2001**, *344*, 699–709. [CrossRef] [PubMed]

19. Ranieri, V.M.; Thompson, B.T.; Barie, P.S.; Dhainaut, J.F.; Douglas, I.S.; Finfer, S.; Gårdlund, B.; Marshall, J.C.; Rhodes, A.; Artigas, A.; et al. PROWESS-SHOCK Study Group. *N. Engl. J. Med.* **2012**, *366*, 2055–2064. [CrossRef] [PubMed]
20. Bonaterra, G.A.; Driscoll, D.; Schwarzbach, H.; Kinscherf, R. Krill oil-in-water emulsion protects against lipopolysaccharide-induced proinflammatory activation of macrophages in vitro. *Mar. Drugs* **2017**, *15*, 74. [CrossRef]
21. Driscoll, D.F. Pharmaceutical and clinical aspects of lipid injectable emulsions. *JPEN* **2017**, *41*, 125–134. [CrossRef] [PubMed]
22. Stanley, J.C.; Elsom, R.L.; Calkder, P.C.; Griffin, B.A.; Harris, W.S.; Jebb, S.A.; Lovegrove, J.A.; Moore, C.S.; Riemersma, R.A.; Sanders, T.A. UK Food Strandards Agency Workshop Report: The effects of the dietary n6/n3 fatty acid ratio on cardiovascular health. *Br. J. Nutr.* **2007**, *98*, 1305–1310. [CrossRef] [PubMed]
23. Heller, A.R.; Rössler, S.; Litz, R.J.; Stehr, S.N.; Heller, S.C.; Koch, R.; Koch, T. Omega-3 fatty acids improve the diagnosis-related outcome. *Crit. Care Med.* **2006**, *34*, 972–979. [CrossRef] [PubMed]
24. Wichmann, M.W.; Thul, P.; Czarnetzki, H.D.; Morlion, B.J.; Kemen, M.; Jauch, K.W. Evaluation of clinical safety and beneficial effects of a fish oil-containing emulsion (Lipoplus, MLF541): Data from a prospective, randomized, multicenter trial. *Crit. Care Med.* **2007**, *35*, 700–706. [CrossRef] [PubMed]
25. Driscoll, D.F.; Nehne, J.; Peterss, H.; Franke, R.; Bistrian, B.R.; Niemann, W. The influence of medium-chain triglycerides on the stability of all-in-one formulations. *Int. J. Pharm.* **2002**, *240*, 1–10. [CrossRef]
26. Hamilton, J.A.; Vural, J.M.; Carpentier, Y.A.; Deckelbaum, R.J. Incorporation of medium chain triacylglycerols into phospholipid bilayers: Effect of long chain triacyglycerols, cholesterol, and cholesterol esters. *J. Lipid Res.* **1996**, *37*, 773–786. [PubMed]
27. Washington, C.; David, S.S. Aging effects in parenteral fat emulsions: The role of fatty acids. *Int. J. Pharm.* **1987**, *39*, 33–37. [CrossRef]
28. Driscoll, D.F. Lipid injectable emulsions: Pharmacopeial and safety issues. *Pharm. Res.* **2006**, *23*, 1959–1969. [CrossRef] [PubMed]

6

A Risk Assessment of Antibiotic Pan-Drug-Resistance in the UK: Bayesian Analysis of an Expert Elicitation Study

Daniel Carter [1], André Charlett [1], Stefano Conti [1], Julie V. Robotham [1], Alan P. Johnson [1,*], David M. Livermore [2], Tom Fowler [1], Mike Sharland [3], Susan Hopkins [4], Neil Woodford [1], Philip Burgess [5] and Stephen Dobra [5] on Behalf of the Expert Panel

1. National Infection Service, Public Health England, London NW9 5EQ, UK; d-carter@dfid.gov.uk (D.C.); andre.charlett@phe.gov.uk (A.C.); stefano.conti@nhs.net (S.C.); julie.robotham@phe.gov.uk (J.V.R.); tom.fowler@phe.gov.uk (T.F.); neil.woodford@phe.gov.uk (N.W.)
2. Norwich Medical School, University of East Anglia, Norwich NR4 7TJ, UK; d.livermore@uea.ac.uk
3. Paediatric Infectious Diseases Research Group, St George's University of London, Cranmer Terrace, London SW17 0RE, UK; mike.sharland@stgeorges.nhs.uk
4. Antimicrobial Resistance Programme, Public Health England, London NW9 5EQ, UK; susan.hopkins@phe.gov.uk
5. Health Protection Analytical Team, Department of Health, Richmond House, 79 Whitehall, London SW1A 2NS, UK; philip.burgess@dh.gsi.gov.uk (P.B.); stephen.dobra@btinternet.com (S.D.)

* Correspondence: alan.johnson@phe.gov.uk

Academic Editor: Christopher C. Butler

Abstract: To inform the UK antimicrobial resistance strategy, a risk assessment was undertaken of the likelihood, over a five-year time-frame, of the emergence and widespread dissemination of pan-drug-resistant (PDR) Gram-negative bacteria that would pose a major public health threat by compromising effective healthcare delivery. Subsequent impact over five- and 20-year time-frames was assessed in terms of morbidity and mortality attributable to PDR Gram-negative bacteraemia. A Bayesian approach, combining available data with expert prior opinion, was used to determine the probability of the emergence, persistence and spread of PDR bacteria. Overall probability was modelled using Monte Carlo simulation. Estimates of impact were also obtained using Bayesian methods. The estimated probability of widespread occurrence of PDR pathogens within five years was 0.2 (95% credibility interval (CrI): 0.07–0.37). Estimated annual numbers of PDR Gram-negative bacteraemias at five and 20 years were 6800 (95% CrI: 400–58,600) and 22,800 (95% CrI: 1500–160,000), respectively; corresponding estimates of excess deaths were 1900 (95% CrI: 0–23,000) and 6400 (95% CrI: 0–64,000). Over 20 years, cumulative estimates indicate 284,000 (95% CrI: 17,000–1,990,000) cases of PDR Gram-negative bacteraemia, leading to an estimated 79,000 (95% CrI: 0–821,000) deaths. This risk assessment reinforces the need for urgent national and international action to tackle antibiotic resistance.

Keywords: antibiotic resistance; risk assessment; Bayesian modelling

---

1. Introduction

The emergence and spread of antibiotic resistance is a major threat to public health. Infections caused by resistant bacteria are associated with increased morbidity, mortality and economic cost [1]. Many advances in medical care have led, as an unintended consequence, to patients becoming more prone to infection involving opportunistic bacteria. Invasive procedures, immunosuppressive drugs, and the use of intravascular or urinary catheters all compromise the body's natural barriers to infection.

As a result, many patients rely on the therapeutic or prophylactic use of antibiotics to minimize the risk of opportunistic healthcare-associated infections. The widespread occurrence of bacteria that are resistant to antibiotics thus threatens the routine management of patients in diverse clinical settings. In a worst-case setting, the proliferation of strains of bacteria resistant to all routinely available antibiotics, hereafter referred to as "pan-drug-resistant" (PDR) bacteria, would severely compromise many aspects of modern medicine.

The global nature of antimicrobial resistance (AMR) and the need for action have been highlighted in recent reports from Europe [2], the USA [3], Australia [4], and the WHO [5]. In the UK, the threat posed by resistance was emphasized in a report by the Chief Medical Officer [6] and led to the publication of a 5-year national strategy [7]. In support of this strategy, a risk assessment was undertaken of the likelihood of emergence and impact of the widespread occurrence of PDR bacteria, using elicitation of expert opinion [8] coupled with Bayesian statistical inference [9,10].

2. Results

2.1. Probability of Occurrence

As outlined in Equation (1) (described in detail in the Materials and Methods), the overall likelihood of the scenario was based on the combined probability that PDR bacteria would emerge in the UK, persist and then become widely disseminated. The consensus view of the expert panel was that PDR Gram-negative bacteria had already emerged in the UK, as evidenced by referral of PDR isolates to the national reference laboratory; therefore, the probability of emergence was set to one. The prior opinion from the expert panel on the two remaining terms in Equation (1), together with summary statistics from corresponding prior Beta distributions, are presented in Figure 1.

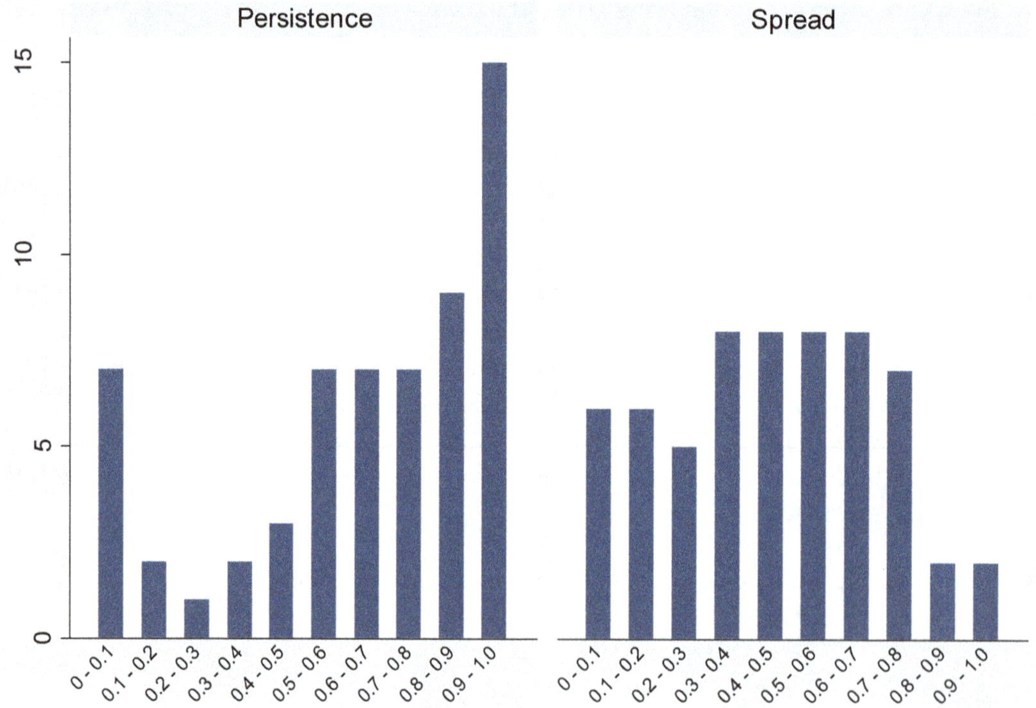

Figure 1. Prior distributions of the expert panel elicitation.

With regard to probability of persistence (given emergence has occurred), analysis of data from the British Society for Antimicrobial Chemotherapy (BSAC) bacteraemia surveillance programme between 2001 and 2012 showed that while emergence of new resistance occurred in four Gram-negative pathogens, only one (carbapenem resistance in *Acinetobacter* spp.) exhibited persistence (Table S3a). In contrast, in 35 instances of pre-existing resistance (inferring persistence), 14 exhibited spread, defined here as a peak annual proportion of resistance of at least 25% (Table S3a). It should be noted that this figure was close to the panel's elicited estimate of 26% for the peak proportion of PDR. Combining this with the prior distributions in Table 1 yields posterior estimates (95% credibility intervals (CrI)) of 0.50 (0.18–0.82), and 0.40 (0.26–0.56) for the probabilities of persistence and spread, respectively. Taking the data on persistence into account led to a downwards revision of the prior estimate of 0.79 elicited from the panel (Table 1) to a posterior estimate of 0.5, whereas the estimate of spread remained largely unaffected by the data. Figure 2 presents the posterior distribution of the probability on the left-hand side of Equation (1), obtained from Monte Carlo simulation. Based on this, the probability of occurrence of the scenario of PDR bacteria emerging, persisting and spreading as agents of bacteraemia within a 5-year interval was estimated to be 0.19 (95% CrI: 0.07–0.37).

Table 1. Prior distributions for persistence and spread elicited from the expert panel.

Parameter	β Distribution				Percentiles		
	α	β	Mean	Variance	50	2.5	97.5
Persistence	2.96	0.99	0.75	0.04	0.79	0.29	0.99
Spread	1.46	1.72	0.46	0.06	0.45	0.05	0.91

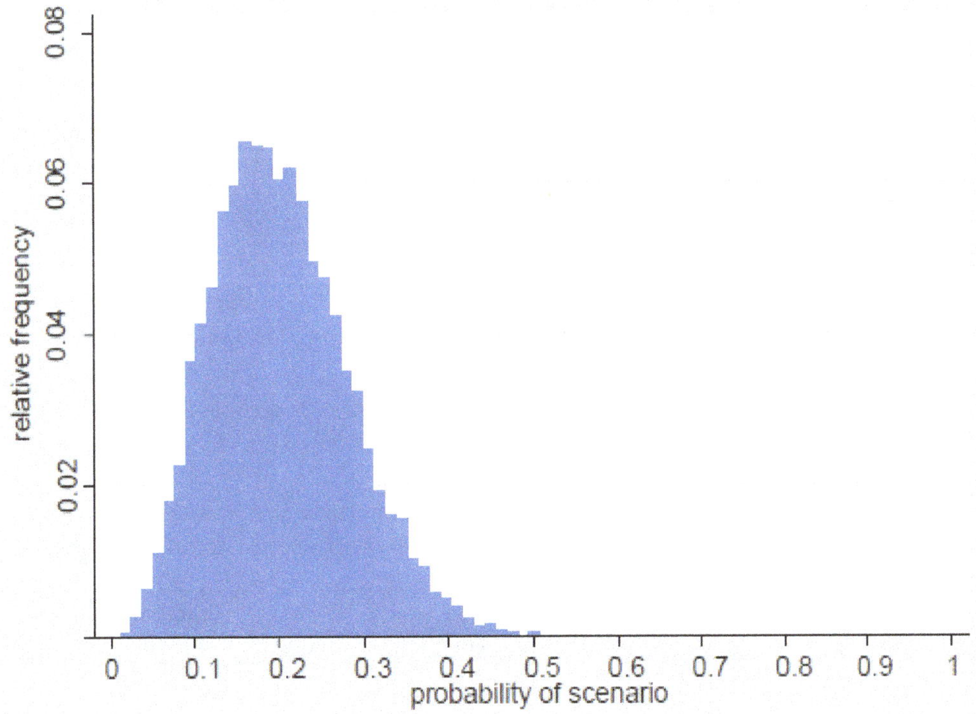

Figure 2. Posterior distribution of the probability of the scenario occurring within five years.

2.2. Impact on Patients

The estimated impact of the widespread occurrence of PDR Gram-negative bacteria using a variety of parameters is shown below.

2.2.1. Number of Bacteraemias

Following occurrence of the scenario, the cumulative numbers of PDR Gram-negative bacteraemias in the UK over five- and 20-year periods were predicted to lie between 1100 and 158,000 and 17,000 and 1,989,000, respectively (Table 2), the interval widths reflecting the combined uncertainty from the expert panel's opinion and the available surveillance data.

Table 2. Point and interval estimates for the annual and cumulative numbers of pan-drug-resistant (PDR) Gram-negative bacteraemia in the UK for selected years of the scenario. CrI, credibility interval.

Year	Median	95% CrI	Median	95% CrI
1	1200	70–7400	1200	70–7400
5	6800	400–58,600	19,600	1100–158,000
10	14,300	800–114,000	77,800	4400–614,000
20	22,800	1500–160,000	283,700	17,000–1,989,000

2.2.2. Mortality

As with the number of PDR bacteraemias, there was considerable uncertainty in the numbers of attributable deaths. These were cumulatively estimated over five and 20-year periods to be 1900 (95% CrI: 0–23,000) and 6400 (95% CrI: 0–64,000), respectively (Table 3).

Table 3. Point and interval estimates for the annual and cumulative numbers of deaths attributable to PDR Gram-negative bacteraemia in the UK for selected years of the scenario.

Year of Scenario	Annual		Cumulative	
	Median	95% CrI	Median	95% CrI
1	300	0–3100	300	0–3100
5	1900	0–23,000	5500	0–63,000
10	4100	0–47,000	22,000	0–248,000
20	6400	0–64,000	79,000	0–821,000

2.2.3. Additional Length of Stay

The expert panel members provided lower and upper limits, lower and upper quartiles and a median estimate of the additional length of stay (LoS) following PDR Gram-negative bacteraemia of 8.0, 17.5, 10.5, 14.5 and 13.0 days respectively. Following occurrence of the scenario, the cumulative numbers of additional LoS days over five- and 20-year periods were estimated to be 60,000 (95% CrI: 2600–875,000) and almost 200,000 days (95% CrI: 10,000–2,400,000), respectively (Table 4).

Table 4. Point and interval estimates for the annual and cumulative additional days length of stay (LoS) attributable to PDR Gram-negative bacteraemia in the UK for selected years of the scenario.

Year of Scenario	Annual		Cumulative	
	Median	95% CrI	Median	95% CrI
1	10,000	500–119,000	10,000	500–119,100
5	60,000	2600–875,000	170,000	8000–2,400,000
10	124,000	5500–1,730,000	676,000	30,000–9,500,000
20	195,000	10,000–2,400,000	2,440,000	120,000–31,900,000

2.2.4. High-Risk Patients

Estimates of the number of PDR infections were made for the groups considered to be at high risk in this scenario. The incidence of surgical site infection (SSI) following large bowel surgery was estimated to rise from 10% in year 0 of the scenario (baseline) to 12% and 18% in years 5 and 20, respectively: it was estimated that about 5000 SSIs from PDR Gram-negative organisms attributable to the scenario would occur over the first five years. For non-elective hip replacement, and repair of fractured neck of femur, it was estimated that about 200 and 400 attributable SSIs involving PDR Gram-negative organisms would occur over the first five years of the scenario.

The impact upon other groups considered the attributable numbers of PDR Gram-negative bacteraemias and so, to some degree, overlapped with previous results. It was estimated that attributable numbers in year 5 of the scenario would be approximately 3700 for patients undergoing flexible cystoscopies, 900 for patients with febrile neutropenia, 900 for renal transplantation, and 90 for renal dialysis patients.

3. Discussion

We describe here a quantitative risk assessment that enabled both the likelihood and impact of a challenging, yet realistic, AMR scenario occurring in the UK to be estimated. The risk assessment focused on infections due to PDR Gram-negative bacteria, as this is the clinical setting where the paucity of new or effective old antibiotics is likely to have the most impact. Evidence to inform the risk assessment was gathered by combining data from existing surveillance systems and expert opinion formally elicited from an expert multi-disciplinary panel of healthcare professionals, chosen for their experience and knowledge of the field of antibiotic resistance. A Bayesian statistical analysis was carried out on the collected body of evidence in a manner designed to take account of both variability in the data and epistemic uncertainty in the expert opinion. Estimates of key measures of the healthcare and economic burden to society following the occurrence of the scenario were obtained over both five and twenty-year projected timeframes.

The approach is not new; for example, Kennedy et al. [11] used a similar approach to quantify the risk of Vero cytotoxin-producing *Escherichia coli* O157 infection from milk. However, to our knowledge, it is the first time such an approach has been used to estimate the risk and impact of the advent of a PDR pathogen. Other recent reviews of AMR [12,13] have used a range of scenarios, including those that are unrealistically at the extremes of 0% and 100% resistance across a range of pathogens. While these reviews concentrated on the global economic impact of AMR, the present UK study has a national focus. Furthermore, although those reviews supplemented available data with expert opinion, the uncertainty surrounding it was not taken into account. While all risk assessments are, by their nature, uncertain, in the present study the capturing of all sources of uncertainty, both within the expert panel elicitation and the available data, and their propagation into final estimates through Bayesian modeling, enabled a comprehensive assessment of the uncertainty surrounding the risk analysis. Consequently, we were able to provide an interval estimate for the likelihood of the selected scenario occurring in the next five years of between 0.07 (~1/14) and 0.37 (~1/3), with a median estimate of 0.2 (~1/5). This likelihood is not negligible, and implies a reasonable expectation that persistence and spread of a PDR Gram-negative organism could occur over five years. In the longer term, this equates to an approximate 4% annual chance of the scenario starting in a given year. This in turn suggests that the likelihood over a 20-year period is around 0.8, highlighting the urgent need to take action and mitigate this risk through a range of measures, such as enhanced antibiotic stewardship and development of new generations of antibiotics, vaccines and effective rapid diagnostics.

Although, from a global perspective, surveillance data on AMR may be somewhat sparse, the UK is better served in this respect than many other nations. The likelihood estimate was derived using data from the BSAC Bacteraemia Surveillance Programme, which have been shown to closely mirror other national surveillance data collected from hospital microbiology laboratories around the UK [14]. These are subject to limitations in the sensitivity and specificity of resistance surveillance, and their use also assumes that historical observations of the persistence and spread of resistance are valid predictors in the context of future PDR. The potential for the rapid proliferation of near pan-resistant clones is well illustrated by the expansion of *Klebsiella pneumoniae* carbapenemase (KPC)-producing

K. pneumoniae of clonal complex (CC) 258. These accounted for most of the early accumulation of carbapenem resistance among *K. pneumoniae* in Italy [15], where the proportion of carbapenem-resistant *K. pneumoniae* rose from 2% in 2008 to 15% in 2010 then to 33% in 2014 [16]. Most representatives of this lineage remain susceptible to gentamicin, polymyxins and tigecycline, though around 16%–22% have acquired resistance to any one of these agents [15]. Although KPC-producing *K. pneumoniae* of CC258 have not yet spread within the UK, despite repeated introduction [17], the pKpQIL plasmids that encode KPC in *K. pneumoniae* of CC258 that have spread widely in Israel [18] are highly related to the plasmids that are spreading among diverse Enterobacteriaceae in north-west England. Additionally, there is growing evidence that KPC carbapenemases are now spreading beyond CC258-related *K. pneumoniae* in Italy, penetrating into a diversity of *Klebsiella* lineages, with an overall colistin resistance rate of 42% [19]. These observations highlight the plausibility of the conclusions reached in the present study.

Point estimates of the cumulative numbers of PDR Gram-negative bacteraemias over the first five and 20 years of the scenario were approximately 20,000 and 280,000, respectively. In the longer term, we estimated approximately 80,000 attributable deaths among the 280,000 cases of bacteraemia. However, the propagation of all the uncertainty in the modeling inputs led to extremely wide credibility intervals around these central estimates.

The estimates of impact necessarily use a number of simplifying assumptions. The projected increase in prevalence of PDR organisms (as a proportion of all Gram-negative bacteraemia isolates) from 0% in year 0 to a peak of approximately 26% in year 20 was determined by modeling the trajectory of increase in prevalence observed with CTX-M extended-spectrum β-lactamases in *E. coli* in the UK and carbapenem-resistant *K. pneumoniae* in Italy and Greece, coupled with expert opinion. An assumption is made that this projected rise in PDR prevalence captures both the spread of pan-resistance and the increased propensity of PDR infections to give rise to bacteraemia as a result of ineffective treatment of underlying infection. The projected baseline number of Gram-negative infections over time, which was required to derive the numbers of PDR Gram-negative bacteraemias from their estimated prevalence, was derived from a simple longitudinal regression model of existing surveillance data.

The numbers of deaths attributable to PDR Gram-negative bacteraemias and of additional hospital LoS days were estimated using data for multidrug-resistant *E. coli* bacteraemias as a proxy for PDR Gram-negative bacteraemias. In particular, estimates of the numbers of attributable deaths will underestimate the true burden of PDR Gram-negative bacteraemias, which is likely to be greater than for multidrug-resistant *E. coli*. Expert elicitation was used to provide a means of assessing this bias and incorporate it into the model. The resulting figures were 1900 (95% CrI: 0–23,000) and 6400 (95% CrI: 0–64,000) over five and 20 years respectively. A lower credibility bound for the 30-day mortality odds ratio of zero might be regarded as implausible, given that the estimated number of PDR cases was never zero. However, this was a reflection of the uncertainty surrounding the opinion elicited from the expert panel on the odds ratio's *actual* lower bound.

Most of the estimates of incidence of infectious complications of medical procedures were based upon published data (though not all from the UK) applied to Hospital Episode Statistics (HES) from a single year. These estimates should be treated with caution, particularly as no credibility intervals around the central estimates were provided, and the range and frequency of medical procedures performed by the NHS may change over the 5–20-year time-scale considered here.

An estimate of the number of cases of PDR infections at anatomical sites other than the bloodstream was projected using a published estimate of the ratio of Gram-negative bacteraemias to other Gram-negative infections [20]. This ratio of 9% would indicate that the total number of PDR infections may be 10-times greater than our estimates of PDR Gram-negative bacteraemia. However, such extrapolations are highly uncertain: this ratio may change as a result of PDR, particularly if bacteraemias become relatively more common due to ineffective treatment of underlying infections at other body sites.

The findings of this risk assessment indicate that there is a measurable risk of PDR pathogens emerging and becoming endemic in a matter of years. The prospect of widespread untreatable infections reinforces the urgent need for action to mitigate the risk of such an event occurring. Moreover, while the outcomes of this risk assessment were derived from an analysis of data and expert opinion relevant to the UK, the risk to public health posed by AMR is global in nature and other counties may face a similar level of risk. Thus, the response to the threat of AMR needs to be international in scope [21]. To this end, it is encouraging that Heads of State came together to commit to fighting the threat posed by AMR at the UN General Assembly meeting in September 2016 [22].

4. Materials and Methods

4.1. Expert Panel and Remit

The panel comprised members from academia, the National Health Service (NHS), Public Health England (PHE) and the UK Department of Health (DH), who variously had expertise in antimicrobial resistance, infectious disease epidemiology, clinical microbiology, pharmacy and patient safety. Their remit was three-fold: firstly, to devise a scenario in which the level of antibiotic resistance in the UK made much of modern medicine untenable due to a high prevalence of untreatable infections; secondly, to assess the likelihood of this scenario occurring within a five-year timeframe; and, lastly, to quantify the impact of this challenge over five- and twenty-year horizons.

The panel considered a range of clinical settings, patient populations and pathogens most relevant to the above scenario. The key features envisioned were that a PDR and highly virulent Gram-negative bacterial strain enters or emerges in the UK, resulting in a loss of clinical utility of all available antibiotics. This resistance pattern would rapidly become geographically widespread, through a combination of strain spread along with intra- and inter-species transfer of a promiscuous plasmid encoding both the multi-resistance and virulence traits. Significant mitigation of the outbreak would not be possible due to failure of prevention and control measures to keep pace with the increasing scale of the problem, insufficient effectiveness of rapid diagnostics and unavailability of new agents for effective treatment.

4.2. Risk Assessment

A Bayesian analytical approach was used, whereby information elicited from the panel was combined with available data (including unpublished surveillance data). The aim was to estimate the likelihood of such a scenario emerging within five years and to assess its subsequent impact over periods of five and twenty years. Aspects considered included affected patient groups, fatalities, excess morbidity and increased LoS in hospital. Outline methods are presented below, with statistical methodology available as Supplementary material.

4.3. Expert Elicitation

During early 2014, opinions on 11 key scenario descriptors (Parameters, Table 5) were formally elicited from expert panel members in the form of probability distributions using the Sheffield Elicitation Framework (SHELF) [23] and the Multidisciplinary Assessment of Technology for Healthcare (MATCH) online elicitation tool [24]. For Parameters 1–5, which are defined as proportions, a "roulette" elicitation method was used, in which each panel member placed ten "chips" amongst as many equally-spaced "bins" spanning the 0 to 1 probability range. For the remaining Parameters, a quartile method was employed, whereby panel members subjectively formulated median, upper and lower quartiles, together with plausible ranges. For each Parameter, distributions elicited from each panel member were thereafter combined into a pooled prior distribution; these distributions were subsequently discussed by all the panel members to reach a consensus prior summarizing the expert panel's beliefs.

Table 5. Parameters elicited from the expert.

Parameter 1: What is the probability that PDR (resulting in loss of susceptibility to all remaining drug classes) in Gram-negative organisms will emerge in or enter the UK within the next five years (i.e., by 2019)?
Parameter 2: In the UK, what proportion of drug class-bug resistance patterns become established, such that they persist over time?
Parameter 3: In the UK, what proportion of established drug class-bug resistance patterns go on to become widespread?
Parameter 4: What is the overall probability that PDR will emerge in or enter the UK within the next five years, and become established and widespread?
Parameter 5: During the scenario, what peak proportion of Gram-negative isolates will demonstrate PDR?
Parameter 6: How many years will elapse from the emergence of PDR, until the peak proportion is reached?
Parameter 7: What cumulative number of PDR Gram-negative bacteraemia will occur during the first five years of the scenario (i.e., 2016–2020)?
Parameter 8: What is the odds ratio for 30-day mortality amongst patients with PDR Gram-negative bacteraemia compared to similar patients with no infection?
Parameter 9: By how many days is length of stay (LoS) greater amongst patients with PDR Gram-negative bacteraemia compared to similar patients with no infection?
Parameter 10: Amongst various potential trajectories for the epidemic curve of PDR Gram-negative bacteraemia (defined in terms of peak prevalence, time to peak prevalence, and the presence or absence of a decline once the peak prevalence is reached), which is considered by the Expert Panel to be the most plausible?
Parameter 11: In addition, panel members were asked to describe the trajectory by which the baseline number of Gram-negative bacteraemias (i.e., non-PDR Gram-negative bacteraemia) may be expected to change over time, to 2035.

4.4. Likelihood of the Scenario

Assessment of the overall likelihood of the scenario was based on the combined probability of three sequential events, as shown in Equation (1), namely the emergence of PDR bacteria in the UK, their persistence and their subsequent widespread dissemination:

$$Pr(scenario) = Pr(emergence) \times Pr(persistence/emergence) \times Pr(spread/emergence, persistence) \quad (1)$$

where *Pr(emergence)* is the probability that a PDR organism enters or emerges in the UK at some point within five years and *Pr(persistence/emergence)* is the probability that, following such an event, the organism persists within the UK (i.e., it becomes endemic within a geographical area or setting). Once persistence is established, the final step is spread of the organism (*Pr(spread/emergence, persistence)*) such that it becomes widespread in the population, defined here as a peak annual proportion of resistance of at least 25%. The overall likelihood of the scenario is the product of the likelihood of each of these steps.

Components of the likelihood were considered separately, combining the panel's prior belief with data obtained from the bacteraemia arm of the BSAC Resistance Surveillance Project [25]. A Monte Carlo simulation approach was adopted to estimate the statistical models for the three above components to finally obtain the overall probability of the proposed scenario.

4.5. Impact Assessment

Evaluation of the impact of PDR Gram-negative bacteraemia in terms of morbidity and mortality required two inputs for each year: the projected proportion of Gram-negative infections that were PDR, and the baseline number of Gram-negative bacteraemias. The expert panel's view was that PDR Gram-negative bacteraemias would independently add to the baseline number of non-PDR Gram-negative bacteraemias. The proportion of PDR cases was informed by Parameters 5 and 6 in Table 5, and the baseline number of Gram-negative bacteraemias derived using Parameter 11.

Equation (S3) (see Supplementary Materials) was then used to generate estimates of the number of deaths directly attributable to PDR Gram-negative bacteraemia.

4.6. *Affected Patient Groups*

The impact of PDR infections would be highest in those patients whose vulnerability to infection is increased by aspects of their medical care, such as invasive procedures or immunosuppression. Patient groups included in the risk assessment were therefore those with/undergoing febrile neutropenia, renal dialysis, renal transplantation, flexible cystoscopy, large bowel surgery, hip replacement surgery or repair of fractured neck of femur. Numbers of PDR Gram-negative infections expected in each of these groups were estimated for each year subsequent to the scenario. Projected estimates of the annual number of patients were made using HES [26] for all groups apart from renal dialysis, which used data from the UK Renal Registry [27]. The incidences of Gram-negative infections for large bowel surgery, hip replacement surgery, and repair of fractured neck of femur were obtained from mandatory and voluntary surgical site infection (SSI) surveillance [28]. Incidence estimates from published literature were used for febrile neutropenia [29], renal transplantation [30], and flexible cystoscopy [31]. While no measures of accuracy were calculated, it was recognized that these estimates would exhibit a similar level of uncertainty to that shown by the numbers of PDR Gram-negative bacteraemias.

4.7. *Hospital Length of Stay*

The total additional LoS in days (S_i) attributable to PDR bacteraemias (b_i) in year i was calculated using the formula $S_i = b_i \times L$ proposed by de Kraker [1], where L is the additional LoS attributable to PDR bacteraemia described by Parameter 9 (Table 5).

5. Conclusions

Many medical procedures predispose patients to infection by providing portals of entry for pathogens or by depressing patients' immune responses. Thus, successful management of patients is frequently dependent of effective antibiotic prophylaxis or treatment. Given the paucity of new antibiotics in development, if resistance to currently available antibiotics becomes widespread, this will adversely impact on delivery of effective medical care in a wide range of clinical settings. This study describes a risk assessment that indicated that there is an approximately 20% chance of such a situation arising in the UK over a five-year time frame. The impact of such an event, were it to occur, would be very significant in clinical and public health terms, with marked increases in morbidity and mortality. This finding reinforces the importance of taking immediate action to tackle the rise in antibiotic resistance.

Supplementary Materials: Supplemental material giving detailed statistical methodology is available online at http://www.mdpi.com/2079-6382/6/1/9/s1. The Supplemental material includes: Table S1: Numbers allocated to each elicitation category for the pooled distributions from the expert panel elicitation for parameters denoting proportions, Table S2: Medians of the elicited quantiles from the expert panel elicitation for parameters not denoting proportions, Table S3a: Proportion of resistance in BSAC RSP in antibiotic class-bug combinations between 2001 and 2012 where resistance emerged during this period, Table S3b: Proportion of resistance in BSAC RSP in antibiotic class-bug combinations between 2001 and 2012 where resistant isolate were present in the initial year of surveillance, Table S4: Point and interval estimates for the annual and cumulative numbers of PDR GNB in the UK by year of scenario, Table S5: reports point and interval longitudinal estimates for d_i, both for individual years and cumulative over time, Table S6: Point and interval estimates for the annual and cumulative numbers of additional LHS in the UK attributable to PDR GNB by year of scenario, Table S7: Point and interval estimates for the annual number of prevalent cases each day in the UK attributable to PDR GNB by year of scenario, Table S8: Estimated number of PDR Gram-negative SSIs (PRGNS) in the high risk patient groups by year.

Acknowledgments: No external funding. We thank Michael Fleming, Department of Health, for constructive discussion regarding the statistical analysis. Membership of the Expert Panel comprised: Matthew Fogarty (Head of Patient Safety and Policy, NHS England); Tom Fowler (Consultant Epidemiologist, Public Health England); Alastair Hay (Primary Care, University of Bristol); Susan Hopkins (Consultant in Infectious Disease, Royal Free Hospital. London); Alan Johnson (Consultant Clinical Scientist, PHE); David Livermore (Medical Microbiology, Norwich Medical School); Keith Ridge (Chief Pharmaceutical Officer, NHS England); Mike Sharland (Chair of the

Advisory Committee on Antimicrobial Resistance and Healthcare-Associated Infections (ARHAI)); Bruce Warne (Deputy Chief Pharmaceutical Officer, NHS England).

Author Contributions: Stephen Dobra, David M. Livermore, Alan P. Johnson, Tom Fowler, Mike Sharland, Neil Woodford and Susan Hopkins conceived and designed the risk analysis scenario; Daniel Carter, André Charlett, Stefano Conti, Julie V. Robotham and Philip Burgess analyzed the data; Daniel Carter, André Charlett and Alan P. Johnson wrote the initial draft of the paper which was then reviewed and revised by all the authors.

Conflicts of Interest: Julie V. Robotham, Alan P. Johnson and David M. Livermore are members of the UK government Advisory Committee on Antimicrobial Resistance and Healthcare Associated Infection (ARHAI). Mike Sharland is the Chair of ARHAI. David M. Livermore is a member of Advisory Boards or has undertaken ad-hoc consultancy for Accelerate, Achaogen, Adenium, Allecra, AstraZeneca, Auspherix, Basilea, BioVersys, Cubist, Centauri, Discuva, Meiji, Pfizer, Roche, Shionogi, Tetraphase, VenatoRx, Wockhardt, Zambon, Zealand, Paid lectures—AstraZeneca, Cepheid, Merck and Nordic. Relevant shareholdings in—Dechra, GSK, Merck, Perkin Elmer, Pfizer amounting to <10% of portfolio value. Contract research/grants from Allecra, AstraZeneca, Melinta, Merck, Roche, Wockhardt. All other authors have none to declare.

References

1. De Kraker, M.E.A.; Davey, P.G.; Grundmann, H. on behalf of the BURDEN study group. Mortality and hospital stay associated with resistant *Staphylococcus aureus* and *Escherichia coli* bacteremia: Estimating the burden of antibiotic resistance in Europe. *PLoS Med.* **2011**, *8*, e1001104. [CrossRef] [PubMed]
2. European Centre for Disease Prevention and Control. Antimicrobial Resistance Surveillance in Europe 2014. Available online: http://ecdc.europa.eu/en/publications/_layouts/forms/Publication_DispForm.aspx?List=4f55ad51--4aed-4d32-b960-af70113dbb90&ID=1400 (accessed on 18 November 2016).
3. Centers for Disease Control and Prevention. Antibiotic resistance threats in the United States, 2013. Available online: http://www.cdc.gov/drugresistance/threat-report-2013 (accessed on 18 November 2016).
4. Australian Government. Responding to the Threat of Antimicrobial Resistance. Commonwealth of Australia, 2015. Available online: http://www.health.gov.au/internet/main/publishing.nsf/content/1803C433C71415CACA257C8400121B1F/\protect\T1\textdollarFile/amr-strategy-2015--2019.pdf (accessed on 18 November 2016).
5. WHO. The Evolving Threat of Antimicrobial Resistance. Options for Action. Available online: http://apps.who.int/iris/bitstream/10665/44812/1/9789241503181_eng.pdf (accessed on 18 November 2016).
6. Davies, S.C. Annual Report of the Chief Medical Officer, Volume Two, 2011. Available online: https://www.gov.uk/government/uploads/system/uploads/attachment_data/file/138331/CMO_Annual_Report_Volume_2_2011.pdf (accessed on 18 November 2016).
7. Department of Health. UK Five Year Antimicrobial Resistance Strategy 2013 to 2018. Available online: https://www.gov.uk/government/uploads/system/uploads/attachment_data/file/244058/20130902_UK_5_year_AMR_strategy.pdf (accessed on 18 November 2016).
8. O'Hagan, A.; Buck, C.E.; Daneshkhah, A.; Eiser, J.R.; Garthwaite, P.H.; Jenkinson, D.J.; Oakley, J.E.; Rakow, T. *Uncertain Judgements: Eliciting Experts' Probabilities*; John Wiley & Sons: Chichester, UK, 2006.
9. Bernardo, J.M.; Smith, A.F.M. *Bayesian Theory*, 2nd ed.; John Wiley & Sons: Chicester, UK, 2000.
10. Gelman, A.; Carlin, J.B.; Stern, H.S.; Dunson, D.B.; Vehtari, A.; Rubin, D.B. *Bayesian Data Analysis*, 3rd ed.; Chapman & Hall/CRC: Boca Raton, FL, USA, 2014.
11. Kennedy, M.C.; Clough, H.E.; Turner, J. Case studies in Bayesian microbial risk assessment. *Environ. Health* **2009**, *8*. [CrossRef] [PubMed]
12. The Global Economic Impact of Anti-Microbial Resistance. Available online: https://www.kpmg.com/UK/en/IssuesAndInsights/ArticlesPublications/Documents/PDF/Issues%20and%20Insights/amr-report-final.pdf (accessed on 18 November 2016).
13. Estimating the Economic Costs of Antimicrobial Resistance. Model and Results. Available online: http://www.rand.org/content/dam/rand/pubs/research_reports/RR900/RR911/RAND_RR911.pdf (accessed on 18 November 2016).
14. Livermore, D.M.; Hope, R.; Reynolds, R.; Blackburn, R.; Johnson, A.P.; Woodford, N. Declining cephalosporin and fluoroquinolone non-susceptibility among bloodstream Enterobacteriaceae from the UK: Links to prescribing change? *J. Antimicrob. Chemother.* **2013**, *68*, 2667–2674. [CrossRef] [PubMed]

15. Giani, T.; Pini, B.; Arena, F.; Conte, V.; Bracco, S.; Migliavacca, R. Epidemic diffusion of KPC carbapenemase-producing *Klebsiella pneumoniae* in Italy: Results of the first countrywide survey, 15 May to 30 June 2011. *Euro. Surveill.* **2013**, *30*, 2–10.
16. ECDC. Surveillance Atlas of Infectious Disease. Available online: http://atlas.ecdc.europa.eu/public/index.aspx?Instance=GeneralAtlas (accessed on 18 November 2016).
17. Findlay, J.; Hopkins, K.L.; Doumith, M.; Meunier, D.; Wiuff, C.; Hill, R.; Pike, R.; Loy, R.; Mustafa, S.; Livermore, D.M.; et al. KPC enzymes in the UK: An analysis of the first 160 cases outside the North-West region. *J. Antimicrob. Chemother.* **2016**, *71*, 1199–1206. [CrossRef] [PubMed]
18. Leavitt, A.; Chmelnitsky, I.; Carmeli, Y.; Navon-Venezia, S. Complete nucleotide sequence of KPC-3-encoding plasmid pKpQIL in the epidemic *Klebsiella pneumoniae* sequence type 258. *Antimicrob. Agents Chemother.* **2010**, *54*, 4493–4496. [CrossRef] [PubMed]
19. Bonura, C.; Giuffrè, M.; Aleo, A.; Fasciana, T.; Di Bernardo, F.; Stampone, T.; Giammanco, A. An update of the evolving epidemic of blaKPC carrying *Klebsiella pneumoniae* in Sicily, Italy, 2014: Emergence of multiple non-ST258 clones. *PLoS ONE* **2015**, *10*, e0132936. [CrossRef] [PubMed]
20. European Centre for Disease Prevention and Control/European Medicines Agency. The Bacterial Challenge: Time to React. European Centre for Disease Prevention and Control: Stockholm, 2009. Available online: http://ecdc.europa.eu/en/publications/Publications/0909_TER_The_Bacterial_Challenge_Time_to_React.pdf (accessed on 18 November 2016).
21. Shallcross, L.J.; Davies, S.C. The World Health Assembly resolution on antimicrobial resistance. *J. Antimicrob. Chemother.* **2014**, *69*, 2883–2885. [CrossRef] [PubMed]
22. WHO. High-Level Meeting on Antimicrobial Resistance. Available online: http://www.un.org/pga/71/2016/09/21/press-release-hl-meeting-on-antimicrobial-resistance/ (accessed on 18 November 2016).
23. Oakley, J.E.; O'Hagan, A. SHELF: The Sheffield Elicitation Framework (version 2.0), School of Mathematics and Statistics, University of Sheffield, UK, 2010. Available online: http://tonyohagan.co.uk/shelf (accessed on 18 November 2016).
24. Morris, D.E.; Oakley, J.E.; Crowe, J.A. A web-based tool for eliciting probability distributions from experts. *Environ. Model. Softw.* **2014**, *52*, 1–4. [CrossRef]
25. British Society for Antimicrobial Chemotherapy Resistance Surveillance Project. Available online: http://www.bsacsurv.org/reports/bacteraemia (accessed on 18 November 2016).
26. Hospital Episode Statistics: Admitted Patient Care, England—2012-13. Available online: http://content.digital.nhs.uk/catalogue/PUB12566/hosp-epis-stat-admi-summ-rep-2012--13-rep.pdf (accessed on 18 November 2016).
27. Crowley, L.; Pitcher, D.; Wilson, J.; Guy, R.; Fluck, R. UK Renal Registry 16th Annual Report: Chapter 15 Epidemiology of Reported Infections amongst Patients Receiving Dialysis for Established Renal Failure in England from May 2011 to April 2012: A Joint Report from Public Health England and the UK Renal Registry. UK Renal Registry: Bristol, 2013. Available online: http://www.renalreg.com/Reports/2013.html (accessed on 18 November 2016).
28. Public Health England. Surgical Site Infection Reports. Available online: http://webarchive.nationalarchives.gov.uk/20140722091854/http://www.hpa.org.uk/Publications/InfectiousDiseases/SurgicalSiteInfectionReports/ (accessed on 18 November 2016).
29. Reuter, S.; Kern, W.V.; Sigge, A.; Dohner, H.; Marre, R.; Kerm, P.; von Baum, H. Impact of fluoroquinolone prophylaxis on reduced infection-related mortality among patients with neutropenia and hematologic malignancies. *Clin. Infect. Dis.* **2005**, *40*, 1087–1093. [CrossRef] [PubMed]
30. Maraha, B.; Bonten, H.; van Hooff, H.; Fiolet, H.; Buiting, A.G.; Stobberingh, E.E. Infectious complications and antibiotic use in renal transplant recipients during a 1-year follow-up. *Clin. Microbiol. Infect.* **2001**, *7*, 619–625. [CrossRef] [PubMed]
31. Almallah, Y.Z.; Rennie, C.D.; Stone, J.; Lancashire, M.J. Urinary tract infection and patient satisfaction after flexible cystoscopy and urodynamic evaluation. *Urology* **2000**, *56*, 37–39. [CrossRef]

7

Neisseria gonorrhoeae Aggregation Reduces Its Ceftriaxone Susceptibility

Liang-Chun Wang *, Madeline Litwin, Zahraossadat Sahiholnasab, Wenxia Song and Daniel C. Stein

Department of Cell Biology and Molecular Genetics, University of Maryland College Park, College Park, MD 20904, USA; mlitwin@terpmail.umd.edu (M.L.); nz.sahiholnasab@gmail.com (Z.S.); wenxsong@umd.edu (W.S.); dcstein@umd.edu (D.C.S.)
* Correspondence: marknjoy@umd.edu

Abstract: Antibiotic resistance in *Neisseria gonorrhoeae* (GC) has become an emerging threat worldwide and heightens the need for monitoring treatment failures. *N. gonorrhoeae*, a gram-negative bacterium responsible for gonorrhea, infects humans exclusively and can form aggregates during infection. While minimal inhibitory concentration (MIC) tests are often used for determining antibiotic resistance development and treatment, the knowledge of the true MIC in individual patients and how it relates to this laboratory measure is not known. We examined the effect of aggregation on GC antibiotic susceptibility and the relationship between bacterial aggregate size and their antibiotic susceptibility. Aggregated GC have a higher survival rate when treated with ceftriaxone than non-aggregated GC, with bacteria in the core of the aggregates surviving the treatment. GC lacking opacity-associated protein or pili, or expressing a truncated lipooligosaccharide, three surface molecules that mediate GC-GC interactions, reduce both aggregation and ceftriaxone survival. This study demonstrates that the aggregation of *N. gonorrhoeae* can reduce the susceptibility to antibiotics, and suggests that antibiotic utilization can select for GC surface molecules that promote aggregation which in turn drive pathogen evolution. Inhibiting aggregation may be a potential way of increasing the efficacy of ceftriaxone treatment, consequently reducing treatment failure.

Keywords: gonorrhea; antibiotic resistance; increased susceptibility; biofilm; treatment failure; recurrence

---

1. Introduction

Gonorrhea is the second most commonly reported sexually transmitted infection (STI) in the United States [1]. It is caused by *Neisseria gonorrhoeae* (GC), a gram-negative diplococcal bacterium. GC colonizes and infects the human genital tract but can also infect rectal and pharyngeal mucosal tissue in both men and women [2]. Symptoms of genital infection include painful urination, genital pain, and abnormal discharge. Nonetheless, the infection is often asymptomatic [3,4], with the asymptomatic rates as high as 56% in men [5] and 80% in women [6]. Asymptomatic infections cause extended colonization without treatment. Such untreated infections raise major concerns on the transmittance of gonorrhea and other STIs. In women, if left untreated, GC infection can lead to complications such as pelvic inflammatory disease (PID) and disseminated gonococcal infection (DGI) [7]. Consequences of PID include scarring of the reproductive organs, which may result in chronic pelvic pain, predisposition to ectopic pregnancy, and/or infertility. DGI can cause arthritis, tenosynovitis, dermatitis, and skin lesions [8]. The significance of gonorrhea is further highlighted by the findings that GC infection increases the risk of HIV infection and co-infections of other sexually transmitted pathogens [9].

Emerging antibiotic resistance of GC has become a public health crisis and a social-economic burden [10]. Declining susceptibility to cephalosporin resulted in a change in the treatment regimen from a single antibiotic to dual therapy, combining ceftriaxone with either azithromycin or doxycycline [11]. The emerging threat of cephalosporin resistance, in combination with subclinical gonorrhea, highlights the need for further understanding gonorrhea treatment failures.

The minimal inhibitory concentration (MIC) test has been the standard test for bacterial antibiotic resistance. However, whether this test reflects bacterial antibiotic resistance in vivo is unclear. For example, it has been well documented that pharyngeal gonococcal infections persist after antibiotic treatment [12]. Nonetheless, GC isolates from pharyngeal infections are sensitive to the antibiotics using the minimal inhibitory concentration test data. These findings suggest that unknown factors contribute to GC survival of antibiotic treatment in patients. Identifying these unknown factors might permit the development of more effective antimicrobial therapies.

The formation of bacterial biofilms has been shown to be a significant contributor to the survival of bacteria. Bacteria in biofilms are significantly more resistant to antimicrobials than bacteria in the planktonic phase of growth [13]. While GC can form biofilms [14], their contribution to antibiotic resistance and/or treatment failure in GC infections has not yet been examined. The GC biofilm progresses from an intimately associated aggregation of microcolonies to an organized biofilm. Pili, opacity-associated protein (Opa), and lipooligosaccharides (LOS), three well-characterized phase variable surface molecules of GC, have been shown to mediate inter-bacterium interactions to form aggregates [15–17]. How phase variations in their expression contribute to different GC-GC interactions and whether these interactions affect GC susceptibility to antibiotics is unknown. This study examines the role of GC aggregation, modulated by surface molecules, in bacterial survival in the presence of antibiotics. The reduced susceptibility of GC aggregates to antibiotics may contribute to treatment failure and recurrent gonorrhea.

2. Results

2.1. GC Aggregation Promotes Survival through Limiting Ceftriaxone Penetration

2.1.1. GC Aggregation Promotes Survival under Ceftriaxone Treatment

To examine if GC aggregation enhances resistance to ceftriaxone killing, we allowed a suspension of MS11Opa+Pil+ to either not aggregate, aggregate for 6 h, or aggregate for 6 h before disrupting the suspension. We then treated these aggregates with various concentrations of ceftriaxone for 24 h and measured the level of ATP production as an indication of GC viability by the BacTiter assay (Figure 1a). We found that the survival of non-aggregated, pre-aggregated, and aggregation-disrupted GC decreased as the concentration of ceftriaxone increased. However, the percentage of survival of pre-aggregated GC was significantly higher than non-aggregated and aggregation-disrupted GC when ceftriaxone concentrations approached the broth MIC of 0.125 μg/mL. To verify the results from the BacTiter assay, we quantified the cultivable CFU with and without pre-aggregation for 6 h in the absence or presence of 0.015, 0.03, and 1 μg/mL ceftriaxone (Figure 1b). Pre-aggregated and non-aggregated GC showed significant differences in the ATP production at these concentrations of ceftriaxone. We found the total cultivable CFU decreased >100 fold at both 0.015 and 0.03 μg/mL ceftriaxone and >10,000 fold at 1 μg/mL ceftriaxone compared to non-treatment control. Compared to non-aggregated GC, the number of cultivable CFU of pre-aggregated GC increased significantly at 0.015 and 0.03 μg/mL ceftriaxone. Furthermore, at 1 μg/mL ceftriaxone, there were still cultivable GC from the pre-aggregated group whereas non-aggregated GC had no growth. These data suggest GC aggregation promotes survival in the presence of ceftriaxone.

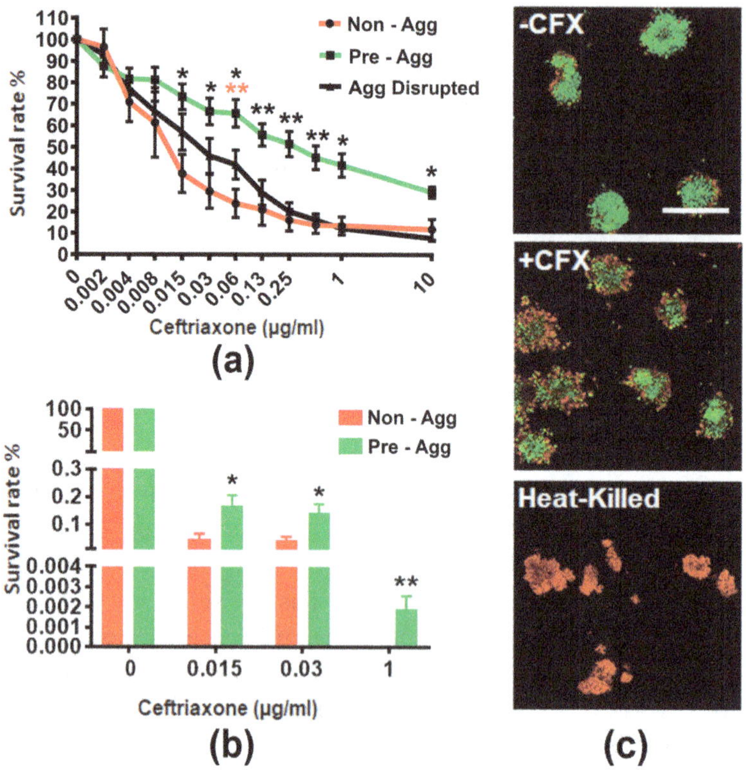

Figure 1. Survival rate and distribution of pre-aggregated MS11Opa+Pil+ *Neisseria gonorrhoeae* (GC) under ceftriaxone treatment. MS11Opa+Pil+ were inoculated in a 96-well plate and the suspensions were either not allowed to aggregate, allowed to pre-aggregate for 6 h, or allowed to pre-aggregate for 6 h before disrupting the suspension. Various concentrations of ceftriaxone were added into different aggregation conditions and incubated for 24 h. (**a**) BacTiter assay was performed to measure total ATP. (**b**) GC suspensions treated with 0, 0.015, 0.03, and 1 μg/mL ceftriaxone were plated onto a GCK plate. Colony forming units (CFU) were counted after 24 h incubation, and survival rates were calculated by dividing CFU from each condition to that with no ceftriaxone treatment. Shown are the average values (±SD) obtained from three independent experiments. *** $p < 0.001$; ** $p < 0.01$; * $p < 0.05$. (**c**) Pre-aggregated and heat-killed GC were incubated with or without 1 μg/mL ceftriaxone for 2 h, stained with Live/Dead BacLight stain to visualize viable (Green) and dead (Red) GC, and analyzed using a confocal fluorescence microscope. Shown are representative images from three independent experiments. +CFX: 1 μg/mL ceftriaxone; -CFX: mock control. Scale bar: 50 μm.

2.1.2. GC Aggregation Limits Ceftriaxone Penetration

To investigate how aggregation enhances GC survival in the presence of antibiotics, we examined the distribution of live and dead GC within aggregates. We allowed MS11Opa+Pil+ to pre-aggregate for 6 h, treated with or without 1 μg/mL ceftriaxone for 2 h, and stained the resulting cultures with BacLight viability stain with heat-killed aggregates as our control (Figure 1c). Our confocal fluorescent microscopy analysis showed that after ceftriaxone treatment, dead bacteria (red) were mostly located at the outer layers whereas viable GC (green) were mostly located in the core of the MS11Opa+Pil+ aggregates. Taken together, our results indicate that GC aggregation reduces susceptibility to antibiotic treatment by limiting antibiotic penetration.

2.2. GC Strains Lacking Opa or Pili or Expressing Truncated LOS Showed a Reduced Survivability against Ceftriaxone Due to Decreased Aggregation

Opa, pili, and LOS, three major surface molecules of GC, play critical roles in promoting GC-GC interactions. To further investigate the role of GC aggregation in antibiotic susceptibility, we compared

GC that switch off pili expression (Pil-), GC that had all 11 *opa* genes deleted (ΔOpa), or GC that cannot express the terminal Lacto-*N*-tetrose (ΔLgtE) with the wildtype phase variable strain. We allowed MS11Opa+Pil+, MS11ΔopaPil+, MS11Opa+Pil- and MS11ΔLgtEPil+ to pre-aggregate for 6 h and treated aggregates with or without 1 μg/mL ceftriaxone for 2 h. We then stained the resulting cultures with BacLight and analyzed the bacteria using confocal fluorescence microscopy (Figure 2a). We quantified the size of GC aggregates by measuring the area of individual aggregate and the survival rate of GC by determining the fluorescence intensity ratio (FIR) of live to dead bacteria in GC aggregates. Our images show that MS11Opa+Pil+ formed the largest and MS11Opa+Pil- formed smallest aggregates among all strains tested. The lack of Opa, complete LOS, or pili progressively and significantly reduced the size of GC aggregates (Figure 2a,b). GC in the outer layers of the large MS11Opa+Pil+ aggregates were dead while those in the core were still alive. In contrast, most of GC in the small loose aggregates of MS11ΔOpaPil+, MS11Opa+Pil-, and MS11ΔLgtEPil+ were mostly dead. Interestingly, MS11Opa+Pil- and MS11ΔLgtEPil+, forming similar sizes of aggregation, displayed a mixed distribution of live and dead GC; note the presence of yellow GC, indicating the uptake of both dyes (Figure 2a). We then compared the live to dead FIR of treated GC to those of untreated GC to measure the percentage of survival. MS11Opa+Pil+ had the highest surviving rate while MS11Opa+Pil- had the lowest among the four strains. Compared to MS11Opa+Pil+, the surviving levels of MS11ΔopaPil+ MS11ΔLgtEPil+, and MS11Opa+Pil- all were significantly decreased (Figure 2c). By plotting the number of GC surviving with the size of GC aggregates, we found a positive correlation ($R = 0.67$) between the two, with statistical significance (Figure 2d). We further confirmed this finding by measuring the ATP production. We found that without aggregation, all of the strains had similar and decreased levels of ATP (Figure 2e). However, with aggregation, MS11Opa+Pil+ aggregates had the highest ATP level post ceftriaxone treatment (0.015–0.125 μg/mL) while other strains significantly decreased the levels of ATP (Figure 2f). Taken together, these results indicate that the ability of GC surface molecules to promote aggregation is responsible for the decreased susceptibility of GC to ceftriaxone treatment.

2.3. GC Aggregation on Human Epithelial Cells also Increases Ceftriaxone Survivability

To determine if GC aggregation also increases the antibiotic survivability of GC that are associated with human epithelial cells, we compared the survival of Opa+Pil+ and Opa+Pil- GC that were pre-incubated with the human cervical epithelial cells ME180. We incubated ME180 cells with MS11Opa+Pil+ or MS11Opa+Pil- for 6 h to let GC attach to epithelial cells and treated the co-culture with or without 1 μg/mL ceftriaxone for 2 h. The resulting cultures were stained with BacLight dye and analyzed by confocal fluorescence microscopy (Figure 3a). Similar to pre-aggregated GC in the absence of epithelial cells, MS11Opa+Pil+ formed larger and tighter aggregates than MS11Opa+Pil-. In ceftriaxone treated MS11Opa+Pil+ aggregates, only bacteria in the outer layer were dead whereas those in the core of the aggregates and at the side of the aggregates that attached to ME180 cells remained viable (yellow arrow). In the small aggregates of MS11Opa+Pil-, live and dead GC were mixed together (white arrow) no matter if they attached to ME180 cells or not. By comparing the live to dead FIRs, we found that after attaching to ME180 cells, MS11Opa+Pil+ still had a higher surviving rate of antibiotic treatment than MS11Opa+Pil- (Figure 3b), similar to what we observed in the absence of epithelial cells. These results support that aggregation helps GC that colonize human epithelial cells to survive ceftriaxone treatments.

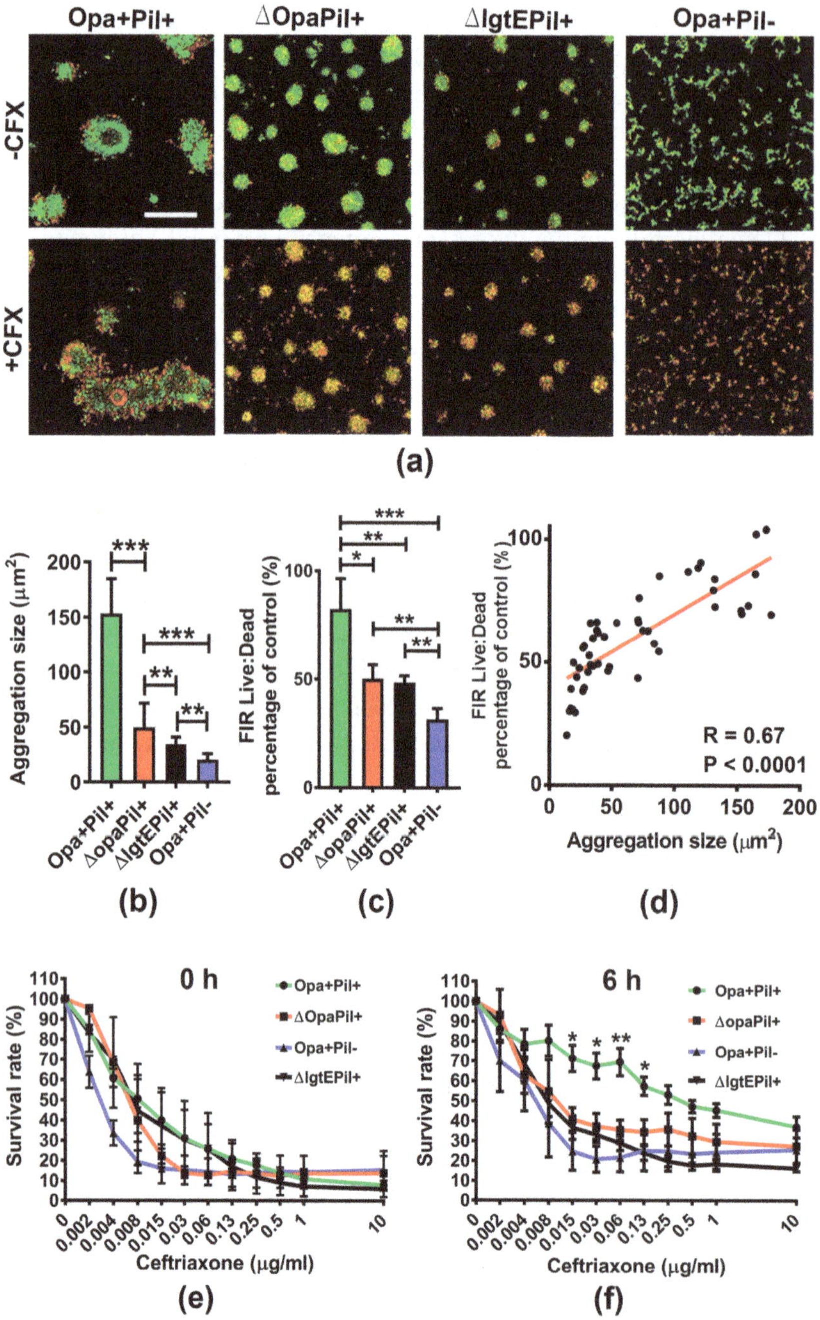

Figure 2. Comparison of survival rate and distribution in GC aggregates that lack Opa or Pili or express truncated lipooligosaccharides (LOS) under ceftriaxone treatment. MS11Opa+Pil+, MS11ΔOpaPil+, MS11Opa+Pil-, or MS11ΔLgtEPil+ were allowed to aggregate for 6 h. (**a**) Pre-aggregated GC were incubated with 1 μg/mL ceftriaxone (+CFX) or mock treated (-CFX) for 2 h, stained with Live/Dead BacLight stain for visualizing live (Green) and dead (Red) GC, and analyzed using a confocal fluorescence microscope. Scale bar: 50 μm. (**b**) The sizes of GC aggregates were quantified by the area of each aggregate. (**c**) The live to dead GC ratios were quantified by the fluorescence intensity ratio (FIR) of green to red staining. The average size of aggregation and live to dead ratio (±SD) were obtained from >40 images of three independent experiments. (**d**) The relation between GC aggregation and their susceptibility to antibiotics was analyzed by plotting the sizes of GC aggregates versus their survival rates and linear regression. (**e**,**f**) 0 h non- and 6 h pre-aggregated GC were incubated with serial concentrations of ceftriaxone for 24 h. The ATP production under each condition was measured. Shown are the average values (±SD) obtained from three independent experiments. *** $p < 0.001$; ** $p < 0.01$; * $p < 0.05$.

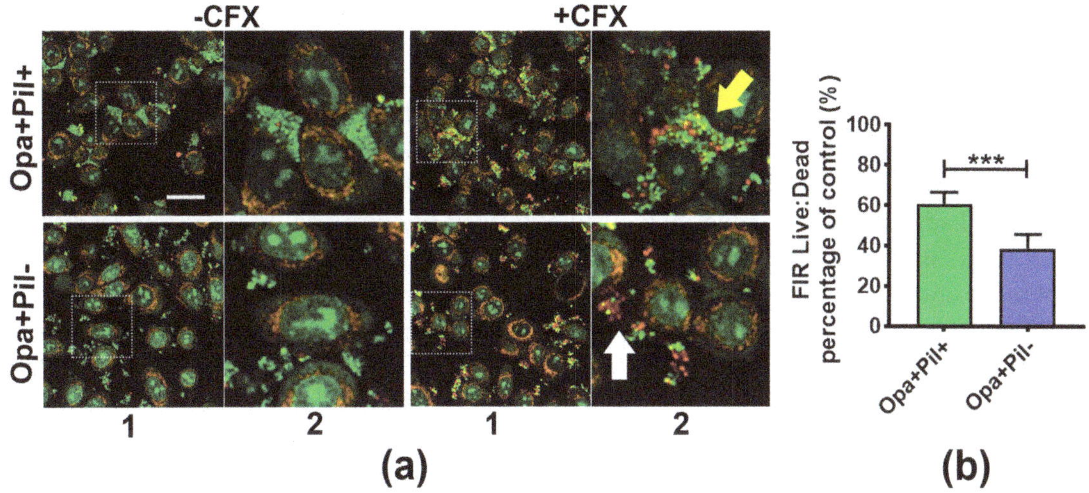

Figure 3. Survival and distribution of GC aggregates on human cervical epithelial cells. MS11Opa+Pil+ or MS11Opa+Pil- were inoculated and incubated with ME180 cells for 6 h. (**a**) GC- epithelial cell co-cultures were treated with 1 μg/mL ceftriaxone (+CFX) or mock treated (-CFX) for 2 h, stained with Live/Dead BacLight stain for visualizing live (Green) and dead (Red) GC, and analyzed using a confocal fluorescence microscope. The images shown in panel (1) reflect the overall distribution of cells and the image in panel (2) is an enlargement of the inset, shown as a dotted box. Yellow arrow, a large aggregate of Opa+Pil+ GC; White arrow, a small aggregate of Opa+Pil- GC. (**b**) The live to dead GC ratios were quantified by the FIR of green to red staining. The average ratio (±SD) was obtained from >30 images of three independent experiments. *** $p < 0.001$; ** $p < 0.01$; * $p < 0.05$. Scale bar, 30 μm.

3. Discussion

The results of this study demonstrate that the ability to form aggregates significantly increased GC survival in the presence of ceftriaxone. Furthermore, the expression of GC surface molecules, Opa, pili, and LOS, enhances GC survival by promoting bacterial aggregation. While there is accumulating evidence for the importance of gonococcal aggregation in infection, this study is the first to reveal the contribution of GC aggregation to its reduced susceptibility to ceftriaxone.

The association of GC aggregation with their survivability in the presence of ceftriaxone suggests an additional mechanism by which GC increase their resistance to clinically relevant antibiotics. GC aggregation has been observed in patient biopsies and exudates where GC aggregates were found on ectocervical epithelium from displaying cervicitis and phagocytic immune cells from patients displaying urethritis [18,19]. Our ex vivo infection study using endocervical tissue explants found GC aggregates on the endocervical epithelium and GC biofilm on the ectocervical epithelium [20,21]. We also noticed that GC form aggregates not only on the surface of epithelium but also on exfoliated cervical epithelial cells even in the absence of Opa or pili expression (data not shown), suggesting the presence of unknown host factors that facilitate GC aggregation. Thus, GC aggregation and the increased antibiotic susceptibility of GC aggregation are likely to happen in vivo.

The surface molecules Opa, pili, and LOS are well-known for their roles in GC pathogenesis [22], but their roles in GC survival with antibiotic treatment have not been examined. This study shows that these molecules decrease GC susceptibility to antibiotic treatment mainly by forming aggregates through mediating bacterium-bacterium interaction. However, Opa, pili, and LOS also interact with host epithelial cells during infections in addition to mediating bacterium-bacterium interactions. GC aggregation and adherence to host cells through these molecules may influence each other, therefore changing both the infectivity and antibiotic resistance of GC in the reproductive tract of women. Indeed, we have previously shown that Opa expression facilitates GC adherence to host cells and GC aggregation, but reduces GC penetration into both polarized epithelial cell monolayers and the endocervical epithelium in the tissue explant model [16,20]. The functions of Opa in both GC-GC and

GC-epithelial interactions enable Opa-expressing GC to survive better in the presence of antibiotic agents and dominate the colonization of the epithelial surface.

Analysis of *opa* and *pil* genes across geographical locations, species, and strains suggests that the host immune system drives sequence polymorphisms within these variable genes [23]. Based on the results presented here, we can extend this model by postulating that antibiotic therapy applies an additional pressure on the gonococcus to select variants expressing surface molecules that promote inter-bacterial adhesion. Combining previously published findings and our results presented here together allows us to propose a working model: the more invasive but less aggregated GC are more susceptible to antibiotic killing. Antibiotic utilization will select for GC that can form strong GC-GC interactions but are less invasive. This model can also be correlated with the fact that DGI strains have been found to be hyper-susceptible to penicillin [24,25]. Our data also predict that as treatment failures accumulate, the resulting strains will be less able to cause disseminated/invasive diseases. From an epidemiological perspective, we should see an increase in the incidence of asymptomatic infection and a decrease in pelvic inflammatory disease, which are currently happening (4, 5 https://www.cdc.gov/std/stats16/womenandinf.htm#pid).

In addition to aggregation, GC may also escape from antibiotic killing by invading into host cells. In men, it is suggested that GC use asialoglycoprotein receptor to invade into urethral epithelial cells [26]. In females, GC preferentially use human complement protein CR3 to adhere and invade ecto- and endo-cervix [27]. GC have also been shown to be capable of surviving and replicating inside neutrophils in vivo and in vitro [28], and the expression of different isoforms of Opa impacts GC survival fitness within neutrophils [29]. Moreover, penetrated GC may also invade into fibroblasts in order to escape contact with antibiotics. Grassme et al. have shown that GC can invade into human fibroblasts through Opa binding to heparan sulfate proteoglycans [30].

Taken together, the multifunctional roles of Opa, pili, LOS molecules in GC aggregation and invasion into host cells maximize the chance of GC survival of antibiotic treatment. Inhibiting the interactions of Opa, pili, and LOS with each other as well as with host cells potentially increase antibiotic treatment efficacy, thereby reducing the frequency of treatment failure and recurrence.

4. Materials and Methods

4.1. Bacteria Strains

N. gonorrhoeae strain MS11 that expressed phase-variable Opa and pili (MS11Opa+ Pil+) was obtained from Dr. Herman Schneider, Walter Reed Army Institute for Research. MS11ΔOpa and MS11ΔLgtE were previously described [17,31]. Pili negative colonies were identified based on colony morphology using a dissecting light microscope. GC was grown on plates with GC media (Difco, BD Bioscience, Franklin Lakes, NJ, USA) and 1% Kellogg's supplement [32] at 37 °C with 5% CO_2 for 16–18 h before use in experiments.

Epithelial cell line—ME180 cells, a human cervical epidermal carcinoma cell line (ATCC# HTB-33), were maintained in RPMI1640 supplemented with 10% heat-inactivated fetal bovine serum and 1% Penicillin-Streptomycin. ME180 cells were seeded at 1×10^5 into 12 mm diameter round glass coverslips (VWR, Radnor, PA, USA) in a 24 well plate (Corning, Lowell, MA, USA) and incubated at 37 °C with 5% CO_2. After 24 h, cells were switched into antibiotic-free medium overnight for aggregation assay.

4.2. BacTiter Assay

GC suspended in GC media with Kellogg's supplement and $NaHCO_3$ were seeded in a 96 well plate (10^7 in 99 µL per well). The GC suspension was allowed to either not aggregate, aggregate for 6 h, or aggregate for 6 h before being disrupted by vortex. Serial dilutions of ceftriaxone (1 µL aliquots) were added into each well within each aggregation condition and incubated for 24 h. An equal volume of BacTiter glow reagent (Promega, Madison, WI, USA) was then added and incubated for

15 min. Optical absorbance was determined at the wavelength 560 nm using a Glomax Illuminamintor (Promega, Madison, WI, USA), and the survival rate was calculated by the ratio of the reading obtained after antibiotic treatment to the reading from untreated wells.

4.3. Fluorescence Microscopic Analysis of Live and Dead Bacteria in Aggregates

GC (10^7/mL/well) were incubated in 8-well coverslip-bottom chambers (Sigma, St. Louis, MO, USA) or on ME180 cells in the coverslip for 6 h to allow the bacteria to form aggregates. Aggregated bacteria were treated with or without 1 μg/mL ceftriaxone for 2 h, or heat-killed at 65 °C for 15 min. These aggregates were then stained with Live/Dead BacLight Stain (Life Technology, Frederick, MD, USA) for 15 min. Z-series images were acquired using a confocal microscope (Leica SP5X). Images were analyzed using NIH ImageJ software to measure the size of GC aggregates and the fluorescence intensity ratio (FIR) of live to dead staining in each aggregate.

4.4. Statistical Analysis

Data were plotted and statistically analyzed using the two-tailed Student's *t*-test and Linear Regression by Prism software (GraphPad Software, La Jolla, CA, USA).

5. Conclusions

This study demonstrates that the aggregation of *N. gonorrhoeae* can reduce the susceptibility to antibiotics, and suggests that antibiotic utilization can select for surface molecules that promote aggregation. This can drive pathogen evolution for better colonization but with reduced invasive capabilities. Moreover, inhibiting aggregation may be a potential way of increasing the efficacy of antibiotic treatment, consequently reducing treatment failure.

Author Contributions: L.-C.W., D.C.S., and W.S. conceived and designed the experiments; L.-C.W., M.L., and Z.S. performed the experiments; L.-C.W., M.L., and Z.S. analyzed the data; D.C.S. and L.-C.W. contributed reagents/materials/analysis tools; L.-C.W., D.C.S., and W.S. wrote the paper.

Acknowledgments: This work was supported by a grant from National Institute of Health to D.C.S. and W.S. AI123340. L.-C.W., M.L., and Z.S. were supported in part/participate in "The First-Year Innovation & Research Experience" program funded by the University of Maryland. The funders had no role in study design, data collection, and analysis, decision to publish, or preparation of the manuscript. We acknowledge the UMD CBMG Imaging Core for all microscopy experiments.

References

1. CDC. STD Facts. Available online: http://www.cdc.gov/std/gonorrhea/STDFact-gonorrhea-detailed.htm (accessed on 5 October 2017).
2. Handsfield, H.H. *Gonorrhea and Uncomplicated Gonococcal Infection*; McGraw-Hill Book Co.: New York, NY, USA, 1984.
3. Den Heijer, C.D.J.; Hoebe, C.; van Liere, G.; van Bergen, J.; Cals, J.W.L.; Stals, F.S.; Dukers-Muijrers, N. A comprehensive overview of urogenital, anorectal and oropharyngeal Neisseria gonorrhoeae testing and diagnoses among different STI care providers: A cross-sectional study. *BMC Infect. Dis.* **2017**, *17*. [CrossRef] [PubMed]
4. Hein, K.; Marks, A.; Cohen, M.I. Asymptomatic gonorrhea: Prevalence in a population of urban adolescents. *J. Pediatr.* **1977**, *90*, 634–635. [CrossRef]
5. Hananta, I.P.; van Dam, A.P.; Bruisten, S.M.; Schim van der Loeff, M.F.; Soebono, H.; de Vries, H.J. Gonorrhea in Indonesia: High Prevalence of Asymptomatic Urogenital Gonorrhea but No Circulating Extended Spectrum Cephalosporins-Resistant *Neisseria gonorrhoeae* Strains in Jakarta, Yogyakarta, and Denpasar, Indonesia. *Sex. Transm. Dis.* **2016**, *43*, 608–616. [CrossRef] [PubMed]
6. WHO. *Chlamydia trachomatis, Neisseria gonorrhoeae, Syphilis and Trichomonas vaginalis. Methods and Results Used by WHO to Generate 2005 Estimates*; Prevalence and Incidence of Selected Sexually Transmitted Infections; World Health Organisation: Geneva, Switzerland, 2011.

7. Mayor, M.T.; Roett, M.A.; Uduhiri, K.A. Diagnosis and management of gonococcal infections. *Am. Fam. Physician* **2012**, *86*, 931–938. [PubMed]
8. Silva, J., Jr.; Wilson, K. Disseminated gonococcal infections (DGI). *Cutis* **1979**, *24*, 601–606. [PubMed]
9. Jarvis, G.A.; Chang, T.L. Modulation of HIV transmission by Neisseria gonorrhoeae: molecular and immunological aspects. *Curr. HIV Res.* **2012**, *10*, 211–217. [CrossRef] [PubMed]
10. Alirol, E.; Wi, T.E.; Bala, M.; Bazzo, M.L.; Chen, X.S.; Deal, C.; Dillon, J.R.; Kularatne, R.; Heim, J.; Hooft van Huijsduijnen, R.; et al. Multidrug-resistant gonorrhea: A research and development roadmap to discover new medicines. *PLoS Med.* **2017**, *14*, e1002366. [CrossRef] [PubMed]
11. Workowski, K.A.; Bolan, G.A. Sexually Transmitted Diseases Treatment Guidelines, 2015. *Morb. Mortal. Wkly. Rep.* **2015**, *64*, 1–138.
12. Hananta, I.P.Y.; De Vries, H.J.C.; van Dam, A.P.; van Rooijen, M.S.; Soebono, H.; Schim van der Loeff, M.F. Persistence after treatment of pharyngeal gonococcal infections in patients of the STI clinic, Amsterdam, the Netherlands, 2012–2015: A retrospective cohort study. *Sex. Transm. Infect.* **2017**, *19*. [CrossRef] [PubMed]
13. Singh, S.; Singh, S.K.; Chowdhury, I.; Singh, R. Understanding the Mechanism of Bacterial Biofilms Resistance to Antimicrobial Agents. *Open Microbiol. J.* **2017**, *11*, 53–62. [CrossRef] [PubMed]
14. Greiner, L.L.; Edwards, J.L.; Shao, J.; Rabinak, C.; Entz, D.; Apicella, M.A. Biofilm Formation by *Neisseria gonorrhoeae*. *Infect. Immun.* **2005**, *73*, 1964–1970. [CrossRef] [PubMed]
15. Zollner, R.; Oldewurtel, E.R.; Kouzel, N.; Maier, B. Phase and antigenic variation govern competition dynamics through positioning in bacterial colonies. *Sci. Rep.* **2017**, *7*, 017–12472. [CrossRef] [PubMed]
16. Stein, D.C.; LeVan, A.; Wang, L.-C.; Zimmerman, L.; Song, W. Expression of opacity proteins interferes with the transmigration of *Neisseria gonorrhoeae* across polarized epithelial cells. *PLoS ONE* **2015**, *10*, e0134342. [CrossRef] [PubMed]
17. LeVan, A.; Zimmerman, L.I.; Mahle, A.C.; Swanson, K.V.; DeShong, P.; Park, J.; Edwards, V.L.; Song, W.; Stein, D.C. Construction and characterization of a derivative of *Neisseria gonorrhoeae* strain MS11 devoid of all *opa* genes. *J. Bacteriol.* **2012**, *194*, 6468–6478. [CrossRef] [PubMed]
18. Steichen, C.T.; Shao, J.Q.; Ketterer, M.R.; Apicella, M.A. Gonococcal cervicitis: A role for biofilm in pathogenesis. *J. Infect. Dis.* **2008**, *198*, 1856–1861. [CrossRef] [PubMed]
19. Novotny, P.; Short, J.A.; Walker, P.D. An electron-microscope study of naturally occurring and cultured cells of Neisseria Gonorrhoeae. *J. Med. Microbiol.* **1975**, *8*, 413–427. [CrossRef] [PubMed]
20. Wang, L.C.; Yu, Q.; Edwards, V.; Lin, B.; Qiu, J.; Turner, J.R.; Stein, D.C.; Song, W. Neisseria gonorrhoeae infects the human endocervix by activating non-muscle myosin II-mediated epithelial exfoliation. *PLoS Pathog.* **2017**, *13*, e1006269. [CrossRef] [PubMed]
21. Bhoopalan, S.V.; Piekarowicz, A.; Lenz, J.D.; Dillard, J.P.; Stein, D.C. nagZ Triggers Gonococcal Biofilm Disassembly. *Sci. Rep.* **2016**, *6*, 22372. [CrossRef] [PubMed]
22. Edwards, J.L.; Butler, E.K. The Pathobiology of Neisseria gonorrhoeae Lower Female Genital Tract Infection. *Front. Microbiol.* **2011**, *2*, 102. [CrossRef] [PubMed]
23. Wachter, J.; Hill, S. Positive Selection Pressure Drives Variation on the Surface-Exposed Variable Proteins of the Pathogenic Neisseria. *PLoS ONE* **2016**, *11*, e0161348. [CrossRef] [PubMed]
24. Eisenstein, B.I.; Lee, T.J.; Sparling, P.F. Penicillin sensitivity and serum resistance are independent attributes of strains of Neisseria gonorrhoeae causing disseminated gonococcal infection. *Infect. Immun.* **1977**, *15*, 834–841. [PubMed]
25. Wiesner, P.J.; Handsfield, H.H.; Holmes, K.K. Low antibiotic resistance of gonococci causing disseminated infection. *N. Engl. J. Med.* **1973**, *288*, 1221–1222. [CrossRef] [PubMed]
26. Harvey, H.A.; Jennings, M.P.; Campbell, C.A.; Williams, R.; Apicella, M.A. Receptor-mediated endocytosis of *Neisseria gonorrhoeae* into primary human urethral epithelial cells: The role of the asialoglycoprotein receptor. *Mol. Microbiol.* **2001**, *42*, 659–672. [CrossRef] [PubMed]
27. Edwards, J.L.; Brown, E.J.; Uk-Nham, S.; Cannon, J.G.; Blake, M.S.; Apicella, M.A. A co-operative interaction between *Neisseria gonorrhoeae* and complement receptor 3 mediates infection of primary cervical epithelial cells. *Cell. Microbiol.* **2002**, *4*, 571–584. [CrossRef] [PubMed]
28. Johnson, M.B.; Criss, A.K. Resistance of *Neisseria gonorrhoeae* to neutrophils. *Front. Microbiol.* **2011**, *2*, 77. [CrossRef] [PubMed]

29. Ball, L.M.; Criss, A.K. Constitutively Opa-expressing and Opa-deficient *Neisseria gonorrhoeae* strains differentially stimulate and survive exposure to human neutrophils. *J. Bacteriol.* **2013**, *195*, 2982–2990. [CrossRef] [PubMed]
30. Grassme, H.; Gulbins, E.; Brenner, B.; Ferlinz, K.; Sandhoff, K.; Harzer, K.; Lang, F.; Meyer, T.F. Acidic sphingomyelinase mediates entry of *N. gonorrhoeae* into nonphagocytic cells. *Cell* **1997**, *91*, 605–615. [CrossRef]
31. Minor, S.Y.; Banerjee, A.; Gotschlich, E.C. Effect of alpha-oligosaccharide phenotype of Neisseria gonorrhoeae strain MS11 on invasion of Chang conjunctival, HEC-1-B endometrial, and ME-180 cervical cells. *Infect. Immun.* **2000**, *68*, 6526–6534. [CrossRef] [PubMed]
32. White, L.A.; Kellogg, D.S. An improved fermentation medium for Neisseria gonorrhoeae and other Neisseria. *Health Lab. Sci.* **1965**, *2*, 238–241. [PubMed]

8

Potential for Bacteriophage Endolysins to Supplement or Replace Antibiotics in Food Production and Clinical Care

Michael J. Love [1], Dinesh Bhandari [1,2], Renwick C. J. Dobson [1,3] and Craig Billington [1,2,*]

1 Biomolecular Interaction Centre and School of Biological Sciences, University of Canterbury, Christchurch 8041, New Zealand; michael.love@pg.canterbury.ac.nz (M.J.L.); dinesh.bhandari@esr.cri.nz (D.B.); renwick.dobson@canterbury.ac.nz (R.C.J.D.)
2 Institute of Environmental Science and Research, Christchurch 8041, New Zealand
3 Department of Biochemistry and Molecular Biology, University of Melbourne, Melbourne 3052, Australia
* Correspondence: craig.billington@esr.cri.nz

Abstract: There is growing concern about the emergence of bacterial strains showing resistance to all classes of antibiotics commonly used in human medicine. Despite the broad range of available antibiotics, bacterial resistance has been identified for every antimicrobial drug developed to date. Alarmingly, there is also an increasing prevalence of multidrug-resistant bacterial strains, rendering some patients effectively untreatable. Therefore, there is an urgent need to develop alternatives to conventional antibiotics for use in the treatment of both humans and food-producing animals. Bacteriophage-encoded lytic enzymes (endolysins), which degrade the cell wall of the bacterial host to release progeny virions, are potential alternatives to antibiotics. Preliminary studies show that endolysins can disrupt the cell wall when applied exogenously, though this has so far proven more effective in Gram-positive bacteria compared with Gram-negative bacteria. Their potential for development is furthered by the prospect of bioengineering, and aided by the modular domain structure of many endolysins, which separates the binding and catalytic activities into distinct subunits. These subunits can be rearranged to create novel, chimeric enzymes with optimized functionality. Furthermore, there is evidence that the development of resistance to these enzymes may be more difficult compared with conventional antibiotics due to their targeting of highly conserved bonds.

Keywords: endolysin; antibiotics; antimicrobial resistance; one health; protein engineering

---

1. Introduction

In 2014, the World Health Organization (WHO) calculated the global prevalence of seven antibiotic-resistant bacteria of international concern, and noted very high rates of resistance (up to 84% of all isolates for methicillin, 81% for third-generation cephalosporins, 49% for fluoroquinolones, and 60% for penicillin) in all WHO regions [1]. In response to this unprecedented crisis, in late 2016 the United Nations General Assembly called upon the WHO, the Food and Agriculture Organization of the United Nations, and the World Organisation for Animal Health to develop a global development and stewardship framework [2]. This request recognized that there was a need to co-ordinate action against antimicrobial resistance in humans, agriculture, animals, and the environment by using a One Health [3] approach. One of the key recommendations in the draft framework was to develop new antimicrobial agents for use in these key sectors.

Here, we discuss the potential of cell wall lysis proteins (endolysins) derived from bacteriophages for use as a new class of antimicrobial agents, and evaluate whether they could replace, or supplement, some of the conventional antibiotics used to treat animals and humans, and perhaps even find use in food production and environmental decontamination processes.

Endolysins are enzymes encoded by bacteriophages (phage; obligate viruses of bacteria) which lyse the host bacterial cell. Endolysins degrade the main structural component of the cell wall (peptidoglycan) at the conclusion of the replicative cycle to release newly assembled progeny phage [4] (Figure 1). Recombinantly expressed endolysins display similarly effective lytic abilities to their native counterparts when applied exogenously to susceptible bacteria [5]. This feature underpins the application of endolysins in medicine, food and agriculture.

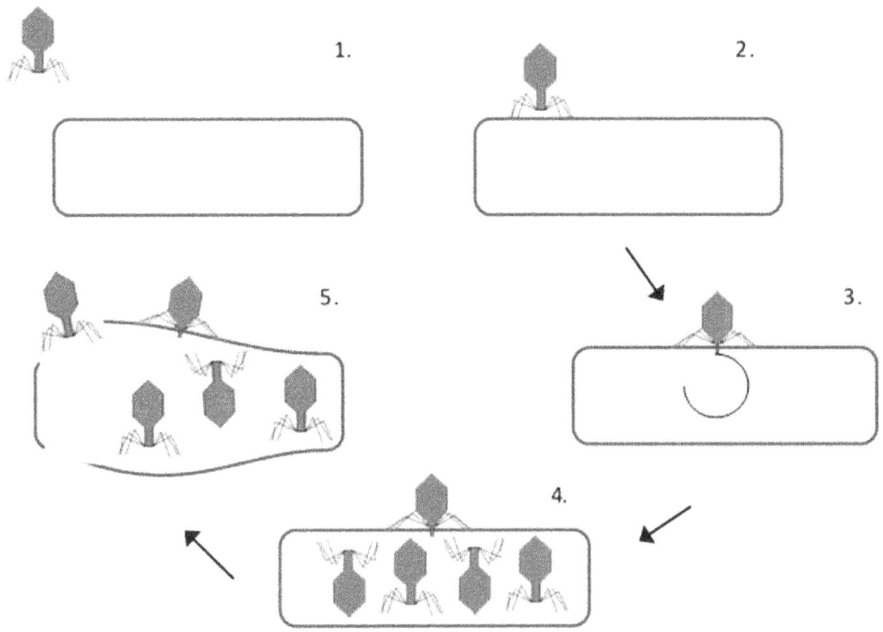

Figure 1. Life cycle of a virulent tailed phage (not to scale). (1) The phage collides with the bacterial cell; (2) the phage binds to cell receptors; (3) the phage is irreversibly bound and injects nucleic acid into the cell via the tail tube, where it is transcribed and translated; (4) many progeny phages are produced within intact cells; (5) endolysins degrade the host bacterial cell wall, which loses its structural integrity and ruptures due to the osmotic pressure, releasing the progeny phages.

Endolysins are predominantly more effective against Gram-positive bacteria than Gram-negative bacteria when applied in this way. The outer membrane of Gram-negative bacteria presents a physical protective barrier against the activity of endolysins [6]. Therefore, endolysin research has mainly focused on Gram-positive bacteria. However, recent work on outer membrane permeabilizers (chemicals and engineered peptides) should increase the prospects of endolysins for treating Gram-negative bacteria.

Numerous types of endolysins have been described, and are typically categorized by the structural bonds in the peptidoglycan that are cleaved by the enzyme [7] (Figure 2). The two alternating glycosidic bonds between the amino sugar moieties, *N*-acetylglucosamine and *N*-acetylmuramic acid (MurNAc), are targeted by different endolysin classes. The *N*-acetylmuramoyl-β-1,4-*N*-acetylglucosamine bond is cleaved by lytic transglycosylases and *N*-acetyl-β-D-muramidases, which are commonly known as lysozymes, while the *N*-acetylglucosaminyl-β-1,4-*N*-acetylmuramine bond is hydrolysed by *N*-acetyl-glucosaminyl-β-D-glucosaminidases. The cleavage of the amide linkage between MurNAc and L-alanine is catalyzed by *N*-acetylmuramoyl-L-alanine amidases. There are different endopeptidases depending on the chemical structure of the peptidoglycan, which is dependent on species and growth conditions. Generally, endopeptidases hydrolyze the peptide bonds between the amino acids that form the cross-linking peptide stems [8–10].

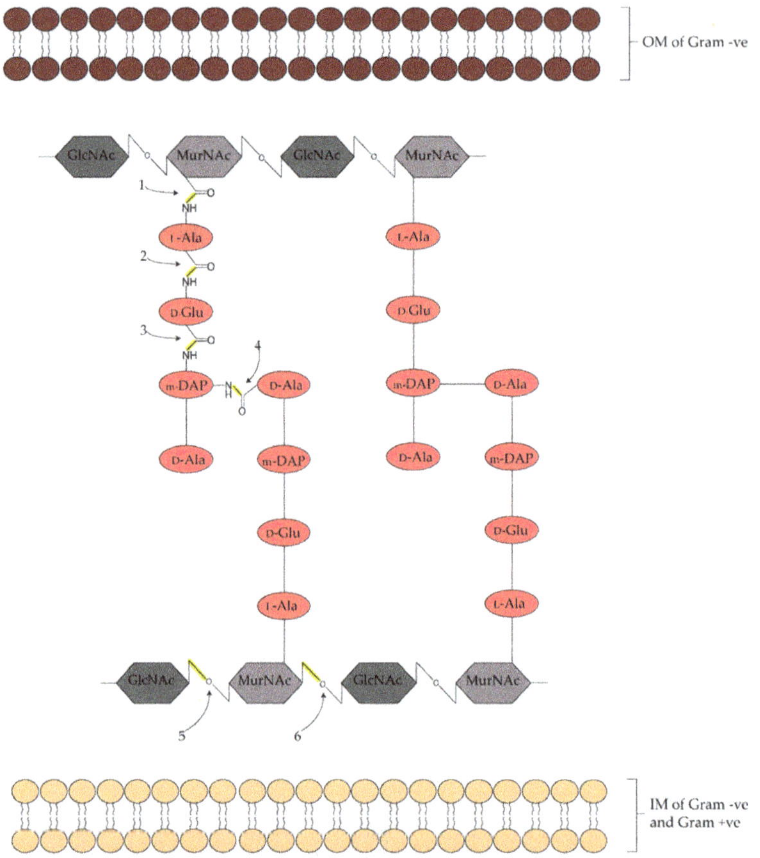

Figure 2. Diagram of the typical cell wall and peptidoglycan structure of bacteria, including the endolysin cleavage sites. The peptidoglycan is composed of repeating sugar units, *N*-acetylglucosamine (GlcNAc) and *N*-acetylmuramic acid (MurNAc), which are cross-linked via an interpeptide bridge between the *meso*-diaminopimelic acid (m-DAP) and D-alanine (D-Ala) residues of adjacent tetrapeptide chains. The chains also contain L-alanine (L-Ala) and D-glutamic acid (D-Glu). Gram-negative bacteria contain an outer membrane (OM) structure not present in Gram-positive bacteria. Both contain an inner membrane (IM) structure. The cleaved bonds and major classifications of endolysin are indicated: (1) *N*-acetylmuramoyl-L-alanine amidase; (2–4) various endopeptidases; (5) N-acetyl-β-D-glucosaminidase; (6) N-acetyl-β-D-muramidase (lysozyme).

A number of promising endolysins have been isolated from phage for application as antimicrobial agents, as described in this review and others [5–9]. However, the bioengineering of modified or novel endolysins also holds promise for the future development of effective tools to kill or detect bacteria. The prospects for engineering are facilitated by the enzymes' structures. The domain structure of endolysins can be modular (Gram-positive bacteria and some Gram-negative species) or globular (most Gram-negative bacteria), with most bioengineering strategies exploiting the modular endolysins. These enzymes usually comprise two distinct domains: an N-terminal enzymatically-active domain and a C-terminal cell wall-binding domain, connected by short, flexible linker regions. N-terminal enzymatically-active domains are responsible for catalyzing the breakdown of specific peptidoglycan bonds, while the C-terminal cell wall-binding domains recognize and bind non-covalently to substrate within the cell wall, resulting in the specificity of the lytic enzymes for the target host [5,8]. In addition, the C-terminal cell wall-binding domain is often required to maintain full lytic activity [11–13]. Interestingly, truncation or deletion of the C-terminal cell wall-binding domain can also result in equal or increased lytic activity [14–16]. In contrast, globular endolysins only contain catalytic domains.

The modular endolysin arrangement can be exploited for bioengineering, as the different domains can be shuffled within the protein, or domains from different endolysins can be combined to generate new enzymes [17,18]. Directed mutagenesis is also an effective strategy, as different amino acids may support improved lytic or binding properties [5,8,17,18]. The seemingly limitless possible permutations of endolysin modular arrangements allow for the development of new enzymes with specific functions or features. Some potential bioengineering strategies and examples of endolysin constructs are shown in Table 1.

Table 1. Possible molecular engineering strategies with potential application(s).

Modification	Property	Example	Reference
Truncation of full-length enzyme	Increased catalytic ability and solubility	CHAPk	Horgan et al. [19]
Fusion of EADs with CBDs of different endolysins	Increased catalytic ability and solubility	ClyS	Daniel et al. [20]
	Increased catalytic ability and broader lytic spectrum	SA2-E-Lyso-SH3b, SA2-E-LysK-SH3b	Schmelcher et al. [21]
	Thermostability	PlyGVE2CpCWB	Swift et al. [22]
Fusion of virion-associated lysin with CBD of endolysin	Increased efficacy	EC300	Proença et al. [23]
Endolysin fusion with OMP	Increased efficacy towards Gram-negative bacteria	OBPgp279, PVP-SE1g-146	Briers et al. [24]
Endolysin fusion with AMP	Increased efficacy towards Gram-negative bacteria	Art-175	Briers et al. [25]
Truncation and site-directed mutagenesis	AMP development	LysAB2	Peng et al. [26]

EAD: enzymatically-active domain; CBD: cell wall-binding domain; OMP: outer-membrane permeabilizer; AMP: antimicrobial peptide.

Both bioengineered and phage-isolated endolysins are promising alternatives to antibiotics. Their specificity allows them to target specific bacterial pathogens without affecting the microflora [11], or alternatively, target a larger spectrum for broader efficacy [27]. At the moment, developed resistance to the activity of the endolysins has not been widely reported, meaning these enzymes could be a long-term solution to antibiotics [28–30]. Endolysins may also have potential as diagnostic tools for bacterial identification [31]. In the following sections, we provide an overview of native and chimeric endolysins with potential therapeutic applications.

2. Endolysins as Human Therapeutics

As the efficacy of antibiotics decreases, once easily-treated bacterial infections will become potentially fatal. This will also have secondary effects in clinical care, such as changing risk-benefit considerations for invasive surgeries. Phage-encoded lytic enzymes have the potential to fulfil the need for novel antibacterial therapeutic agents for use in humans. This new class of antimicrobials has been recognized by the United States of America in the National Action Plan for Combating Antibiotic-resistant Bacteria [32], which identified the use of "phage-derived lysins to kill specific bacteria while preserving the microbiota" as a key strategy to reduce the development of antimicrobial resistance.

Methicillin-resistant *Staphylococcus aureus* (MRSA) is a significant public health concern, causing a range of skin and respiratory infections, as well as food-borne illnesses that are not easily treatable with currently available antibiotics [33]. O'Flaherty et al. [27] treated a human-derived MRSA strain with *Lactococcus lactis* cell lysate containing recombinantly overexpressed endolysin LysK, and observed a 99% reduction in colony-forming units at 1 h post-exposure. However, the researchers had difficulties obtaining soluble protein, which would hinder future applications of LysK, a difficulty that was also encountered in subsequent studies [34,35]. A stability study was conducted on LysK, as medical application requires a stable enzyme [34]. LysK was stabilized in the presence of low molecular weight polyols such as sucrose and glycerol, for example, stability increased 100-fold at 30 °C, and LysK retained 100% activity after storage up to 1 month at room temperature. This stability, under simple condition changes, is useful for developing treatment strategies [34]. LysK contains two catalytic domains: a cysteine- and histidine-dependent amidohydrolase/peptidase (CHAP) domain, and an *N*-acetylmuramoyl-L-alanine amidase domain. In an attempt to overcome the solubility issue, Horgan et al. [19] generated a single-domain truncated LysK mutant, designated CHAPk, containing only the CHAP domain. Soluble CHAPk was easier to obtain than full-length LysK, and displayed at least a two-fold increase in lytic activity against both heat-killed and live staphylococcal cells in vitro. Subsequent studies demonstrated that CHAPk was also effective in vivo, and that the loss of the C-terminal cell wall-binding domain, which directs specificity, resulted in activity against a broader range of targets compared with full-length CHAPk [36,37].

Jun et al. [38] compared LysK with SAL-1, an endolysin that differs by three residues. They also produced six derivatives of SAL-1 containing mutations in each of the three residues to investigate the impact of each mutation. SAL-1 displayed cell-wall hydrolytic activity approximately two-fold greater than that of LysK. The mutation of residue 114 from glutamatic acid in LysK to glutamine in SAL-1 had the largest impact on activity. This residue is located inside the catalytic CHAP domain, and the structurally minor sequence change corresponded to enhanced activity. The combination of such enhanced activity with the identification and mechanistic characterization of key residues of different enzymes is important for rational design and engineering of new endolysins with optimized activity [38]. Compared with LysK, SAL-1 had increased catalytic activity, and high yields of soluble protein were easier to obtain; therefore, SAL-1 may be a more promising antibiotic alternative than LysK [39]. The therapeutic application of SAL-1 is currently being trialed by iNtRON Biotechnology in the form of SAL200, an endolysin-based candidate drug for the treatment of *S. aureus*. A preclinical safety study of SAL200 observed no toxicity in rodent intravenous single- and repeat-dose studies [40]. A repeat-dose experiment was also performed in dogs, with each dog receiving four doses of 0, 0.5, 12.5 and 25 mg/kg in 1-week intervals over four weeks. After ten days, short-lived (i.e., lasting only 30 minutes to 1 hour) and mild clinical signs were observed including, vomiting, subdued behavior and irregular respiration. The transient response of the dogs to SAL200 administration was linked to complement system activation that resulted from antibody production [40]. A follow-up study in monkeys investigated the impact of single-dose escalation (up to 80 mg/kg) or 5-day multiple-dose (up to 40 mg/kg/day) administration of SAL200, with no adverse effects observed [41] SAL200 was further evaluated in a human single dose-escalating (up to 10 mg/kg) study. This study was the first in-human clinical study of a intravenously administered endolysin-based drug [42]. The volunteers had a reasonable tolerability to SAL200, with no significant adverse effects and most of the adverse effects were mild and self-limited. Although an increased concentration of antibodies was observed, the antibody concentration of participants administered 3.0 mg/kg was greater than that of those administered 10 mg/kg, with large variation within the different cohorts. The immunogenicity of SAL200 should, therefore, be a focus of future studies in order to better develop treatment regimes [42]. A phase II clinical study is now being conducted on patients with persistent *S. aureus* bacteremia, with results expected in 2018. Overall, the current evaluations shows a promising future for not just SAL200, but also for the development of other endolysin-based drug treatments.

Biofilm formation in clinical environments and on medical devices can have significant medical implications, as biofilms can harbor pathogenic and multidrug-resistant bacteria. Microorganisms within biofilms are protected by extracellular polymeric substances (EPS), which are a source of environmental contamination when partially dislodged. EPS can contain polysaccharides, proteins, phospholipids, teichoic acids, nucleic acids, and polymers, and protect the biofilm inhabitants by concentrating nutrients, preventing access of biocides, sequestering metals and toxins, and preventing desiccation [43]. Linden et al. [44] found that recombinantly-expressed PlyGRCS (from the phage GRCS) effectively lysed *S. aureus* in a biofilm, as well as in stationary phase. PlyGRCS contains a single enzymatically-active domain that can cleave two different bonds in peptidoglycan. This bifunctional domain could be highly useful in developing endolysins with effective lytic activity.

Rashel et al. [45] found that a dose of the phage ϕMR11-derived lysin MV-L rescued mice from fatal levels of MRSA exposure. In addition, MV-L in combination with vancomycin killed vancomycin-resistant strains. MV-L was specific for *S. aureus* and *Staphylococcus simulans*, with no lytic activity observed against other staphylococcal strains or bacterial species, including *Staphylococcus epidermidis* and *Escherichia coli*. Although excessive exposure to MV-L induced the production of antibodies, no adverse effects on the mice or impact on the efficacy of MV-L was observed.

Daniel et al. [20] demonstrated the potential of bioengineering to generate enzymes with novel and specific lytic activity against MRSA. The endolysin ClyS was constructed from the enzymatically active domain of a *S. aureus* Twort phage lysin fused with the cell wall-binding domain of phiNM3. Mice were exposed to MRSA strains that were resistant to the antibiotic oxacillin. A dose of ClyS increased survival rates to 88%, compared with the 0% survival rate for untreated mice. Treatment of infected mice with a sub-therapeutic concentration of ClyS in combination with oxacillin increased survival rates when compared with each treatment alone. This synergistic relationship with antibiotics may have widespread potential, and reinitiate the use of historical antibiotics that have been discontinued due to resistance concerns.

Schuch et al. [46] further showed this synergistic potential with the lysin CF-301. Mice with staphylococcal-induced bacteremia had a survival time of less than 24 h without treatment. Following individual treatments with CF-301 and daptomycin at 4 h post-inoculation, survival rates after 72 h were measured at 13% and 23%, respectively. Combination therapy yielded a survival rate of 73%. The study further confirmed the efficacy of co-therapy in 16 individual experiments including the antibiotics oxacillin and vancomycin. The immunogenicity of CF-301 was briefly evaluated in vitro; rabbit antisera raised against CF-301 did not inhibit the activity of CF-301 [46]. Despite the in vitro results, the immunogenic nature of CF-301 needs to be studied in a range of model organisms in vivo, because there may be clinically relevant adverse effects. CF-301 also has anti-biofilm activity [47], and clinical phase I trials are now underway to evaluate CF-301 as an alternative to traditional antibiotics, with an expected study completion in late 2018.

Thermal injury patients are usually also immunocompromised, meaning they are more susceptible to bacterial infection, including drug-resistant *S. aureus* strains [48]. Chopra et al. [49] investigated the use of endolysin MR-10 alone and in combination with minocycline to treat burn wound infections in mice. The control mice, inoculated with *S. aureus* and receiving no medical treatment, had a 100% mortality rate within 5 days. Individually, MR-10 (50 μg/ml) and minocycline (50 mg/kg) both resulted in a survival rate of 35% at 5 days post-inoculation, but 100% mortality was observed by day 7. In contrast, 100% survival was observed following treatment with a combination of the therapeutic agents at the same concentrations. These findings further support the future use of endolysins in medicine, especially in co-therapy with existing antibiotics.

Staphefekt is an endolysin bioengineered to selectively target *S. aureus* strains, including MRSA. It is currently available as a component of gels and creams for over-the-counter treatment of infections [50,51]. Its specificity for *S. aureus* is an important feature in the treatment of skin infections, as it prevents the disturbance of commensal bacteria, which can cause further health complications [52]. Evidence for the efficacy of Staphefekt is limited; there are few available publications describing the rationale of engineering or the in vitro properties and structure of the endolysin. However, a recent report by Totté et al. [51] demonstrated the efficacy of Staphefekt in treating three different patients with recurrent *S. aureus*-related dermatoses that had previously been unsuccessfully treated with antibiotics. Despite the limited published evidence, these brief findings suggest a promising future for Staphefekt as a long-term alternative to antibiotics.

Enterococcus faecalis is the third most common cause of life-threatening nosocomial infections [53], and is intrinsically resistant to antibiotics [54]. Although vancomycin is considered a drug of last resort, a growing number of vancomycin-resistant *E. faecalis* strains have been isolated. [55,56].

An endolysin isolated from phage ϕ1, PlyV12, kills a variety of *E. faecalis* strains in vitro, including vancomycin-resistant isolates. PlyV12 also showed a broad spectrum of lethality against a variety of streptococcal and staphylococcal strains, highlighting it as a promising candidate in antibacterial medicine [57]. Son et al. [58] also identified a novel phage, EFAP-1, which was not significantly similar to any previously identified phages. The endolysin of EFAP-1, EFAL-1, exhibited lytic activity against 24 different strains of bacteria, including vancomycin-resistant *E. faecalis* strains and four streptococcal strains, whereas the phage itself only showed activity against *E. faecalis*. There is a lack of in vivo studies of *E. faecalis* endolysins. Such studies are important because *E. faecalis* is also a commensal bacterium found in the human gut, and therefore the potential impact of endolysins on the gut microbiota needs to be understood [52]. Zhang et al. [59] isolated phage IME-EF1 and its endolysin from hospital sewage, and investigated their ability to rescue mice from lethal challenge with *E. faecalis*. Individually, both the phage and the endolysin reduced the bacterial count in the blood of infected animals. However, a 200-μg dose of the endolysin at 30 min post-bacterial inoculation supported a higher survival rate (80%) than that observed following phage treatment alone (60%) [59].

The endolysin LysEF-P10, derived from *E. faecalis* phage EF-P10, has also been studied in a mouse model. A single dose of just 5 μg was enough to protect mice from vancomycin-resistant *E. faecalis* infection, suggesting promising protective efficacy of LysEF-P10 against vancomycin-resistant *E. faecalis* strains. Furthermore, when the mice were subjected to a large dose of 5 mg, no side effects were observed. The administration of EF-P10 stimulated specific antibody production, however, there was no impact on the bactericidal activity of the enzyme. Treatment with EF-P10 did not negatively affect the gut microbiota, owing to the specificity of the lysin. Although *E. faecalis* in the normal gut microbiota may have been targeted, no significant health impact on the mice was observed [60]. Proença et al. [23] constructed a bacteriolysin-like enzyme to target *E. faecalis*. The construct, EC300, was created from the fusion of the peptidase domain from a virion-associated lysin and the cell wall-binding domain of Lys170, both found in phage F170/08. EC300 inhibited the growth of *E. faecalis* in bacterial culture media, whereas the parental endolysin Lys170 showed limited inhibition. The enhanced lytic and killing ability of EC300 highlights the potential for engineered endolysins compared with wild-type enzymes.

Streptococcal infections are associated with a range of clinical manifestations, including strep throat, pneumonia, skin infections, and meningitis [61,62]. Drug resistant streptococcal strains are also increasing in prevalence. Loeffler et al. [28] examined the potential of the endolysin Pal to kill *S. pneumoniae* that had colonized the nasopharynx of mice. Pal was effective against 15 different strains of pneumococci, including some drug-resistant strains, reducing *S. pneumoniae* to undetectable levels within 5 h of treatment. The same research group [63] then examined the antibacterial ability of a previously described lytic enzyme, Cpl-1 [64]. Rabbit antiserum was raised against Cpl-1 and the impact on bacterial lysis measured. Only a small amount of inhibition was measured, showing the antibodies had little effect on the enzymatic activity [63]. In the same study, these findings were corroborated in vivo. Mice that were subjected to several doses of Cpl-1 tested positive for IgG. These immunized mice along with naïve mice were challenged with *S. pneumoniae*. Comparatively, no significant difference was measured with regards to the reduction of bacteria numbers by the enzyme [64]. Mice intravenously infected with *S. pneumoniae* and treated only with buffer had a median survival time of 30.75 h, with no mice surviving at 72 h post-infection. Mice treated with Cpl-1 at 5 and 10 h post-infection had a median survival time of 60 h, although after 96 h, only one mouse survived. Although the potential for complete eradication of the bacteria was shown, the dosage used in the experiments was not high enough, meaning that all animals eventually succumbed to infection. Therefore, for greater efficacy of Cpl-1, a higher dose would be required [63].

Subsequent studies demonstrated the effectiveness of Cpl-1 combination therapy with lytic enzyme Pal, or with antibiotics [65–67]. In vivo mouse model studies demonstrated these Cpl-1 treatments were effective in the treatment of pneumococcal diseases such as sepsis [68], endocarditis [69], meningitis [70], and pneumonia [71,72]. Despite its demonstrable antibacterial activity, a key limitation of Cpl-1 is its half-life in blood of only 20.5 min in mice [63,69]. Resch et al. [72] introduced specific cysteine residues into Cpl-1 to promote disulfide bond formation and subsequent dimerization. Dimerization is required for full activity of LytA, a pneumococcal autolysin [73], with which Cpl-1 shares extensive sequence similarity. Dimerized Cpl-1 displayed a two-fold increase in antimicrobial activity and had a nearly ten-fold decrease in plasma clearance, resulting in an increased half-life. These enhanced properties not only increase the prospects for Cpl-1 application, but also highlight the potential for enhanced activity through structural changes and engineering.

The exogenous treatment of Gram-negative bacteria with endolysins has been limited because of the presence of the outer membrane, which prevents access to the peptidoglycan layer [74]. Overcoming this protective layer is a major obstacle in developing endolysin-based treatments. Most studies have focused on nosocomial pathogens *Acinetobacter baumannii* and *Pseudomonas aeruginosa*, both of which are Gram-negative and capable of forming biofilms. Multidrug-resistant strains of both pathogens are also being increasingly isolated [75–78]. Some endolysins can intrinsically permeate the outer membrane [79–81]. Lai et al. [79] recombinantly expressed LysAB2 from ϕAB2 and applied it to *A. baumannii*. The C-terminus of LysAB2 contains an amphipathic α-helix that interacts with the negatively charged elements of the outer membrane, facilitating the formation of a transmembrane pore [82]. This allows the N-terminus catalytic domain to interact with the peptidoglycan layer and lyse the cell, achieving antibacterial activity. Lood et al. [80] identified and screened 21 different endolysins for sequence diversity and *A. baumannii*-killing activity. The endolysins displayed varying degrees of antibacterial activity, with the lysin PlyF307 exhibiting the greatest activity. The C-terminus of PlyF307 contains a highly positively charged region, which may interact with the outer membrane. PlyF307 successfully killed both planktonic cells and, more importantly, those within biofilms, providing an advantage over antibiotics. PlyF307 also functioned under physiological conditions, rescuing mice treated with lethal doses of *A. baumannii*. There remains a library of lysins for structural and biochemical characterization from this research.

Walmagh et al. [81] showed that OBPgp279, from the phage OBP, can permeate the outer membrane of *P. aeruginosa*. It does not appear to contain an amphipathic helix, and thus the mechanism of permeabilization is unclear. OBPgp279 may therefore contain novel structural elements that could lend themselves to the engineering of new endolysins to target Gram-negative bacteria [81]. The lysin LysPA26 from phage JD010 has antibacterial activity against both planktonic and biofilm-contained *P. aeruginosa* cells, as well as other Gram-negative species such as *E. coli* and *Klebsiella pneumoniae*. However, LysPA26 was ineffective against Gram-positive species, including *S. aureus*. This specificity may allow for selective targeting of Gram-negative species in medical treatments [83].

Strategies employing endolysins in conjunction with antibiotics or outer membrane-permeabilizing agents have been explored. Thummeepak et al. [84] investigated the use of LysABP-01 in combination with colistin for treatment of hospital-isolated strains of *A. baumannii*. Although LysABP-01 alone prevented growth, elevated levels of antibacterial activity were observed in combination with colistin. Additionally, the minimum inhibitory concentrations of LysABP-01 and colistin were reduced 32-fold and by up to eight-fold, respectively, when used in combination, compared with individual application. Endolysin EL188, from phage EL, combined with EDTA reduced *P. aeruginosa* cell counts by up to four log units, whereas EL188 on its own exhibited no antibacterial activity [85]. However, the use of EDTA would be restricted to topical applications because of its ability to inhibit blood coagulation [86].

Artilysin bioengineering has also shown promise in targeting Gram-negative bacteria. Artilysins are created through the fusion of outer membrane-permeabilizing peptides, which interfere with the stabilizing forces within the outer membrane, with endolysins. These fusion proteins allow the uptake of an endolysin across the outer membrane, providing access to the peptidoglycan layer [87]. Initially, two endolysins, OBPgp279 and PVP-SE1g-146, fused with one of seven different peptides were investigated for their antibacterial activity. Although the endolysins exhibited limited antibacterial activity on their own, fusion with polycationic nonapeptide correlated with up to a 2.6 log reduction of *P. aeruginosa* in only 30 min. Moderate antibacterial activity against *A. baumannii*, *E. coli*, and *Salmonella* Typhimurium was also observed. The mode of action was examined using time-lapse microscopy, confirming that the artilysins were passing through the outer membrane and degrading the peptidoglycan [24].

Briers et al. [25] developed Art-175, composed of the antimicrobial peptide (AMP) sheep myeloid 29-amino acid peptide (SMAP-29) fused with endolysin KZ144, to target *P. aeruginosa*. AMPs are involved in the innate immune response, and can move across the outer membrane [88]. Art-175 reduced the *P. aeruginosa* cell count by up to 4 log units compared with untreated controls, and continuous exposure to Art-175 to exert a selection pressure did not elicit the development of resistance. On its own, SMAP-29 is cytotoxic to mammalian cells [89]; however, Art-175 exhibited little toxicity in L-292 mouse connective tissue. As a result of these findings, Peng et al. [26] developed AMPs based on the amino acid sequence of LysAB2. The synthesized AMPs killed *A. baumannii* cells by permeating the outer membrane in vitro. Treatment with the AMPs also increased the survival rate of mice infected with a lethal dose of *A. baumannii* by 60%. This research highlights a novel method of bioengineering endolysins for use as antimicrobials.

3. Endolysins as Veterinary Treatments

In response to widespread concern regarding the overuse of antibiotics in food-producing animals, many major food suppliers are now committed to phasing out prophylactic antibiotic use and the tighter control of therapeutic treatments. This presents obvious challenges for the animal-husbandry industry, which may be overcome by the use of endolysins. Companion and working animals can also be susceptible to recalcitrant microbial infections, including those caused by multidrug-resistant microorganisms, and so may also benefit from endolysin treatment.

Clostridium perfringens is a leading cause of necrotic enteritis and sub-clinical disease in poultry, and can lead to significant economic losses [90]. Swift et al. [22] constructed recombinant endolysin PlyGVE2CpCWB, which shows enhanced thermostability, an important feature for surviving feed heat treatments. The recombinant endolysin contains an amidase domain from an endolysin derived from a thermophilic phage fused with the cell wall-recognition domain from *C. perfringens*-specific phage endolysin PlyCP26F, which is not resistant to high temperatures. PlyGVE2CpCWB inactivated *C. perfringens* in both liquid and solid media at temperatures up to 50 °C, and so may be a promising antimicrobial feed treatment for controlling necrotic enteritis in poultry. This thermostable construct demonstrates the potential for other thermophilic bacteriophage endolysins to be utilized in bioengineering. A different approach to *C. perfringens* control was taken by Gervasi et al. [91,92], whereby an amidase endolysin (CP25L) was cloned and expressed in a *Lactobacillus johnsonii* strain isolated from poultry. In co-cultures, reductions of up to 2.6 $\log_{10}$ CFU·ml^{-1} *C. perfringens* were noted; however, the reduction was inconsistent between experiments, and the effect declined significantly over time. This reduced activity was attributed to a loss in stability of the endolysin in culture, and a reduction in the viability of *L. johnsonii.* Other researchers [93,94] have also performed detailed analyses, including X-ray crystallography, on another *C. perfringens* endolysin, Psm, which may have applications in poultry. Psm is an *N*-acetylmuramidase endolysin with wide activity against *C. perfringens* strains.

Another economically significant disease in animal husbandry is bovine mastitis, which is caused by a variety of bacteria, of which staphylococci and streptococci account for 75% of cases [95]. In studies aimed at treating bovine mastitis caused by *S. aureus*, Schmelcher et al. [21] demonstrated that fusion of an endopeptidase endolysin domain from a *Streptococcus* lambda phage (SA2) with either lysostaphin (SA2-E-Lyso-SH3b) or staphylococcal phage endolysin LysK (SA2-E-LysK-SH3b) could inhibit staphylococci in a murine mammary mastitis model. The extended lytic spectrum targeting multiple genera would be particularly useful for efficiently treating bovine mastitis [96]. Infusion of 25 μg of SA2-E-Lyso-SH3b or SA2-E-LysK-SH3b into the mammary glands reduced *S. aureus* counts by 0.63 and 0.81 $\log_{10}$ CFU·mg^{-1}, respectively. Additional testing of SA2-E-LysK-SH3b and lysostaphin in combination (12.5 μg/gland) revealed a 3.36 $\log_{10}$ CFU·mg^{-1} reduction in the concentration of *S. aureus* compared with the control [21]. Further work by the same group [97], determined the potential of the lambda SA2 and phage B30 (a CHAP endopeptidase) endolysins in combination as a therapeutic treatment of *Streptococcus*-induced mastitis, again in a murine mastitis model. The best results obtained by the study were reductions of 1.5 $\log_{10}$ CFU·mg^{-1} against *Streptococcus uberis* (SA2), 4.6 $\log_{10}$ CFU·mg^{-1} against *Streptococcus agalactiae* (B30), and 2.2 $\log_{10}$ CFU·mg^{-1} against *Streptococcus dysgalactiae* (SA2). More recently, purified endolysin Trx-SA1, isolated from *S. aureus* phage IME-SA1, was used to treat naturally infected cow udders [98]. Udder quarters received an intramammary infusion of 20 mg of Trx-SA1 once per day, and qualitative reductions in somatic cell counts and *S. aureus* numbers were noted over the three-day regime.

Anthrax, a potentially fatal zoonotic disease affecting a wide variety of species, is a threat to wild and farmed animals as well as humans, especially as a biological weapon [99,100]. Schuch et al. [29] reported the usefulness of PlyG lysin, isolated from the γ-phage of *Bacillus anthracis*, in killing vegetative cells and germinating spores of *B. anthracis* and streptomycin-resistant *Bacillus cereus* RSVF1. The researchers screened an expression library of cloned γ-phage DNA sequences and identified a 702-bp open reading frame (ORF) encoding a protein with homology to an amidase-type endolysin. When PlyG was injected intraperitoneally (50 U in 0.5 mL) into mice infected with 6 $\log_{10}$ CFU RSVF1, a notable therapeutic effect was observed, with 68.4% (13/19) of mice showing full recovery. Furthermore, the survival time of the remaining mice was prolonged to 21 h post-infection.

Equine strangles is a highly contagious disease of horses caused by *Streptococcus equi*. The disease progresses as an inflammation of the upper respiratory tract, and leads to abscess formation in the retropharyngeal lymph node [101]. Strangles is a significant economic threat to the horse racing industry, where many high value animals are typically housed in close proximity. Hoopes et al. [102] used PlyC, an unusual multimeric amidase-type endolysin [17], as a disinfectant against *S. equi* and reported it to be 1000 times more active on a per weight basis than the widely used disinfectant Virkon-S. PlyC was effective against >20 clinical isolates of *S. equi*, including both *S. equi* subsp. *equi* and *S. equi* subsp. *zooepidemicus*, demonstrating its sterilizing ability against an eight log CFU·ml^{-1} culture of *S. equi* within 30 min of exposure.

The clinical efficacy of a muramidase as a veterinary treatment for companion animals was demonstrated in a trial by Junjappa et al. [103], where they successfully treated 17 dogs suffering from pyoderma (bacterial skin lesions) caused by MRSA. The skin lesions were treated with a hydrogel containing a chimeric endolysin composed of the cell wall-targeting domain (SH3b) of lysostaphin and the phage K ORF56 muralytic domain [104]. Another important zoonotic pathogen, *Streptococcus suis*, has been linked to arthritis, meningitis, septicemia, and endocarditis in pigs, as well as in humans who have come into contact with infected animals or their byproducts. Wang et al. [105] isolated a phage from *S. suis* (SMP), and then expressed the endolysin LySMP in *E. coli* BL21. The resultant product, following chromatography and treatment with β-mercaptoethanol, killing 15 out of 17 clinical *S. suis* serotype 2 isolates from diseased pigs in China, and had demonstrated activity against *S. suis* serotype 7 and 9 strains, *S. equi* subsp. *zooepidemicus*, and *S. aureus* [105].

There is growing evidence to suggest that food-producing animals are an important global reservoir of vancomycin-resistant enterococci (VRE) [106,107]. This group of potentially invasive microorganisms is resistant to almost all of the available antibiotic regimens recommended for treatment of Gram-positive bacterial infections. In an attempt to combat VRE in food-producing animals, Yoong et al. [57] cloned the PlyV12-encoding gene from enterococcal phage Φ1 into the *E. coli-Bacillus* shuttle vector pDG148, followed by its expression in *Bacillus megaterium* strain WH320. The resultant product, an amidase-type endolysin, had lytic activity against 14 clinical and laboratory *E. faecalis* and *Enterococcus faecium* strains, including two vancomycin-resistant *E. faecalis* and three vancomycin-resistant *E. faecium* strains, in addition to its host, *E. faecalis* V12. Intriguingly, PlyV12 also had a significant killing effect on pathogenic streptococcal strains, including *Streptococcus pyogenes* (group A streptococcus) and group C streptococci.

Diarrheal outbreaks caused by *Clostridium difficile* have frequently been reported in animals, including cattle, horses, and pigs [108,109]. Treatment of *C. difficile* diarrhea with antibiotics is not recommended as it can further exacerbate the disease condition [110]. In a quest for an alternative approach to treat infections caused by *C. difficile*, Mayer et al. [111] sequenced the genome of a temperate phage from *C. difficile*. They identified endolysin gene *cd27l* and cloned it into vectors pET15b and pUK200 to express the gene product in *E. coli* and *L. lactis*, respectively. The purified endolysin was active against 30 diverse strains of *C. difficile*, including those belonging to the major epidemic ribotype, 027 (B1/NAP1). Unlike antibiotics, the endolysin was selective for *C. difficile*, demonstrating no activity against a range of commensal species from within the gastrointestinal tract, including other clostridia, bifidobacteria, and lactobacilli.

Paenibacillus larvae subsp. *larvae* causes American Foulbrood disease in honey bees, which are important insect pollinators of agricultural crops. The disease occurs in honeybee larvae as a result of *P. larvae* spores germinating in the larval midgut and subsequently causing sepsis and death. The use of antibiotics to treat the disease in the USA now requires supervision by a veterinarian, and a withholding period of 4–6 weeks is recommended for honey from treated hives prior to sale (https://www.fda.gov/AnimalVeterinary/ResourcesforYou/AnimalHealthLiteracy/ucm309134.htm). In the European Union, no veterinary medicines containing antibiotics are permitted in beekeeping (http://europroxima.com/european-legislation-regarding-antibiotics-in-honey-an-overview/). For these reasons, endolysins are being investigated as a potential alternative control tool. An amidase endolysin, PlyPl23, has been cloned from a *P. larvae* phage and subsequently expressed [112]. In bee larvae experimentally infected with spores, PlyPl23 effectively decreased the rate of *P. larvae* infection, and no toxic side effects were noted in the larvae. However, the endolysin was not effective until the spores had germinated.

4. Endolysins as Food and Environmental Decontaminants

During post-harvest processing, food is vulnerable to cross-contamination from microbial pathogens, which pose a risk to food safety, as well as from microorganisms that can cause quality or shelf-life defects. Effective interventions for foods and the food processing environment are therefore vital to maintain the integrity of the food supply chain. Endolysins have the potential to be key intervention tools for this purpose.

The use of endolysins to prevent contamination of ready-to-eat foods by the common food and environmental pathogen *Listeria monocytogenes* has been established by groups from around the world [16,113–117]. Zhang et al. [113] cloned an endolysin gene (*lysZ5*) from the genome of *L. monocytogenes* phage FWLLm3 into *E. coli* and tested the sterilization efficacy of the expressed protein (a murine hydrolase) in soya milk contaminated with *L. monocytogenes*. The purified protein had a bactericidal effect on *L. monocytogenes* growing in soya milk, with the pathogen concentration reduced by more than 4 $\log_{10}$ CFU·ml^{-1} after 3 h of incubation at 4 °C. Furthermore, the protein displayed a broad host spectrum, lysing lawn cultures of *L. monocytogenes*, *Listeria innocua*, and *Listeria welshimeri*. In a different approach, van Nassau et al. [114] tested the combined effect of previously characterized endolysins (PlyP40, Ply511, or PlyP825) and high hydrostatic pressure on the survival of *L. monocytogenes*. They reported that the combination of treatments had a synergistic effect, capable of reducing viable cell counts of *L. monocytogenes* by up to 5.5 $\log_{10}$, compared with 0.3 and 0.2 $\log_{10}$ CFU reductions, respectively, when used alone.

Turner et al. [115] and Gaeng et al. [16] demonstrated that the *L. monocytogenes* endolysin gene *ply511* can be cloned and expressed in *Lactobacillus* spp., which have potential as biopreservatives in foods and as a starter culture for fermented milk products. Further to this, Turner et al. [115] combined the cloned A511 phage *ply511* gene with a lysostaphin-encoding *lss* gene from *S. simulans* biovar *staphylolyticus* in-frame with a Sep secretion signal. The resulting construct, Sep-6_His-Ply511, was able to secrete both Ply511 and lysostaphin from *Lactobacillus lactis*, indicating that this recombinant organism could be used for industrial applications as a preservative to prevent contamination of foods with *Staphylococcus* spp. and *L. monocytogenes*.

Staphylococcal food poisoning caused by heat stable enterotoxins produced by *S. aureus* is frequently reported following the consumption of contaminated food and milk products [118]. Chang et al. [119] tested LysSA11, a *S. aureus* phage SA11-derived endolysin, to determine its bactericidal activity in food and on food utensils artificially contaminated with MRSA. Treatment of artificially contaminated ham and pasteurized milk with endolysin for 15 min resulted in 3.1 $\log_{10}$ CFU·cm^{-3} and 1.4 $\log_{10}$ CFU·ml^{-1} reductions in viable MRSA, respectively, at refrigeration temperature (4 °C), and 3.4 $\log_{10}$ CFU·cm^{-3} and 2.0 $\log_{10}$ CFU·ml^{-1} reductions, respectively, at room temperature (25 °C). The same group [120] tested the antibacterial potential of LysSA97 in combination with several active compounds derived from essential oils used by the food industry against *S. aureus*. They reported the superior activity of carvacrol in combination with LysSA97, compared with that of the endolysin alone, in food products including beef and milk contaminated with *S. aureus*. When used alone, LysSA97 and carvacrol reduced *S. aureus* concentrations by 0.8 and 1.0 $\log_{10}$ CFU·ml^{-1}, respectively; however, a synergistic reduction of 4.5 $\log_{10}$ CFU·ml^{-1} was observed when the treatments were combined. Similarly, Obeso et al. [121] and Rodriguez-Rubio et al. [122] demonstrated the potential of phage-derived endolysins LysH5 and HydH5 (a hydrolase), respectively, to protect milk products from *S. aureus* contamination.

Salmonella species are the leading cause of bacterial foodborne illness in the USA and many other countries [123]. *Salmonella* disease outbreaks are associated with a wide variety of food products, including red meats, poultry, and produce [124]. Several recombinant endolysins derived from *Salmonella* phages have been characterized [125–127]. Interestingly, many of these endolysins have activity outside of the host species of the parental phage, particularly when cell membrane-disrupting chemicals are used in conjunction with the enzymes. Lim et al. [125] expressed the endolysins and spanin proteins from *Salmonella* phage SPN1S and observed activity against both *Salmonella* Typhimurium and *E. coli* isolates in buffer containing EDTA to destabilize the cell membranes. Furthermore, some activity was also noted against typhoidal salmonellae, *Shigella*, *Cronobacter*, *Pseudomonas*, and *Vibrio* species. Oliveira et al. [126] characterized a thermostable *Salmonella* endolysin, Lys68, that displayed better activity at neutral pH and a wide temperature tolerance, maintaining 76.7% of its activity after 2 months at 4°C and partial activity following exposure to 100 °C for 30 min. Thermostability is a useful feature for diverse application, such as in heat treatment of food When Lys68 was tested in combination with citric or malic acid against *S.* Typhimurium LT2, up to 5 $\log_{10}$ CFU reductions were achieved, with cells in stationary phase or in biofilms also reduced by up to 1 $\log_{10}$ CFU [126]. More recently, Rodriguez-Rubio et al. [127] reported a *Salmonella* phage endolysin, Gp110, that possessed both a novel enzyme structure and N-acetylmuramidase lysis domain, and had unusually high in vitro activity against *Salmonella* and other Gram-negative pathogens [127].

Around the turn of the century, a rare but frequently fatal disease of neonatal infants was first reported to be associated with contamination of powdered infant milk formula with *Enterobacter* (now *Cronobacter*) *sakazakii* [128]. It is now known that several species of *Cronobacter* can cause a variety of diseases, including sepsis and severe meningitis, in neonates, as well as respiratory and urinary tract infections in elderly and immunocompromised individuals. These opportunistic pathogens are now under much scrutiny because of their ability to survive heat, desiccation, and acid stress, which poses a risk of contamination of various milk powders, herbal teas, and other dried products (https://www.cdc.gov/cronobacter/technical.html). Enderson et al. [129,130] expressed and purified a peptidoglycan hydrolase (LysCs4) from *C. sakazakii* that had the highest sequence similarity to a putative lysozyme from the temperate *Cronobacter* phage ES2. The purified lysozyme could degrade the peptidoglycan from both Gram-negative and Gram-positive bacteria belonging to six different genera, and could lyse outer membrane-permeabilized *C. sakazakii*. Similarly, the previously discussed endolysins SPN1S [125] and Lys68 [126] are active against permeabilized *C. sakazakii* cells.

Several groups have investigated the potential of endolysins active against *B. cereus* as biocides and preservatives for use in the food industry [131–133]. *B. cereus*, a Gram-positive spore-forming bacterium, is known for its ability to cause food poisoning by producing both an emetic toxin and a diarrheal toxin [131]. Loessner et al. [132] isolated and characterized three endolysins (PlyBa, Ply12, and Ply21) from the *B. cereus* phages Bastille, TP21, and 12826, respectively, and tested their efficacy against a range of Gram-positive and Gram-negative bacteria. They reported that all three endolysins were effective against 24 strains of *B. cereus*, along with several strains of *B. thuringiensis*. Ply12 and Ply21 were found to be *N*-acetylmuramoyl-L-alanine amidases, while PlyBa could not be classified at the time, but is also likely to be an amidase (http://www.uniprot.org/uniprot/P89927). Park et al. [133] isolated a putative endolysin gene from the genome of *B. cereus* phage BPS13, and expressed it in *E. coli*. The purified LysBPS13 protein, an amidase, retained its lytic activity against *B. cereus* ATCC 10876 even after incubation at 100 °C for 30 min, demonstrating its potential as a decontaminant in food processing applications. In contrast, Son et al. [131] proposed *L*-alanoyl-D-glutamate endopeptidase LysB4 as a potential biocontrol agent against *B. cereus* and other pathogenic bacteria. They confirmed the endopeptidase had a broad range of bactericidal activity against Gram-positive bacteria, including *B. cereus*, *B. subtilis*, and *L. monocytogenes*, and also a few Gram-negative bacteria. The endolysin showed optimum lytic activity at pH 8–10 and at 50 °C, making it a suitable candidate for use in the food industry.

In addition to causing diseases in poultry, clostridial species are linked to food spoilage. In the dairy industry, germinated *Clostridium sporogenes* and *Clostridium tyrobutyricum* can contribute to the production of gases and acids that change the structural and sensory qualities of cheeses [134]. Mayer et al. [135] isolated an *N*-acetylmuramoyl-L-alanine amidase, CS74L, from *C. sporogenes* and reported that the purified protein effectively lysed *C. sporogenes* cells when added exogenously. Using the turbidity assay and fresh bacterial cells, the authors also demonstrated that CS74L was active against *C. tyrobutyricum* and *Clostridium acetobutylicum*, making it a candidate biopreservative for use in cheese. The same group also characterized another endolysin isolated from a virulent phage, CPT1l, but this enzyme had a more limited host range [134].

The dairy industry has a long-held interest in utilizing endolysins to control the cheese maturation process. Vasala et al. [136] isolated a muramidase, Mur, from the LL-H phage of *Lactobacillus delbrueckii* subsp. *lactis* that had activity against cell wall preparations of *L. delbrueckii* subsp. *lactis*, *L. delbrueckii* subsp. *bulgaricus*, *Lactobacillus acidophilus*, *Lactobacillus helveticus*, and *Pediococcus damnosus*. Similarly, Deutsch et al. [137] purified endolysin Mur-LH from a phage infecting the Swiss cheese starter *L. helveticus*. This muramidase had activity against other lactobacilli, *Leuconostoc lactis*, *P. acidilactici*, and, surprisingly, against *B. subtilis*. Kashige et al. [138] isolated an *N*-acetylmuramoyl-L-alanine amidase from phage PL-1, which was originally isolated from an abnormal fermentation of a lactic acid beverage produced using a *Lactobacillus casei* strain. There are also many examples of endolysins isolated from lactococci, including from phages P001, C2 US3, and TUC2009 [136]. A survey of 18 *L. lactis* phage endolysins revealed that muramidases and amidases predominate [139].

In addition to the aforementioned enzymes, several other endolysins with potential to be used against a range of foodborne microorganisms in different food types have been identified, and selected examples of these are illustrated in Table 2.

Table 2. Examples of other potential uses of endolysins in foods.

Food	Organism	Endolysin	Reference
Fish	*Shewanella putrefaciens*	ORF62	Han et al. [140]
Vegetable fermentation	*Leuconostoc mesenteroides*	ORF35	Lu et al. [141]
Kimchi	*Lactobacillus plantarum*	SC921 lysin	Yoon et al. [142]
Pears	*Erwinia amylovora*	ΦEa1h lysozyme	Kim et al. [143]
Banana juice	*Salmonella* Typhimurium, *Yersinia enterocolitica*, *Escherichia coli O157:H7*, *Shigella flexneri*	λ lysozyme (with high pressure treatment)	Nakimbugwe et al. [144]

Table 2. *Cont.*

Food	Organism	Endolysin	Reference
Shellfish	*Vibrio parahaemolyticus*	Lysqdvp001	Wang et al. [145]
Lettuce	*Listeria innocua*	Ply500 (with packaging film)	Solanki et al. [146]
Milk	*Listeria monocytogenes*	PlyP825 (with high pressure treatment)	Misiou et al. [147]
Mozzarella cheese	*L. monocytogenes*	PlyP825 (with high pressure treatment)	Misiou et al. [147]

The growth of biofilms in food processing environments leads to an increased risk of microbial contamination of foods [148]. There are some examples of endolysins being used to disrupt biofilms with relevance to the food industry. Gutierrez et al. [149] investigated the activity of three endolysins (LysH5, CHAP-SH3b, and HydH5-SH3b) against biofilms formed by two *S. aureus* isolates from food. Preformed biofilms were treated with 7 μM of the enzymes, with LysH5 and CHAP-SH3b most effective against strains IPLA1 and Sa9, respectively. In another study, an *N*-acetylmuramoyl-L-alanine amidase was used to disrupt *Listeria* biofilms in vitro, but was found to be most effective when used in combination with a protease [150]. The *Salmonella*-phage endolysin Lys68 also reduced the concentration of cells in a *S.* Typhimurium LT2 biofilm by up to 1.2 $\log_{10}$ CFU [128], but this required the presence of either citric or maleic acid to permeabilize the cell membranes.

Phytopathogenic bacteria have a significant global economic cost, and are the cause of multiple food security issues [151]. The use of antibiotics in plant agriculture is controversial because its contribution to the development of antibiotic resistance in human pathogens is undetermined [152] Although its impact may be small, ideally, an alternative strategy to control phytopathogenic bacteria will be developed. As such, the use of endolysins to protect plants from bacterial diseases has been proposed [16]. Widespread implementation of these endolysins will, however, be a significant challenge because of the vast number of crops that would require treatment, and the presence of beneficial soil-borne bacteria. A proposed strategy is the development of transgenic crops that express endolysins, providing protection against the pathogenic bacteria. The potential of this approach has been demonstrated by Düring et al. [153], who produced transgenic potato plants expressing T4 lysozyme. These engineered plants displayed resistance to *Pectobacterium carotovora* (formerly *Erwinia carotovora*) species, which are the cause soft rot [153,154]. Wittmann et al. [155] produced transgenic tomato plants expressing the endolysins from bacteriophage CMP1 in an attempt to prevent *Clavibacter michiganensis* subsp. *michiganensis* infection, the causative agent of bacterial wilt and canker [156]. No symptoms of bacterial infection were observed in the transgenic plants; however, the bacteria were not completely eliminated [155]. A key limitation of this research was that the bacterial infection model may not be representative of natural infection, and therefore the efficacy of these transgenic tomato plants should to be evaluated under more natural conditions. It is also unknown whether *C. michiganensis* subsp. *michiganensis* could acquire resistance to these transgenic plants. However, this is a promising advancement in the development of transgenic plants. As new endolysins are characterized, more opportunities for bioengineering to optimize the activity of the protection mechanism will be possible.

Xanthmonas oryzae pv. *oryzae* causes bacterial leaf blight in rice [157], with a number of antibiotic resistant strains having been isolated [158]. In 2006, Lee et al. [159] identified Lys411 from ΦXo411, which exhibited strong lytic activity against *Xanthmonas.* Additionally, it displayed activity against the multidrug-resistant bacterium *Stenotrophomonas maltophilia* [159], which has growing clinical significance with regards to nosocomial infections and immunocompromised patients [160]. However, no follow-up studies investigating Lys411 have been published, which means the potential of this enzyme for medical or agriculture applications is unknown.

Attai et al. [161] recently characterized an endolysin from bacteriophages Atu_ph02 and Atu_ph03 for the biocontrol of *Agrobacterium tumefaciens. A. tumefaciens* is a Gram-negative soil-borne bacterium that is the etiologic agent of crown gall disease in a variety of orchard and vineyard crops [162].

Its severity and widespread impact has contributed to it to becoming the subject of many recent studies [163]. The lytic protein displayed interesting properties, with the ability to not only rapidly lyse the cell, but to also block cell division, ensuring potent antimicrobial activity [161]. Therefore, the enzyme is a candidate for biocontrol of *A. tumefaciens*; however, the method of implementation needs to be researched before a viable strategy for crop protection can be developed. The practicalities of implementing these endolysins on a global scale for individual phytobacteria may be a significant challenge, and may contribute to the limited information currently available on the use of endolysins for treatment of plant bacterial diseases. However, the cost to society of plant bacterial disease as current strategies become ineffective means that endolysin research should be an important focus.

5. Challenges of Endolysin Development and Engineering

The potential for endolysins to supplement, or replace antibiotics is exciting. However, this field is still emerging, with very few clinical trials on endolysin-based drugs being conducted. There are a number of challenges and considerations which researchers still face to bring these to market. As highlighted by several studies, the immunogenicity of endolysins must be considered and fully assessed. Undesirable immune responses to these foreign proteins could result in decreased efficacy of the enzymes, or possibly anaphylaxis and autoimmunity [164,165]. While there are studies that have reported on the immunogenicity in the application of endolysins [40–42,45,60,63] assessing the degree of immunogenicity in humans using traditional animal models has so far proven unreliable [166]. This was highlighted in studies of SAL200, which showed varying degrees of antibody production between rats, dogs, monkeys and humans [40–42]. Although the efficacy of the endolysin may not be observably impacted in vitro or in vivo, the clinical effects may be more significant. Until more human and animal-specific (for animal husbandry applications) clinical trials are conducted, the immunogenic nature of endolysins will remain unpredicatable.

In light of the current antibiotic resistance crisis, new antibacterials should be rigorously assessed for their potential susceptibility to developed resistance by bacteria. Promisingly, bacterial mutants resistant to endolysins are very infrequent [28–30,167]. Fischetti [167] proposed the lack of developed resistance to endolysins has resulted from the evolution of the interactions between bacteriophage and bacteria. The endolysins have evolved to target essential, immutable, molecules within the cell wall, thereby reducing the likelihood of the bacteria developing resistance mechanisms [167]. However, there are also reports of resistance to other peptidoglycan-cleaving enzymes including lysozymes and lysostaphin [168–173]. In the event of bacterial adaptation, enzyme engineering may prove useful to combat changes to bacteria in order to maintain the efficacy of endolysins.

The potential for endolysin bioengineering are seemingly endless, including optimizing or changing the catalytic abilities, modifying the lytic spectrum, improving its ability to permeate outer membranes and increasing stability (Table 1). Designing new enzymes requires an understanding of the structure and function of individual domains, the interactions between domains, the placement and composition of linker regions, and elucidation of key residues involved in catalysis. Bioinformatics and structural characterization studies are integral in this process [174]. Often, structural characterization can be achieved by X-ray crystallography, a powerful and effective technique for elucidating high resolution 3-D structures of proteins [11]; however, the limited ability to crystallize endolysins is a major challenge. The majority of endolysin crystal structures published to date are of single domains, with very few full-length endolysin crystal structures having been solved. This is attributed to the short flexible linker regions between domains [8], as protein flexibility is a common hindrance of crystal formation [175]. It is important to study full-length proteins to get a better understanding of the potential synergistic/antagonistic interactions between domains. Because of the difficulties in obtaining endolysin crystals, alternative structural characterization strategies need to be considered. These include the fusion of endolysins to proteins to decrease their flexibility, thereby allowing for crystallography, and other structural elucidation techniques such as nuclear magnetic resonance [176,177] and cryo-electron microscopy [178]. Although these approaches also have limitations, such as physiological relevance or size restrictions, exploration of these techniques may advance the structural characterization of endolysins.

6. Conclusions

The field of endolysin research is dynamic, with many potential applications being investigated in the medical, veterinary, and food sectors. The current global crisis of antimicrobial resistance is driving much of this work, with endolysins showing great promise to replace or supplement antibiotics. Engineering endolysins with optimized or new properties provides an opportunity to create even more effective tools. As more bacteriophage endolysins are biochemically and structurally characterized, the ability to design new enzymes improves, therefore expanding the arsenal of lytic tools. However, there are still many challenges that need to be addressed before this technology can be widely adopted by practitioners and industry. While many researchers have described the isolation and in vitro characterization of endolysins, establishing the in vivo efficacy and operating parameters of endolysins for human clinical use, food protection and supplementation, animal husbandry and welfare, and in the environment will be of great importance over the coming years. New technology to cost-effectively scale up endolysin production is also required, as this is currently a significant barrier to implementation. Finally, regulatory pathways need to be established for the use of endolysins in each of the various fields of application, and this can only be achieved by early and effective dialogue with the relevant authorities.

Acknowledgments: This article is supported by ESR SSIF funding. M.L. is supported by an UC Connect scholarship. R.C.J.D. acknowledges the following for funding support, in part: (1) the New Zealand Royal Society Marsden Fund (UOC1506); (2) a Ministry of Business, Innovation and Employment Smart Ideas grant (UOCX1706) the Biomolecular Interactions Centre, University of Canterbury.

Author Contributions: M.J.L., D.B., R.C.J.D. and C.B. wrote the paper.

References

1. World Health Organization. *Antimicrobial Resistance: Global Report on Surveillance*; World Health Organization: Geneva, Switzerland, 2014.
2. World Health Organization. *Global Framework for Development & Stewardship to Combat Antimicrobial Resistance—Draft Roadmap*; World Health Organization: Geneva, Switzerland, 2017.
3. Mwangi, W.; de Figueiredo, P.; Criscitiello, M.F. One health: Addressing global challenges at the nexus of human, animal, and environmental health. *PLoS Pathog.* **2016**, *12*, e1005731. [CrossRef] [PubMed]
4. Young, R. Bacteriophage lysis: Mechanism and regulation. *Microbiol. Rev.* **1992**, *56*, 430–481. [PubMed]
5. Loessner, M.J. Bacteriophage endolysins—Current state of research and applications. *Curr. Opin. Microbiol.* **2005**, *8*, 480–487. [CrossRef] [PubMed]
6. Fischetti, V.A. Bacteriophage endolysins: A novel anti-infective to control Gram-positive pathogens. *Int. J. Med. Microbiol.* **2010**, *300*, 357–362. [CrossRef] [PubMed]
7. Borysowski, J.; Weber-Dabrowska, B.; Gorski, A. Bacteriophage endolysins as a novel class of antibacterial agents. *Exp. Biol. Med. (Maywood)* **2006**, *231*, 366–377. [CrossRef] [PubMed]
8. Schmelcher, M.; Donovan, D.M.; Loessner, M.J. Bacteriophage endolysins as novel antimicrobials. *Future Microbiol.* **2012**, *7*, 1147–1171. [CrossRef] [PubMed]
9. Nelson, D.C.; Schmelcher, M.; Rodriguez-Rubio, L.; Klumpp, J.; Pritchard, D.G. Endolysins as antimicrobials. *Adv. Virus Res.* **2012**, *83*, 299–365. [PubMed]
10. Vollmer, W.; Bertsche, U. Murein (peptidoglycan) structure, architecture and biosynthesis in *Escherichia coli*. *Biochim. Biophys. Acta. Biomembr.* **2008**, *1778*, 1714–1734. [CrossRef] [PubMed]
11. Donovan, D.M.; Lardeo, M.; Foster-Frey, J. Lysis of Staphylococcal mastitis pathogens by bacteriophage Phi11 endolysin. *FEMS Microbiol. Lett.* **2006**, *265*, 133–139. [CrossRef] [PubMed]

12. Korndorfer, I.P.; Danzer, J.; Schmelcher, M.; Zimmer, M.; Skerra, A.; Loessner, M.J. The crystal structure of the bacteriophage PSA endolysin reveals a unique fold responsible for specific recognition of *Listeria* cell walls. *J. Mol. Biol.* **2006**, *364*, 678–689. [CrossRef] [PubMed]
13. Sass, P.; Bierbaum, G. Lytic activity of recombinant bacteriophage phi11 and phi12 endolysins on whole cells and biofilms of *Staphylococcus aureus*. *Appl. Environ. Microbiol.* **2007**, *73*, 347–352. [CrossRef] [PubMed]
14. Low, L.Y.; Yang, C.; Perego, M.; Osterman, A.; Liddington, R.C. Structure and lytic activity of a *Bacillus anthracis* prophage endolysin. *J. Biol. Chem.* **2005**, *280*, 35433–35439. [CrossRef] [PubMed]
15. Mayer, M.J.; Garefalaki, V.; Spoerl, R.; Narbad, A.; Meijers, R. Structure-based modification of a *Clostridium difficile*-targeting endolysin affects activity and host range. *J. Bacteriol.* **2011**, *193*, 5477–5486. [CrossRef] [PubMed]
16. Gaeng, S.; Scherer, S.; Neve, H.; Loessner, M.J. Gene cloning and expression and secretion of *Listeria monocytogenes* bacteriophage-lytic enzymes in *Lactococcus lactis*. *Appl. Environ. Microbiol.* **2000**, *66*, 2951–2958. [CrossRef] [PubMed]
17. Schmelcher, M.; Tchang, V.S.; Loessner, M.J. Domain shuffling and module engineering of *Listeria* phage endolysins for enhanced lytic activity and binding affinity. *Microb. Biotechnol.* **2011**, *4*, 651–662. [CrossRef] [PubMed]
18. Gerstmans, H.; Criel, B.; Briers, Y. Synthetic biology of modular endolysins. *Biotechnol. Adv.* **2017**, in press. [CrossRef] [PubMed]
19. Horgan, M.; O'Flynn, G.; Garry, J.; Cooney, J.; Coffey, A.; Fitzgerald, G.F.; Ross, R.P.; McAuliffe, O. Phage lysin Lysk can be truncated to its chap domain and retain lytic activity against live antibiotic-resistant staphylococci. *Appl. Environ. Microbiol.* **2009**, *75*, 872–874. [CrossRef] [PubMed]
20. Daniel, A.; Euler, C.; Collin, M.; Chahales, P.; Gorelick, K.J.; Fischetti, V.A. Synergism between a novel chimeric lysin and oxacillin protects against infection by methicillin-resistant *Staphylococcus aureus*. *Antimicrob. Agents Chemother.* **2010**, *54*, 1603–1612. [CrossRef] [PubMed]
21. Schmelcher, M.; Powell, A.M.; Becker, S.C.; Camp, M.J.; Donovan, D.M. Chimeric phage lysins act synergistically with lysostaphin to kill mastitis-causing *Staphylococcus aureus* in murine mammary glands. *Appl. Environ. Microbiol.* **2012**, *78*, 2297–2305. [CrossRef] [PubMed]
22. Swift, S.; Seal, B.; Garrish, J.; Oakley, B.; Hiett, K.; Yeh, H.-Y.; Woolsey, R.; Schegg, K.; Line, J.; Donovan, D. A thermophilic phage endolysin fusion to a *Clostridium perfringens*-specific cell wall binding domain creates an anti-clostridium antimicrobial with improved thermostability. *Viruses* **2015**, *7*, 3019–3034. [CrossRef] [PubMed]
23. Proença, D.; Leandro, C.; Garcia, M.; Pimentel, M.; São-José, C. EC300: A phage-based, bacteriolysin-like protein with enhanced antibacterial activity against *Enterococcus faecalis*. *Appl. Microbiol. Biotechnol.* **2015**, *99*, 5137–5149. [CrossRef] [PubMed]
24. Briers, Y.; Walmagh, M.; Van Puyenbroeck, V.; Cornelissen, A.; Cenens, W.; Aertsen, A.; Oliveira, H.; Azeredo, J.; Verween, G.; Pirnay, J.-P.; et al. Engineered endolysin-based "Artilysins" to combat multidrug-resistant Gram-negative pathogens. *mBio* **2014**, *5*. [CrossRef] [PubMed]
25. Briers, Y.; Walmagh, M.; Grymonprez, B.; Biebl, M.; Pirnay, J.-P.; Defraine, V.; Michiels, J.; Cenens, W.; Aertsen, A.; Miller, S.; et al. Art-175 is a highly efficient antibacterial against multidrug-resistant strains and persisters of *Pseudomonas aeruginosa*. *Antimicrob. Agents Chemother.* **2014**, *58*, 3774–3784. [CrossRef] [PubMed]
26. Peng, S.-Y.; You, R.-I.; Lai, M.-J.; Lin, N.-T.; Chen, L.-K.; Chang, K.-C. Highly potent antimicrobial modified peptides derived from the *Acinetobacter baumannii* phage endolysin LysAB2. *Sci. Rep.* **2017**, *7*, 11477. [CrossRef] [PubMed]
27. O'Flaherty, S.; Coffey, A.; Meaney, W.; Fitzgerald, G.F.; Ross, R.P. The recombinant phage lysin LysK has a broad spectrum of lytic activity against clinically relevant staphylococci, including methicillin-resistant *Staphylococcus aureus*. *J. Bacteriol.* **2005**, *187*, 7161–7164. [CrossRef] [PubMed]
28. Loeffler, J.M.; Nelson, D.; Fischetti, V.A. Rapid killing of *Streptococcus pneumoniae* with a bacteriophage cell wall hydrolase. *Science* **2001**, *294*, 2170–2172. [CrossRef] [PubMed]
29. Schuch, R.; Nelson, D.; Fischetti, V.A. A bacteriolytic agent that detects and kills *Bacillus anthracis*. *Nature* **2002**, *418*, 884–889. [CrossRef] [PubMed]
30. Pastagia, M.; Euler, C.; Chahales, P.; Fuentes-Duculan, J.; Krueger, J.G.; Fischetti, V.A. A novel chimeric lysin shows superiority to mupirocin for skin decolonization of methicillin-resistant and -sensitive *Staphylococcus aureus* strains. *Antimicrob. Agents Chemother.* **2011**, *55*, 738–744. [CrossRef] [PubMed]

31. Kretzer, J.W.; Lehmann, R.; Schmelcher, M.; Banz, M.; Kim, K.P.; Korn, C.; Loessner, M.J. Use of high-affinity cell wall-binding domains of bacteriophage endolysins for immobilization and separation of bacterial cells. *Appl. Environ. Microbiol.* **2007**, *73*, 1992–2000. [CrossRef] [PubMed]
32. Enright, M.C.; Robinson, D.A.; Randle, G.; Feil, E.J.; Grundmann, H.; Spratt, B.G. The evolutionary history of methicillin-resistant *Staphylococcus aureus* (MRSA). *Proc. Natl. Acad. Sci. USA* **2002**, *99*, 7687–7692. [CrossRef] [PubMed]
33. The White House. *National Action Plan for Combating Antibiotic-Resistant Bacteria. Interagency Task Force for Combating Antibiotic-Resistant Bacteria*; U.S. Office of the Press Secretary: Washington, DC, USA, 2015.
34. Filatova, L.Y.; Becker, S.C.; Donovan, D.M.; Gladilin, A.K.; Klyachko, N.L. Lysk, the enzyme lysing *Staphylococcus aureus* cells: Specific kinetic features and approaches towards stabilization. *Biochimie* **2010**, *92*, 507–513. [CrossRef] [PubMed]
35. Becker, S.C.; Foster-Frey, J.; Donovan, D.M. The phage K lytic enzyme LysK and lysostaphin act synergistically to kill MRSA. *FEMS Micriobiol. Lett.* **2008**, *287*, 185–191. [CrossRef] [PubMed]
36. Fenton, M.; Casey, P.G.; Hill, C.; Gahan, C.G.M.; Ross, R.P.; McAuliffe, O.; O'Mahony, J.; Maher, F.; Coffey, A. The truncated phage lysin CHAP(k) eliminates *Staphylococcus aureus* in the nares of mice. *Bioeng. Bugs* **2010**, *1*, 404–407. [CrossRef] [PubMed]
37. Fenton, M.; Ross, R.P.; McAuliffe, O.; O'Mahony, J.; Coffey, A. Characterization of the staphylococcal bacteriophage lysin CHAP(k). *J. Appl. Microbiol.* **2011**, *111*, 1025–1035. [CrossRef] [PubMed]
38. Jun, S.Y.; Jung, G.M.; Son, J.-S.; Yoon, S.J.; Choi, Y.-J.; Kang, S.H. Comparison of the antibacterial properties of phage endolysins SAL-1 and Lysk. *Antimicrob. Agents Chemother.* **2011**, *55*, 1764–1767. [CrossRef] [PubMed]
39. Jun, S.Y.; Jung, G.M.; Yoon, S.J.; Oh, M.-D.; Choi, Y.-J.; Lee, W.J.; Kong, J.-C.; Seol, J.G.; Kang, S.H. Antibacterial properties of a pre-formulated recombinant phage endolysin, SAL-1. *Int. J. Antimicrob. Agents* **2013**, *41*, 156–161. [CrossRef] [PubMed]
40. Jun, S.Y.; Jung, G.M.; Yoon, S.J.; Choi, Y.-J.; Koh, W.S.; Moon, K.S.; Kang, S.H. Preclinical safety evaluation of intravenously administered SAL200 containing the recombinant phage endolysin SAL-1 as a pharmaceutical ingredient. *Antimicrob. Agents Chemother.* **2014**, *58*, 2084–2088. [CrossRef] [PubMed]
41. Jun, S.Y.; Jung, G.M.; Yoon, S.J.; Youm, S.Y.; Han, H.-Y.; Lee, J.-H.; Kang, S.H. Pharmacokinetics of the phage endolysin-based candidate drug SAL200 in monkeys and its appropriate intravenous dosing period. *Clin. Exp. Pharmacol. Physiol.* **2016**, *43*, 1013–1016. [CrossRef] [PubMed]
42. Jun, S.Y.; Jang, I.J.; Yoon, S.; Jang, K.; Yu, K.S.; Cho, J.Y.; Seong, M.W.; Jung, G.M.; Yoon, S.J.; Kang, S.H. Pharmacokinetics and tolerance of the phage endolysin-based candidate drug SAL200 after a single intravenous administration among healthy volunteers. *Antimicrob. Agents Chemother.* **2017**, *61*. [CrossRef] [PubMed]
43. Bryers, J.D. Medical biofilms. *Biotechnol. Bioeng.* **2008**, *100*, 1–18. [CrossRef] [PubMed]
44. Linden, S.B.; Zhang, H.; Heselpoth, R.D.; Shen, Y.; Schmelcher, M.; Eichenseher, F.; Nelson, D.C. Biochemical and biophysical characterization of PlyGRCS, a bacteriophage endolysin active against methicillin-resistant *Staphylococcus aureus*. *Appl. Microbiol. Biotechnol.* **2015**, *99*, 741–752. [CrossRef] [PubMed]
45. Rashel, M.; Uchiyama, J.; Ujihara, T.; Uehara, Y.; Kuramoto, S.; Sugihara, S.; Yagyu, K.-I.; Muraoka, A.; Sugai, M.; Hiramatsu, K.; et al. Efficient elimination of multidrug-resistant *Staphylococcus aureus* by cloned lysin derived from bacteriophage ϕMR11. *J. Infect. Dis.* **2007**, *196*, 1237–1247. [CrossRef] [PubMed]
46. Schuch, R.; Lee, H.M.; Schneider, B.C.; Sauve, K.L.; Law, C.; Khan, B.K.; Rotolo, J.A.; Horiuchi, Y.; Couto, D.E.; Raz, A.; et al. Combination therapy with lysin CF-301 and antibiotic is superior to antibiotic alone for treating methicillin-resistant *Staphylococcus aureus*—induced murine bacteremia. *J. Infect. Dis.* **2014**, *209*, 1469–1478. [CrossRef] [PubMed]
47. Schuch, R.; Khan, B.K.; Raz, A.; Rotolo, J.A.; Wittekind, M. Bacteriophage lysin CF-301, a potent antistaphylococcal biofilm agent. *Antimicrob. Agents Chemother.* **2017**, *61*. [CrossRef] [PubMed]
48. Altoparlak, U.; Erol, S.; Akcay, M.N.; Celebi, F.; Kadanali, A. The time-related changes of antimicrobial resistance patterns and predominant bacterial profiles of burn wounds and body flora of burned patients. *Burns* **2004**, *30*, 660–664. [CrossRef] [PubMed]
49. Chopra, S.; Harjai, K.; Chhibber, S. Potential of combination therapy of endolysin MR-10 and minocycline in treating MRSA induced systemic and localized burn wound infections in mice. *Int. J. Med. Microbiol.* **2016**, *306*, 707–716. [CrossRef] [PubMed]

50. Herpers, B.; Badoux, P.; Pietersma, F.; Eichenseher, F.; Loessner, M. Specific lysis of methicillin susceptible and resistant *Staphylococcus aureus* by the endolysin staphefekt SA. 100. In Proceedings of the 24th European Congress of Clinical Microbiology and Infectious Diseases (ECCMID), Barcelona, Spain, 10–13 May 2014.
51. Totté, J.E.E.; van Doorn, M.B.; Pasmans, S.G.M.A. Successful treatment of chronic *Staphylococcus aureus*-related dermatoses with the topical endolysin staphefekt sa.100: A report of 3 cases. *Case Rep. Dermatol.* **2017**, *9*, 19–25. [CrossRef] [PubMed]
52. Rafii, F.; Sutherland, J.B.; Cerniglia, C.E. Effects of treatment with antimicrobial agents on the human colonic microflora. *Ther. Clin. Risk Manag.* **2008**, *4*, 1343–1358. [CrossRef] [PubMed]
53. Murray, B.E. The life and times of the Enterococcus. *Clin. Micriobiol. Rev.* **1990**, *3*, 46–65. [CrossRef]
54. Hammerum, A.M. Enterococci of animal origin and their significance for public health. *Clin. Microbiol. Infect.* **2012**, *18*, 619–625. [CrossRef] [PubMed]
55. Courvalin, P. Vancomycin resistance in Gram-positive cocci. *Clin. Infect. Dis.* **2006**, *42*, S25–S34. [CrossRef] [PubMed]
56. Boneca, I.G.; Chiosis, G. Vancomycin resistance: Occurrence, mechanisms and strategies to combat it. *Expert Opin. Ther. Targets* **2003**, *7*, 311–328. [CrossRef] [PubMed]
57. Yoong, P.; Schuch, R.; Nelson, D.; Fischetti, V.A. Identification of a broadly active phage lytic enzyme with lethal activity against antibiotic-resistant *Enterococcus faecalis* and *Enterococcus faecium*. *J. Bacteriol.* **2004**, *186*, 4808–4812. [CrossRef] [PubMed]
58. Son, J.S.; Jun, S.Y.; Kim, E.B.; Park, J.E.; Paik, H.R.; Yoon, S.J.; Kang, S.H.; Choi, Y.J. Complete genome sequence of a newly isolated lytic bacteriophage, EFAP-1 of *Enterococcus faecalis*, and antibacterial activity of its endolysin EFAL-1. *J. Appl. Microbiol.* **2010**, *108*, 1769–1779. [CrossRef] [PubMed]
59. Zhang, W.; Mi, Z.; Yin, X.; Fan, H.; An, X.; Zhang, Z.; Chen, J.; Tong, Y. Characterization of *Enterococcus faecalis* phage IME-EF1 and its endolysin. *PLoS ONE* **2013**, *8*, e80435. [CrossRef] [PubMed]
60. Cheng, M.; Zhang, Y.; Li, X.; Liang, J.; Hu, L.; Gong, P.; Zhang, L.; Cai, R.; Zhang, H.; Ge, J.; et al. Endolysin LysEF-P10 shows potential as an alternative treatment strategy for multidrug-resistant *Enterococcus faecalis* infections. *Sci. Rep.* **2017**, *7*, 10164. [CrossRef] [PubMed]
61. Jedrzejas, M.J. Pneumococcal virulence factors: Structure and function. *Microbiol. Mol. Biol. Rev.* **2001**, *65*, 187–207. [CrossRef] [PubMed]
62. Cunningham, M.W. Pathogenesis of group a streptococcal infections. *Clin. Microbiol. Rev.* **2000**, *13*, 470–511. [CrossRef] [PubMed]
63. Loeffler, J.M.; Djurkovic, S.; Fischetti, V.A. Phage lytic enzyme Cpl-1 as a novel antimicrobial for pneumococcal bacteremia. *Infect. Immun.* **2003**, *71*, 6199–6204. [CrossRef] [PubMed]
64. Garcia, J.L.; Garcia, E.; Arraras, A.; Garcia, P.; Ronda, C.; Lopez, R. Cloning, purification, and biochemical characterization of the pneumococcal bacteriophage Cp-1 lysin. *J. Virol.* **1987**, *61*, 2573–2580. [PubMed]
65. Djurkovic, S.; Loeffler, J.M.; Fischetti, V.A. Synergistic killing of *Streptococcus pneumoniae* with the bacteriophage lytic enzyme Cpl-1 and penicillin or gentamicin depends on the level of penicillin resistance. *Antimicrob. Agents Chemother.* **2005**, *49*, 1225–1228. [CrossRef] [PubMed]
66. Jado, I.; López, R.; García, E.; Fenoll, A.; Casal, J.; García, P. Phage lytic enzymes as therapy for antibiotic-resistant *Streptococcus pneumoniae* infection in a murine sepsis model. *J. Antimicrob. Chemother.* **2003**, *52*, 967–973. [CrossRef] [PubMed]
67. Loeffler, J.M.; Fischetti, V.A. Synergistic lethal effect of a combination of phage lytic enzymes with different activities on penicillin-sensitive and -resistant *Streptococcus pneumoniae* strains. *Antimicrob. Agents Chemother.* **2003**, *47*, 375–377. [CrossRef] [PubMed]
68. Entenza, J.; Loeffler, J.; Grandgirard, D.; Fischetti, V.; Moreillon, P. Therapeutic effects of bacteriophage Cpl-1 lysin against *Streptococcus pneumoniae* endocarditis in rats. *Antimicrob. Agents Chemother.* **2005**, *49*, 4789–4792. [CrossRef] [PubMed]
69. Grandgirard, D.; Loeffler, J.M.; Fischetti, V.A.; Leib, S.L. Phage lytic enzyme Cpl-1 for antibacterial therapy in experimental pneumococcal meningitis. *J. Infect. Dis.* **2008**, *197*, 1519–1522. [CrossRef] [PubMed]
70. Doehn, J.M.; Fischer, K.; Reppe, K.; Gutbier, B.; Tschernig, T.; Hocke, A.C.; Fischetti, V.A.; Löffler, J.; Suttorp, N.; Hippenstiel, S.; et al. Delivery of the endolysin Cpl-1 by inhalation rescues mice with fatal pneumococcal pneumonia. *J. Antimicrob. Chemother.* **2013**, *68*, 2111–2117. [CrossRef] [PubMed]

71. Witzenrath, M.; Schmeck, B.; Doehn, J.M.; Tschernig, T.; Zahlten, J.; Loeffler, J.M.; Zemlin, M.; Müller, H.; Gutbier, B.; Schütte, H. Systemic use of the endolysin Cpl-1 rescues mice with fatal pneumococcal pneumonia. *Crit. Care Med.* **2009**, *37*, 642–649. [CrossRef] [PubMed]
72. Resch, G.; Moreillon, P.; Fischetti, V.A. A stable phage lysin (Cpl-1) dimer with increased antipneumococcal activity and decreased plasma clearance. *Int. J. Antimicrob. Agents* **2011**, *38*, 516–521. [CrossRef] [PubMed]
73. Usobiaga, P.; Medrano, F.J.; Gasset, M.; García, J.L.; Saiz, J.L.; Rivas, G.; Laynez, J.; Menéndez, M. Structural organization of the major autolysin from streptococcus pneumoniae. *J. Biol. Chem.* **1996**, *271*, 6832–6838. [CrossRef] [PubMed]
74. Beveridge, T.J. Structures of Gram-negative cell walls and their derived membrane vesicles. *J. Bacteriol.* **1999**, *181*, 4725–4733. [PubMed]
75. Peleg, A.Y.; Seifert, H.; Paterson, D.L. *Acinetobacter baumannii*: Emergence of a successful pathogen. *Clin. Microbial. Rev.* **2008**, *21*, 538–582. [CrossRef] [PubMed]
76. Dijkshoorn, L.; Nemec, A.; Seifert, H. An increasing threat in hospitals: Multidrug-resistant *Acinetobacter baumannii*. *Nat. Rev. Microbiol.* **2007**, *5*, 939–951. [CrossRef] [PubMed]
77. Bodey, G.P.; Bolivar, R.; Fainstein, V.; Jadeja, L. Infections caused by *Pseudomonas aeruginosa*. *Rev. Infect. Dis.* **1983**, *5*, 279–313. [CrossRef] [PubMed]
78. Lister, P.D.; Wolter, D.J.; Hanson, N.D. Antibacterial-resistant *Pseudomonas aeruginosa*: Clinical impact and complex regulation of chromosomally encoded resistance mechanisms. *Clin. Microbial. Rev.* **2009**, *22*, 582–610. [CrossRef] [PubMed]
79. Lai, M.-J.; Lin, N.-T.; Hu, A.; Soo, P.-C.; Chen, L.-K.; Chen, L.-H.; Chang, K.-C. Antibacterial activity of *Acinetobacter baumannii* phage ϕAB2 endolysin (LysAB2) against both Gram-positive and Gram-negative bacteria. *Appl. Microbiol. Biotechnol.* **2011**, *90*, 529–539. [CrossRef] [PubMed]
80. Lood, R.; Winer, B.Y.; Pelzek, A.J.; Diez-Martinez, R.; Thandar, M.; Euler, C.W.; Schuch, R.; Fischetti, V.A. Novel phage lysin capable of killing the multidrug-resistant Gram-negative bacterium *Acinetobacter baumannii* in a mouse bacteremia model. *Antimicrob. Agents Chemother.* **2015**, *59*, 1983–1991. [CrossRef] [PubMed]
81. Walmagh, M.; Briers, Y.; dos Santos, S.B.; Azeredo, J.; Lavigne, R. Characterization of modular bacteriophage endolysins from *Myoviridae* phages OBP, 201φ2-1 and PVP-SE1. *PLoS ONE* **2012**, *7*, e36991. [CrossRef] [PubMed]
82. Sato, H.; Feix, J.B. Peptide–membrane interactions and mechanisms of membrane destruction by amphipathic α-helical antimicrobial peptides. *Biochim. Biophys. Acta. Biomembr.* **2006**, *1758*, 1245–1256. [CrossRef] [PubMed]
83. Guo, M.; Feng, C.; Ren, J.; Zhuang, X.; Zhang, Y.; Zhu, Y.; Dong, K.; He, P.; Guo, X.; Qin, J. A novel antimicrobial endolysin, LysPA26, against *Pseudomonas aeruginosa*. *Front. Microbiol.* **2017**, *8*. [CrossRef] [PubMed]
84. Thummeepak, R.; Kitti, T.; Kunthalert, D.; Sitthisak, S. Enhanced antibacterial activity of acinetobacter baumannii bacteriophage øABP-01 endolysin (LysABP-01) in combination with colistin. *Front. Microbiol.* **2016**, *7*. [CrossRef] [PubMed]
85. Briers, Y.; Walmagh, M.; Lavigne, R. Use of bacteriophage endolysin EL188 and outer membrane permeabilizers against *Pseudomonas aeruginosa*. *J. Appl. Microbiol.* **2011**, *110*, 778–785. [CrossRef] [PubMed]
86. Triantaphyllopoulos, D.C.; Quick, A.J.; Greenwalt, T.J. Action of disodium ethylenediamine tetracetate on blood coagulation; evidence of the development of heparinoid activity during incubation or aeration of plasma. *Blood* **1955**, *10*, 534–544. [PubMed]
87. Briers, Y.; Lavigne, R. Breaking barriers: Expansion of the use of endolysins as novel antibacterials against Gram-negative bacteria. *Future Microbiol.* **2015**, *10*, 377–390. [CrossRef] [PubMed]
88. Zasloff, M. Antimicrobial peptides of multicellular organisms. *Nature* **2002**, *415*, 389. [CrossRef] [PubMed]
89. Dawson, R.M.; Liu, C.-Q. Cathelicidin peptide SMAP-29: Comprehensive review of its properties and potential as a novel class of antibiotics. *Drug Dev. Res.* **2009**, *70*, 481–498. [CrossRef]
90. Timbermont, L.; Haesebrouck, F.; Ducatelle, R.; Van Immerseel, F. Necrotic enteritis in broilers: An updated review on the pathogenesis. *Avian Pathol.* **2011**, *40*, 341–347. [CrossRef] [PubMed]
91. Gervasi, T.; Lo Curto, R.; Minniti, E.; Narbad, A.; Mayer, M.J. Application of *Lactobacillus johnsonii* expressing phage endolysin for control of *Clostridium perfringens*. *Lett. Appl. Microbiol.* **2014**, *59*, 355–361. [CrossRef] [PubMed]

92. Gervasi, T.; Horn, N.; Wegmann, U.; Dugo, G.; Narbad, A.; Mayer, M.J. Expression and delivery of an endolysin to combat *Clostridium perfringens*. *Appl. Microbiol. Biotechnol.* **2014**, *98*, 2495–2505. [CrossRef] [PubMed]
93. Tamai, E.; Yoshida, H.; Sekiya, H.; Nariya, H.; Miyata, S.; Okabe, A.; Kuwahara, T.; Maki, J.; Kamitori, S. X-ray structure of a novel endolysin encoded by episomal phage phiSM101 of *Clostridium perfringens*. *Mol. Microbiol.* **2014**, *92*, 326–337. [CrossRef] [PubMed]
94. Nariya, H.; Miyata, S.; Tamai, E.; Sekiya, H.; Maki, J.; Okabe, A. Identification and characterization of a putative endolysin encoded by episomal phage phiSM101 of *Clostridium perfringens*. *Appl. Microbiol. Biotechnol.* **2011**, *90*, 1973–1979. [CrossRef] [PubMed]
95. Wilson, D.J.; Gonzalez, R.N.; Das, H.H. Bovine mastitis pathogens in New York and Pennsylvania: Prevalence and effects on somatic cell count and milk production. *J. Dairy Sci.* **1997**, *80*, 2592–2598. [CrossRef]
96. Donovan, D.M.; Dong, S.; Garrett, W.; Rousseau, G.M.; Moineau, S.; Pritchard, D.G. Peptidoglycan hydrolase fusions maintain their parental specificities. *Appl. Environ. Microbiol.* **2006**, *72*, 2988–2996. [CrossRef] [PubMed]
97. Schmelcher, M.; Powell, A.M.; Camp, M.J.; Pohl, C.S.; Donovan, D.M. Synergistic streptococcal phage λSA2 and B30 endolysins kill streptococci in cow milk and in a mouse model of mastitis. *Appl. Microbiol. Biotechnol.* **2015**, *99*, 8475–8486. [CrossRef] [PubMed]
98. Fan, J.; Zeng, Z.; Mai, K.; Yang, Y.; Feng, J.; Bai, Y.; Sun, B.; Xie, Q.; Tong, Y.; Ma, J. Preliminary treatment of bovine mastitis caused by *Staphylococcus aureus*, with Trx-SA1, recombinant endolysin of *S. aureus* bacteriophage IME-SA1. *Vet. Microbiol.* **2016**, *191*, 65–71. [CrossRef] [PubMed]
99. Fasanella, A.; Galante, D.; Garofolo, G.; Jones, M.H. Anthrax undervalued zoonosis. *Vet. Microbiol.* **2010**, *140*, 318–331. [CrossRef] [PubMed]
100. Toole, T.O.; Henderson, D.; Bartlett, J.G.; Ascher, M.S.; Eitzen, E.; Friedlander, A.M.; Gerberding, J.; Hauer, J.; Hughes, J.; McDade, J.; et al. Anthrax as a biological weapon, 2002: Updated recommendations for management. *J. Am. Med. Assoc.* **2002**, *287*, 2236–2253.
101. Sykes, J.E.; Hartmann, K.; Lunn, K.F.; Moore, G.E.; Stoddard, R.; Goldstein, R.E. ACVIM Consensus Statement. *J. Vet. Intern. Med.* **2011**, *19*, 1–13. [CrossRef] [PubMed]
102. Hoopes, J.T.; Stark, C.J.; Kim, H.A.; Sussman, D.J.; Donovan, D.M.; Nelson, D.C. Use of a bacteriophage lysin, PlyC, as an enzyme disinfectant against *Streptococcus equi*. *Appl. Environ. Microbiol.* **2009**, *75*, 1388–1394. [CrossRef] [PubMed]
103. Junjappa, R.P.; Desai, S.N.; Roy, P.; Narasimhaswamy, N.; Raj, J.R.M.; Durgaiah, M.; Vipra, A.; Bhat, U.R.; Satyanarayana, S.K.; Shankara, N.; et al. Efficacy of anti-staphylococcal protein P128 for the treatment of canine pyoderma: Potential applications. *Vet. Res. Commun.* **2013**, *37*, 217–228. [CrossRef] [PubMed]
104. Vipra, A.A.; Desai, S.N.; Roy, P.; Patil, R.; Raj, J.M.; Narasimhaswamy, N.; Paul, V.D.; Chikkamadaiah, R.; Sriram, B. Antistaphylococcal activity of bacteriophage derived chimeric protein P128. *BMC Microbiol.* **2012**, *12*, 41. [CrossRef] [PubMed]
105. Wang, Y.; Sun, J.H.; Lu, C.P. Purified recombinant phage lysin LySMP: An extensive spectrum of lytic activity for swine streptococci. *Curr. Microbiol.* **2009**, *58*, 609–615. [CrossRef] [PubMed]
106. Bates, J.; Jordens, J.; Griffith, D.T. Farm animals as putative reservoir for vancomycin resistant enterococcal infections in man. *J. Antiomicrob. Chemother.* **1994**, *34*, 507–516. [CrossRef]
107. Coque, T.M.; Tomayko, J.F.; Ricke, S.C.; Okhyusen, P.C.; Murray, B.E. Vancomycin-resistant enterococci from nosocomial, community, and animal sources in the United States. *Antimicrob. Agents Chemother.* **1996**, *40*, 2605–2609. [PubMed]
108. Madewell, B.R.; Tang, Y.J.; Jang, S.; Madigan, J.E.; Hirsh, D.C.; Gumerlock, P.H.; Silva, J., Jr. Apparent outbreaks of *Clostridium difficile*-associated diarrhea in horses in a veterinary medical teaching hospital. *J. Vet. Diagn. Invest.* **1995**, *7*, 343–346. [CrossRef] [PubMed]
109. Debast, S.B.; Van Leengoed, L.A.M.G.; Goorhuis, A.; Harmanus, C.; Kuijper, E.J.; Bergwerff, A.A. *Clostridium difficile* PCR ribotype 078 toxinotype V found in diarrhoeal pigs identical to isolates from affected humans. *Environ. Microbiol.* **2009**, *11*, 505–511. [CrossRef] [PubMed]
110. Kelly, C.P.; Pothoulakis, C.; LaMont, J.T. *Clostridium difficile* Colitis. *N. Engl. J. Med.* **1994**, *330*, 257–262. [CrossRef] [PubMed]
111. Mayer, M.J.; Narbad, A.; Gasson, M.J. Molecular characterization of a *Clostridium difficile* bacteriophage and its cloned biologically active endolysin. *J. Bacteriol.* **2008**, *190*, 6734–6740. [CrossRef] [PubMed]

112. Oliveira, A.; Leite, M.; Kluskens, L.D.; Santos, S.B.; Melo, L.D.R.; Azeredo, J. The first *Paenibacillus* larvae bacteriophage endolysin (PlyPl23) with high potential to control American Foulbrood. *PLoS ONE* **2015**, *10*, e0132095.
113. Zhang, H.; Bao, H.; Billington, C.; Hudson, J.A.; Wang, R. Isolation and lytic activity of the *Listeria* bacteriophage endolysin LysZ5 against *Listeria monocytogenes* in soya milk. *Food Microbiol.* **2012**, *31*, 133–136. [CrossRef] [PubMed]
114. van Nassau, T.J.; Lenz, C.A.; Scherzinger, A.S.; Vogel, R.F. Combination of endolysins and high pressure to inactivate *Listeria monocytogenes*. *Food Microbiol.* **2017**, *68*, 81–88. [CrossRef] [PubMed]
115. Turner, M.S.; Waldherr, F.; Loessner, M.J.; Giffard, P.M. Antimicrobial activity of lysostaphin and a *Listeria monocytogenes* bacteriophage endolysin produced and secreted by lactic acid bacteria. *Syst. Appl. Microbiol.* **2007**, *30*, 58–67. [CrossRef] [PubMed]
116. van Tassell, M.L.; Angela Daum, M.; Kim, J.S.; Miller, M.J. Creative lysins: *Listeria* and the engineering of antimicrobial enzymes. *Curr. Opin. Biotechnol.* **2016**, *37*, 88–96. [CrossRef] [PubMed]
117. Schmelcher, M.; Waldherr, F.; Loessner, M.J. *Listeria* bacteriophage peptidoglycan hydrolases feature high thermoresistance and reveal increased activity after divalent metal cation substitution. *Appl. Microbiol. Biotechnol.* **2012**, *93*, 633–643. [CrossRef] [PubMed]
118. Hennekinne, J.A.; De Buyser, M.L.; Dragacci, S. *Staphylococcus aureus* and its food poisoning toxins: Characterization and outbreak investigation. *FEMS. Microbiol. Rev.* **2012**, *36*, 815–836. [CrossRef] [PubMed]
119. Chang, Y.; Kim, M.; Ryu, S. Characterization of a novel endolysin LysSA11 and its utility as a potent biocontrol agent against *Staphylococcus aureus* on food and utensils. *Food. Microbiol.* **2017**, *68*, 112–120. [CrossRef] [PubMed]
120. Chang, Y.; Yoon, H.; Kang, D.H.; Chang, P.S.; Ryu, S. Endolysin LysSA97 is synergistic with carvacrol in controlling *Staphylococcus aureus* in foods. *Int. J. Food Microbiol.* **2017**, *244*, 19–26. [CrossRef] [PubMed]
121. Obeso, J.M.; Martinez, B.; Rodriguez, A.; Garcia, P. Lytic activity of the recombinant staphylococcal bacteriophage ΦH5 endolysin active against *Staphylococcus aureus* in milk. *Int. J. Food Microbiol.* **2008**, *128*, 212–218. [CrossRef] [PubMed]
122. Rodriguez-Rubio, L.; Martinez, B.; Donovan, D.M.; Garcia, P.; Rodriguez, A. Potential of the virion-associated peptidoglycan hydrolase HydH5 and its derivative fusion proteins in milk biopreservation. *PLoS ONE* **2013**, *8*, e54828. [CrossRef] [PubMed]
123. World Health Organization. *WHO Estimates of the Global Burden of Foodborne Diseases: Foodborne Disease Burden Epidemiology Reference Group 2007–2015*; World Health Organization: Geneva, Switzerland, 2015.
124. Interagency Food Safety Analytics Collaboration (IFSAC) Project. Foodborne Illness Source Attribution Estimates for *Salmonella*, *Escherichia coli* O157 (*E. coli* O157), *Listeria monocytogenes* (lm) and *Campylobacter* Using Outbreak Surveillance Data. 2014. Available online: https://www.cdc.gov/foodsafety/pdfs/IFSAC-2013FoodborneillnessSourceEstimates-508.pdf (accessed on 13 March 2015).
125. Lim, J.A.; Shin, H.; Kang, D.H.; Ryu, S. Characterization of endolysin from a *Salmonella* Typhimurium-infecting bacteriophage SPN1S. *Res. Microbiol.* **2012**, *163*, 233–241. [CrossRef] [PubMed]
126. Oliveira, H.; Thiagarajan, V.; Walmagh, M.; Sillankorva, S.; Lavigne, R.; Neves-Petersen, M.T.; Kluskens, L.D.; Azeredo, J. A thermostable *Salmonella* phage endolysin, Lys68, with broad bactericidal properties against Gram-negative pathogens in presence of weak acids. *PLoS ONE* **2014**, *9*, e108376. [CrossRef] [PubMed]
127. Rodríguez-Rubio, L.; Gerstmans, H.; Thorpe, S.; Mesnage, S.; Lavigne, R.; Briers, Y. DUF3380 domain from a *Salmonella* phage endolysin shows potent *N*-acetylmuramidase activity. *Appl. Environ. Microbiol.* **2016**, *82*, 4975–4981. [CrossRef] [PubMed]
128. Drudy, D.; Mullane, N.R.; Quinn, T.; Wall, P.G.; Fanning, S. *Enterobacter sakazakii*: An emerging pathogen in powdered infant formula. *Clin. Infect. Dis.* **2006**, *42*, 996–1002. [CrossRef] [PubMed]
129. Endersen, L.; Guinane, C.M.; Johnston, C.; Neve, H.; Coffey, A.; Ross, R.P.; McAuliffe, O.; O'Mahony, J. Genome analysis of *Cronobacter* phage vB_CsaP_Ss1 reveals an endolysin with potential for biocontrol of Gram-negative bacterial pathogens. *J. Gen. Virol.* **2015**, *96*, 463–477. [CrossRef] [PubMed]
130. Endersen, L.; Coffey, A.; Ross, R.P.; McAuliffe, O.; Hill, C.; O'Mahony, J. Characterisation of the antibacterial properties of a bacterial derived peptidoglycan hydrolase (LysCs4), active against *C. sakazakii* and other Gram-negative food-related pathogens. *Int. J. Food Microbiol.* **2015**, *215*, 79–85. [CrossRef] [PubMed]
131. Son, B.; Yun, J.; Lim, J.-A.; Shin, H.; Heu, S.; Ryu, S. Characterization of LysB4, an endolysin from the *Bacillus cereus*-infecting bacteriophage B4. *BMC Microbiol.* **2012**, *12*, 33. [CrossRef] [PubMed]

132. Loessner, M.J.; Maier, S.K.; Daubek-Puza, H.; Wendlinger, G.; Scherer, S. Three *Bacillus cereus* bacteriophage endolysins are unrelated but reveal high homology to cell wall hydrolases from different bacilli. *J. Bacteriol.* **1997**, *179*, 2845–2851. [CrossRef] [PubMed]
133. Park, J.; Yun, J.; Lim, J.A.; Kang, D.H.; Ryu, S. Characterization of an endolysin, LysBPS13, from a *Bacillus cereus* bacteriophage. *FEMS Microbiol. Lett.* **2012**, *332*, 76–83. [CrossRef] [PubMed]
134. Mayer, M.J.; Payne, J.; Gasson, M.J.; Narbad, A. Genomic sequence and characterization of the virulent bacteriophage *ϕ*CTP1 from *Clostridium tyrobutyricum* and heterologous expression of its endolysin. *Appl. Envrion. Microbiol.* **2010**, *76*, 5415–5422. [CrossRef] [PubMed]
135. Mayer, M.J.; Gasson, M.J.; Narbad, A. Genomic sequence of bacteriophage ATCC 8074-B1 and activity of its endolysin and engineered variants against *Clostridium sporogenes. Appl. Environ. Microbiol.* **2012**, *78*, 3685–3692. [CrossRef] [PubMed]
136. Vasala, A.; Valkkila, M.; Caldentey, J.; Alatossava, T. Genetic and biochemical characterization of the *Lactobacillus delbrueckii* subsp. *Lactis* bacteriophage LL-H lysin. *Appl. Environ. Microbiol.* **1995**, *61*, 4004–4011. [PubMed]
137. Deutsch, S.-M.; Guezenec, S.; Piot, M.; Foster, S.; Lortal, S. Mur-LH, the broad-spectrum endolysin of *Lactobacillus helveticus* temperate bacteriophage φ-0303. *Appl. Environ. Microbiol.* **2004**, *70*, 96–103. [CrossRef] [PubMed]
138. Kashige, N.; Nakashima, Y.; Miake, F.; Watanabe, K. Cloning, sequence analysis, and expression of *Lactobacillus casei* phage PL-1 lysis genes. *Arch. Virol.* **2000**, *145*, 1521–1534. [CrossRef] [PubMed]
139. Labrie, S.; Vukov, N.; Loessner, M.J.; Moineau, S. Distribution and composition of the lysis cassette of *Lactococcus lactis* phages and functional analysis of bacteriophage Ul36 holin. *FEMS Microbiol. Lett.* **2004**, *233*, 37–43. [CrossRef] [PubMed]
140. Han, F.; Li, M.; Lin, H.; Wang, J.; Cao, L.; Khan, M.N. The novel *Shewanella putrefaciens*-infecting bacteriophage Spp001: Genome sequence and lytic enzymes. *J. Ind. Microbiol. Biotechnol.* **2014**, *41*, 1017–1026. [CrossRef] [PubMed]
141. Lu, Z.; Altermann, E.; Breidt, F.; Kozyavkin, S. Sequence analysis of *Leuconostoc mesenteroides* bacteriophage Phi1-A4 isolated from an industrial vegetable fermentation. *Appl. Environ. Microbiol.* **2010**, *76*, 1955–1966. [CrossRef] [PubMed]
142. Yoon, S.S.; Kim, J.W.; Breidt, F.; Fleming, H.P. Characterization of a lytic *Lactobacillus plantarum* bacteriophage and molecular cloning of a lysin gene in *Escherichia coli. Int. J. Food Microbiol.* **2001**, *65*, 63–74. [CrossRef]
143. Kim, W.-S.; Salm, H.; Geider, K. Expression of bacteriophage φEa1h lysozyme in *Escherichia coli* and its activity in growth inhibition of *Erwinia amylovora. Microbiology* **2004**, *150*, 2707–2714. [CrossRef] [PubMed]
144. Nakimbugwe, D.; Masschalck, B.; Anim, G.; Michiels, C.W. Inactivation of Gram-negative bacteria in milk and banana juice by hen egg white and lambda lysozyme under high hydrostatic pressure. *Int. J. Food Microbiol.* **2006**, *112*, 19–25. [CrossRef] [PubMed]
145. Wang, W.; Li, M.; Lin, H.; Wang, J.; Mao, X. The *Vibrio parahaemolyticus*-infecting bacteriophage qdvp001: Genome sequence and endolysin with a modular structure. *Arch. Virol.* **2016**, *161*, 2645–2652. [CrossRef] [PubMed]
146. Solanki, K.; Grover, N.; Downs, P.; Paskaleva, E.E.; Mehta, K.K.; Lillian, L.; Schadler, L.S.; Kane, R.S.; Dordick, J.S. Enzyme-based Listericidal nanocomposites. *Sci. Rep.* **2013**, *3*, 1584. [CrossRef] [PubMed]
147. Misiou, O.; van Nassau, T.J.; Lenz, C.A.; Vogel, R.F. The preservation of listeria-critical foods by a combination of endolysin and high hydrostatic pressure. *Int. J. Food Microbiol.* **2017**, in press. [CrossRef] [PubMed]
148. Chmielewski, R.A.N.; Frank, J.F. Biofilm formation and control in food processing facilities. *Compr. Rev. Food Sci. Food Saf.* **2003**, *2*, 22–32. [CrossRef]
149. Gutiérrez, D.; Fernández, L.; Martínez, B.; Ruas-Madiedo, P.; García, P.; Rodríguez, A. Real-time assessment of *Staphylococcus aureus* biofilm disruption by phage-derived proteins. *Front. Microbiol.* **2017**, *8*. [CrossRef] [PubMed]
150. Simmons, M.; Morales, C.A.; Oakley, B.B.; Seal, B.S. Recombinant expression of a putative amidase cloned from the genome of *Listeria monocytogenes* that lyses the bacterium and its monolayer in conjunction with a protease. *Probiotics Antimicrob. Proteins* **2012**, *4*, 1–10. [CrossRef] [PubMed]
151. Strange, R.N.; Scott, P.R. Plant disease: A threat to global food security. *Annu. Rev. Phytopathol.* **2005**, *43*, 83–116. [CrossRef] [PubMed]

152. McManus, P.S.; Stockwell, V.O.; Sundin, G.W.; Jones, A.L. Antibiotic use in plant agriculture. *Annu. Rev. Phytopathol.* **2002**, *40*, 443–465. [CrossRef] [PubMed]
153. Düring, K.; Porsch, P.; Fladung, M.; Lörz, H. Transgenic potato plants resistant to the phytopathogenic bacterium *Erwinia carotovora*. *Plant J.* **1993**, *3*, 587–598. [CrossRef]
154. De Vries, J.; Harms, K.; Broer, I.; Kriete, G.; Mahn, A.; Düring, K.; Wackernagel, W. The bacteriolytic activity in transgenic potatoes expressing a chimeric T4 lysozyme gene and the effect of T4 lysozyme on soil- and phytopathogenic bacteria. *Syst. Appl. Microbiol.* **1999**, *22*, 280–286. [CrossRef]
155. Wittmann, J.; Brancato, C.; Berendzen, K.W.; Dreiseikelmann, B. Development of a tomato plant resistant to *Clavibacter michiganensis* using the endolysin gene of bacteriophage CMP1 as a transgene. *Plant Pathol.* **2016**, *65*, 496–502. [CrossRef]
156. Hausbeck, M.K.; Bell, J.; Medina-Mora, C.; Podolsky, R.; Fulbright, D.W. Effect of bactericides on population sizes and spread of *Clavibacter michiganensis* subsp. *Michiganensis* on tomatoes in the greenhouse and on disease development and crop yield in the field. *Phytopathology* **2000**, *90*, 38–44. [PubMed]
157. Tang, J.L.; Feng, J.X.; Li, Q.Q.; Wen, H.X.; Zhou, D.L.; Wilson, T.J.; Dow, J.M.; Ma, Q.S.; Daniels, M.J. Cloning and characterization of the rpfc gene of *Xanthomonas oryzae* pv. *Oryzae*: Involvement in exopolysaccharide production and virulence to rice. *Mol. Plant Microbe. Interact.* **1996**, *9*, 664–666. [PubMed]
158. Xu, Y.; Luo, Q.-q.; Zhou, M.-g. Identification and characterization of integron-mediated antibiotic resistance in the phytopathogen *Xanthomonas oryzae* pv. *Oryzae*. *PLoS ONE* **2013**, *8*, e55962. [CrossRef] [PubMed]
159. Lee, C.-N.; Lin, J.-W.; Chow, T.-Y.; Tseng, Y.-H.; Weng, S.-F. A novel lysozyme from *Xanthomonas oryzae* phage ϕxo411 active against *Xanthomonas* and *Stenotrophomonas*. *Protein Expr. Purif.* **2006**, *50*, 229–237. [CrossRef] [PubMed]
160. Brooke, J.S. *Stenotrophomonas maltophilia*: An emerging global opportunistic pathogen. *Clin. Microbiol. Rev.* **2012**, *25*, 2–41. [CrossRef] [PubMed]
161. Attai, H.; Rimbey, J.; Smith, G.P.; Brown, P.J.B. Expression of a peptidoglycan hydrolase from lytic bacteriophages Atu_ph02 and Atu_ph03 triggers lysis of *Agrobacterium tumefaciens*. *Appl. Environ. Microbiol.* **2017**, *83*, 17. [CrossRef] [PubMed]
162. Pulawska, J. Crown gall of stone fruits and nuts, economic significance and diversity of its causal agents: Tumorigenic *Agrobacterium* spp. *J. Plant Pathol.* **2010**, *92*, S87–S98.
163. Mansfield, J.; Genin, S.; Magori, S.; Citovsky, V.; Sriariyanum, M.; Ronald, P.; Dow, M.; Verdier, V.; Beer, S.V.; Machado, M.A.; et al. Top 10 plant pathogenic bacteria in molecular plant pathology. *Mol. Plant Pathol.* **2012**, *13*, 614–629. [CrossRef] [PubMed]
164. Rosenberg, A.S. Immunogenicity of biological therapeutics: A hierarchy of concerns. *Dev. Biol.* **2003**, *112*, 15–21.
165. De Groot, A.S.; Scott, D.W. Immunogenicity of protein therapeutics. *Trends Immunol.* **2007**, *28*, 482–490. [CrossRef] [PubMed]
166. Baker, M.P.; Reynolds, H.M.; Lumicisi, B.; Bryson, C.J. Immunogenicity of protein therapeutics: The key causes, consequences and challenges. *Self Nonself* **2010**, *1*, 314–322. [CrossRef] [PubMed]
167. Fischetti, V.A. Bacteriophage lytic enzymes: Novel anti-infectives. *Trends Microbiol.* **2005**, *13*, 491–496. [CrossRef] [PubMed]
168. DeHart, H.P.; Heath, H.E.; Heath, L.S.; LeBlanc, P.A.; Sloan, G.L. The lysostaphin endopeptidase resistance gene (epr) specifies modification of peptidoglycan cross bridges in *Staphylococcus simulans* and *Staphylococcus aureus*. *Appl. Environ. Microbiol.* **1995**, *61*, 1475–1479. [PubMed]
169. Sugai, M.; Fujiwara, T.; Ohta, K.; Komatsuzawa, H.; Ohara, M.; Suginaka, H. Epr, which encodes glycylglycine endopeptidase resistance, is homologous to femab and affects serine content of peptidoglycan cross bridges in *Staphylococcus capitis* and *Staphylococcus aureus*. *J. Bacteriol.* **1997**, *179*, 4311–4318. [CrossRef] [PubMed]
170. Gründling, A.; Missiakas, D.M.; Schneewind, O. *Staphylococcus aureus* mutants with increased lysostaphin resistance. *J. Bacteriol.* **2006**, *188*, 6286–6297. [CrossRef] [PubMed]
171. Vollmer, W. Structural variation in the glycan strands of bacterial peptidoglycan. *FEMS. Microbiol. Rev.* **2008**, *32*, 287–306. [CrossRef] [PubMed]
172. Guariglia-Oropeza, V.; Helmann, J.D. *Bacillus subtilis* σ(v) confers lysozyme resistance by activation of two cell wall modification pathways, peptidoglycan o-acetylation and d-alanylation of teichoic acids. *J. Bacteriol.* **2011**, *193*, 6223–6232. [CrossRef] [PubMed]

173. Davis, K.M.; Weiser, J.N. Modifications to the peptidoglycan backbone help bacteria to establish infection. *Infect. Immun.* **2011**, *79*, 562–570. [CrossRef] [PubMed]
174. Schmelcher, M.; Shabarova, T.; Eugster, M.R.; Eichenseher, F.; Tchang, V.S.; Banz, M.; Loessner, M.J. Rapid multiplex detection and differentiation of *Listeria* cells by use of fluorescent phage endolysin cell wall binding domains. *Appl. Environ. Microbiol.* **2010**, *76*, 5745–5756. [CrossRef] [PubMed]
175. Buck, M. Crystallography: Embracing conformational flexibility in proteins. *Structure* **2003**, *11*, 735–736. [CrossRef]
176. Kashyap, M.; Jagga, Z.; Das, B.K.; Arockiasamy, A.; Bhavesh, N.S. H-1, C-13 and N-15 NMR assignments of inactive form of P1 endolysin Lyz. *Biomol. NMR Assign.* **2012**, *6*, 87–89. [CrossRef] [PubMed]
177. Kutyshenko, V.P.; Mikoulinskaia, G.V.; Molochkov, N.V.; Prokhorov, D.A.; Taran, S.A.; Uversky, V.N. Structure and dynamics of the retro-form of the bacteriophage T5 endolysin. *Biochim. Biophys. Acta Proteins Proteom.* **2016**, *1864*, 1281–1291. [CrossRef] [PubMed]
178. Topf, M.; Lasker, K.; Webb, B.; Wolfson, H.; Chiu, W.; Sali, A. Protein structure fitting and refinement guided by Cryo-EM density. *Structure* **2008**, *16*, 295–307. [CrossRef] [PubMed]

9

Future Prospects for *Neisseria gonorrhoeae* Treatment

Beatriz Suay-García and María Teresa Pérez-Gracia *

Área de Microbiología, Departamento de Farmacia, Instituto de Ciencias Biomédicas, Facultad de Ciencias de la Salud, Universidad CEU Cardenal Herrera, C/Santiago Ramón y Cajal, 46115 Alfara del Patriarca, Valencia, Spain; bea.suay.ce@ceindo.ceu.es

* Correspondence: teresa@uchceu.es

Abstract: Gonorrhea is a sexually transmitted disease with a high morbidity burden. Incidence of this disease is rising due to the increasing number of antibiotic-resistant strains. *Neisseria gonorrhoeae* has shown an extraordinary ability to develop resistance to all antimicrobials introduced for its treatment. In fact, it was recently classified as a "Priority 2" microorganism in the World Health Organization (WHO) Global Priority List of Antibiotic-Resistant Bacteria to Guide Research, Discovery and Development of New Antibiotics. Seeing as there is no gonococcal vaccine, control of the disease relies entirely on prevention, diagnosis, and, especially, antibiotic treatment. Different health organizations worldwide have established treatment guidelines against gonorrhea, mostly consisting of dual therapy with a single oral or intramuscular dose. However, gonococci continue to develop resistances to all antibiotics introduced for treatment. In fact, the first strain of super-resistant *N. gonorrhoeae* was recently detected in the United Kingdom, which was resistant to ceftriaxone and azithromycin. The increase in the detection of resistant gonococci may lead to a situation where gonorrhea becomes untreatable. Seeing as drug resistance appears to be unstoppable, new treatment options are necessary in order to control the disease. Three approaches are currently being followed for the development of new therapies against drug-resistant gonococci: (1) novel combinations of already existing antibiotics; (2) development of new antibiotics; and (3) development of alternative therapies which might slow down the appearance of resistances. *N. gonorrhoeae* is a public health threat due to the increasing number of antibiotic-resistant strains. Current treatment guidelines are already being challenged by this superbug. This has led the scientific community to develop new antibiotics and alternative therapies in order to control this disease.

Keywords: *Neisseria gonorrhoeae*; antibiotic resistance; gonorrhea; treatment

---

1. Introduction

Gonorrhea is a sexually transmitted disease (STD) caused by the obligate human pathogen *Neisseria gonorrhoeae*. This disease has a high morbidity burden, with more than 106 million new cases being diagnosed every year worldwide [1]. In fact, this morbidity is increasing exponentially due to the fact that gonococci have an extraordinary ability to develop resistances to all antimicrobials introduced for its treatment (Figure 1) [2–4].

The issue with drug-resistant *N. gonorrhoeae* has become such that the Centers for Disease Control (CDC) classified it as a "superbug" in 2012, announcing a near future in which gonorrhea would become untreatable [5]. Furthermore, the World Health Organization (WHO) classified it as a "Priority 2" microorganism in the recently published WHO Global Priority List of Antibiotic-Resistant Bacteria to Guide Research, Discovery, and Development of New antibiotics [6]. This document highlights the importance of developing new antibiotics to treat this disease, seeing as the existence of *N. gonorrhoeae* strains resistant to third generation cephalosporins and fluoroquinolones have already been reported.

In fact, failure of current dual therapy was detected in the United Kingdom in 2016. More importantly, the first "super-resistant" strains were recently reported in the United Kingdom and Australia, showing resistance against the current first line treatment, dual therapy with azithromycin and ceftriaxone [7,8].

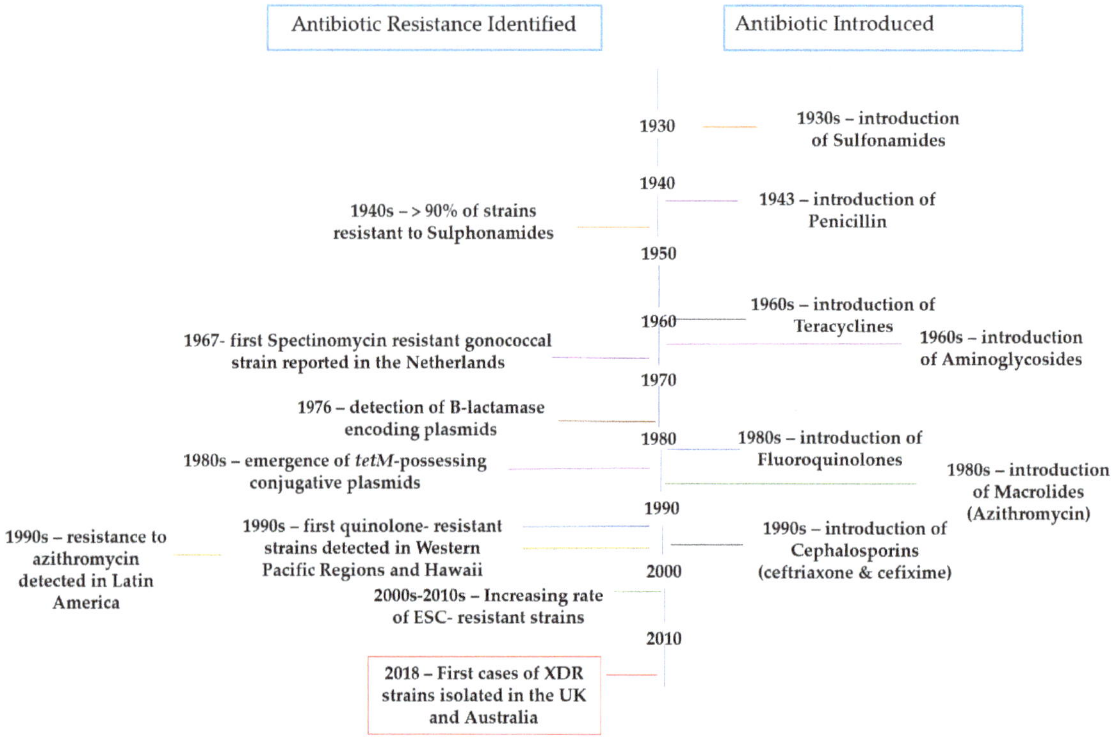

Figure 1. Timeline representing the introduction of treatments used against gonorrhea (right) and the first reports of resistance (left) [4,7,8].

Seeing as there is no gonococcal vaccine, control of the disease relies entirely on prevention, diagnosis, and, especially, antibiotic treatment [9]. It is for this reason that the present review focuses on current treatment options and the future perspectives for the treatment of this disease.

2. Current Treatment

Generally, treatment for gonococcal infection is given at the first clinical visit, which implies that antimicrobial susceptibility is rarely performed prior to prescription. According to WHO guidelines [10], first-line antimicrobial therapy must be highly effective, widely available and affordable, lack toxicity, comprise a single dose, and rapidly cure at least >95% of infected patients.

Different health organizations worldwide have established treatment guidelines against gonorrhea, mostly consisting of dual therapy with a single oral or intramuscular dose of a third-generation cephalosporin (250–500 mg intramuscular (IM) ceftriaxone or 400 mg per os-oral (PO) cefixime) in combination with a single oral dose of 1–2 g of azithromycin [11–17] (Table 1).

However, as it was mentioned earlier, these treatment options will not be useful in the near future, as they have already been reported as ineffective in treating some patients [7,8,18]. With this in mind, it is evident that, in the absence of a vaccine, the future control of this disease relies completely on the development of new antibiotics and alternative treatments.

Table 1. Different treatment guidelines for gonorrhea worldwide (all single dose).

WHO * [11]	Australasia [12]	Canada [13]	USA [14]	UK [15]	EU [16]	New Zealand [17]
Ceftriaxone 250 mg IM + Azithromycin 1 g PO Or ** Cefixime 400 mg PO + Azithromycin 1 g PO	Cetriaxone 500 mg IM + Azithromycin 1 g PO	Ceftriaxone 250 mg IM + Azithromycin 1 g PO	Ceftriaxone 250 mg IM + Azithromycin 1 g PO	Ceftriaxone 500 mg IM + Azithromycin 1 g PO	Ceftriaxone 500 mg IM + Azithromycin 1 g PO	Ceftriaxone 250 mg IM + Azithromycin 1 g PO
Ceftriaxone 500 mg IM + Azithromycin 2 g PO Or ** Cefixime 800 mg PO + Azithromycin 2 g PO Or ** Gentamicin 240 mg IM + Azithromycin 2 g PO Or ** Spectinomycin 2 g IM + Azithromycin 2 g PO		Cefixime 800 mg PO + Azithromycin 1 g PO Or ** Spectinomycin 2 g IM + Azithromycin 1 g PO	Cefixime 400 mg PO + Azithromycin 1 g PO	Cefixime 400 mg PO + Azithromycin 1 g PO Or ** Spectinomycin 2 g IM + Azithromycin 1 g PO Or ** Cefotaxime 500 mg IM + Azithromycin 1 g PO	Cefixime 400 mg PO + Azithromycin 2 g PO Or ** Spectinomycin 2 g IM + Azithromycin 2 g PO	Spectinomycin 2 g IM + Azithromycin 1 g PO Or ** Gentamicin 240 mg IM + Azithromycin 2 g PO

* WHO (World Health Organization); IM (Intramuscular); PO (Per os-oral) ** An "or" between combinations means that any of those combinations may be prescribed.

3. Future Perspectives

Seeing as drug resistance appears to be unstoppable, new treatment options are necessary in order to control the disease [19]. Three approaches are currently being followed for the development of new therapies against drug-resistant gonococci: (1) novel combinations of already existing antibiotics; (2) development of new antibiotics; and (3) development of alternative therapies, which might slow down the appearance of resistances (Table 2).

Table 2. Antigonococcal agents currently under development.

Future Options	Name	Action Mechanism	Structure	Reference
Drug repurposing	Sitafloxacin	DNA gyrase and topoisomerase IV inhibitor	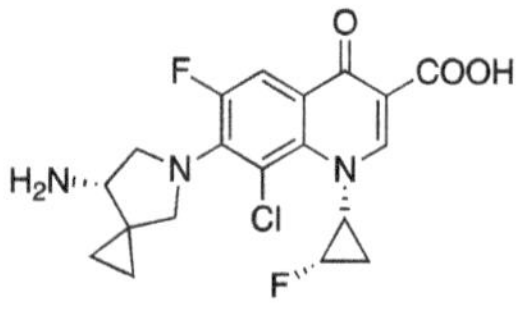	[20,21]
	Delafloxacin	DNA gyrase and topoisomerase IV inhibitor	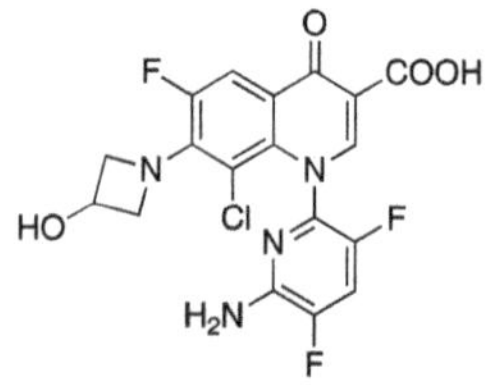	[22]
	Novel dual therapies	-	-	[23,24]
New antibacterial agents	Solithromycin	Protein synthesis inhibitor	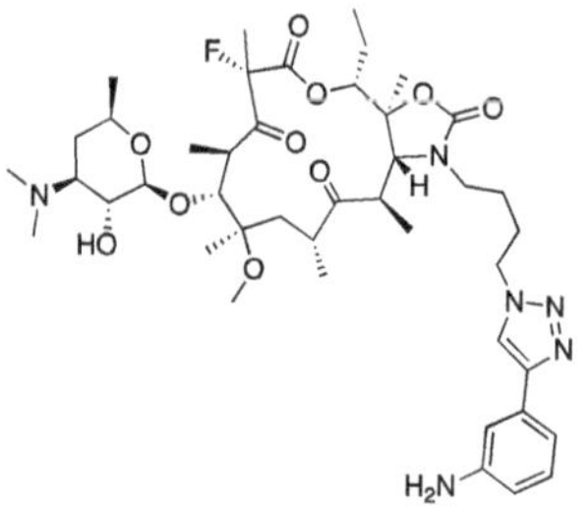	[25–27]
	Zoliflodacin	Spiropyrimidinetrione topoisomerase inhibitor	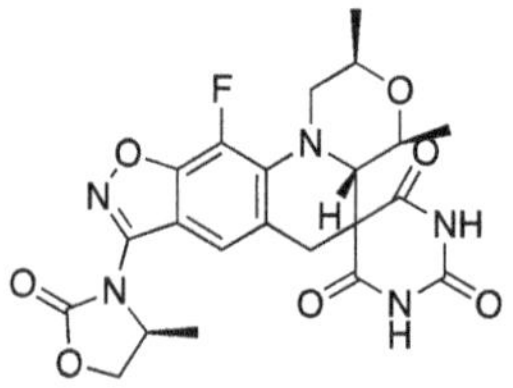	[28,29]
	Gepotidacin	DNA gyrase and topoisomerase IV inhibitor	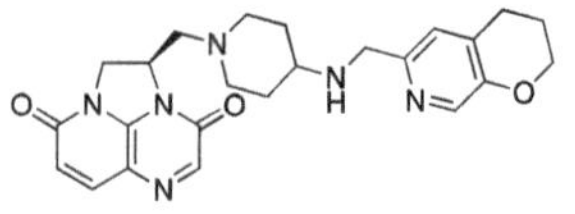	[25,30,31]
	Lefamulin	Protein synthesis inhibitor	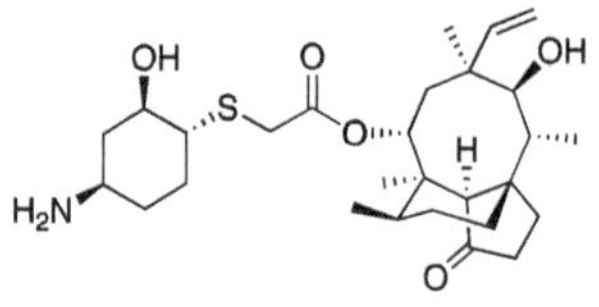	[32,33]
	Aminoethyl spectinomycins	Protein synthesis inhibitor	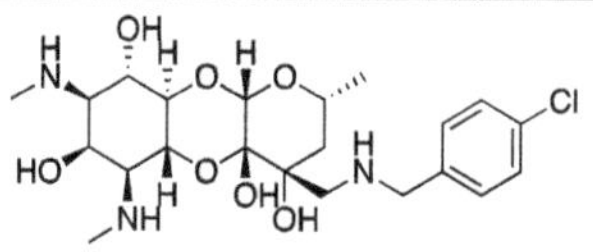	[34]
	PBP2 inhibitors	Inhibition of cell wall synthesis	-	[35]

Table 2. *Cont.*

Future Options	Name	Action Mechanism	Structure	Reference
Alternative therapies	IL-12	Induction of immune response	-	[36]
	Lactobacillus crispatus	Biosurfactant and acidic environment	-	[37]
	Monocaprin Myristoleic acid	Cell membrane disruption	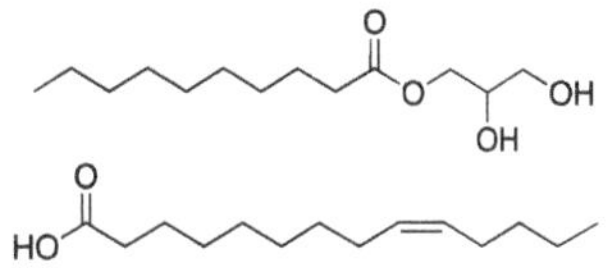	[38,39]
	Bacteriophage therapy	Lysis	-	[40,41]

3.1. Repurposing of Already Existing Antibiotics

Considering the fact that untreatable gonorrhea has indeed become a reality, the need for new treatment options has become a pressing issue. For this reason, the scientific community has turned to trying new combinations of already existing antibiotics as the fastest way to fight multi-resistant superbugs. Along these lines, Jönsson et al. studied the viability of introducing sitafloxacin, a newer-generation broad spectrum fluoroquinolone mostly used for respiratory infections, as part of a dual therapy against gonococci [20]. In the study, sitafloxacin was tested against a global gonococcal panel of 250 isolates, showing a rapid bactericidal effect with a Minimum Inhibitory Concentration (MIC) range of $\leq$0.001–1 mg/L. These results prove that sitafloxacin is a good candidate to be included in dual antimicrobial therapy for gonorrhea in cases with cephalosporin resistance or allergy.

Along these lines, another study focuses on the evaluation of sitafloxacin and five additional fluoroquinolones against ciprofloxacin-resistant *N. gonorrhoeae* isolates [21]. The in vitro potency of sitafloxacin was substantially higher compared with the other five fluoroquinolones, with an MIC range of 0.03–0.5 mg/L against the ciprofloxacin-resistant strains. These results further confirm the utility of sitafloxacin in dual antimicrobial therapy.

Another fluoroquinolone currently being studied for the treatment of gonorrhea is delafloxacin [22]. Soge et al. evaluated the activity of delafloxacin against 117 strains of *N. gonorrhoeae*. The results showed an MIC range of $\leq$0.001–0.25 μg/mL, which is higher than that of ciprofloxacin, penicillin, tetracycline, azithromycin, and spectinomycin. Further studies are required to correlate these promising in vitro results with clinical treatment outcomes.

On a similar note, Singh et al. assayed the potent utility of in vitro interactions of 21 dual therapy combinations against 95 *N. gonorrhoeae* strains [23]. Of these 21 combinations, five were novel introductions that are not included in any existing guidelines: gentamicin + ertapenem, moxifloxacin + ertapenem, spectinomycin + ertapenem, azithromycin + moxifloxacin, and cefixime + gentamicin. All five novel combinations produced high synergistic effects against the studied strains, which suggests that further in vivo evaluation in clinical trials should be performed in order to include these combinations for future treatment of gonorrhea.

Gentamicin is already included in several guidelines in combination with azithromycin as an alternative treatment option when main treatment options fail. A recent study examines the synergistic effect of this combination along with gentamicin combined with five other antimicrobials (cefixime, ceftriaxone, spectinomycin, azithromycin, moxifloxacin, and ertapenem) [24]. The study concludes that gentamicin in combination with ertapenem or cefixime could be introduced as new antimicrobial dual therapy seeing as these combinations showed maximum efficacy and synergism against 75 gonococcal strains.

3.2. New Antibiotics

However, seeing as gonococci have proven to be able to develop resistances to all antibiotics introduced for their treatment, the long-term solution includes the development of new antibiotics. Ideally, these new antibiotics should belong to antibacterial families different to the ones already included in treatment guidelines in order to delay the appearance of resistances as much as possible.

Along these lines, WHO launched the Global Antibiotic Research and Development Partnership (GARDP) in order to work with experts to draw a plan to meet the urgent need for new drugs to treat gonorrhea [25]. Within this partnership, experts analyze current drugs in clinical development for the treatment of this disease. Currently, only three molecules have reached clinical trials: Solithromycin, Zoliflodacin, and Gepotidacin.

Solithromycin is a broad-spectrum oral fluoroketolide which targets three prokaryotic ribosomal sites [26]. In vitro studies against 246 clinical isolates and international reference strains of N. gonorrhoeae showed promising results, with an MIC range of 0.001–32 μg/mL, showing more activity than the antimicrobials currently recommended for its treatment. Phase II clinical trials concluded with 100% efficacy for infection in men and women for all studied sites (genital, oral, and rectal) [27]. This drug is currently in Phase III trials.

As for Zoliflodacin, it has a novel action mechanism by which it inhibits the spiropyrimidinetrione topoisomerase [28]. Early in vitro studies showed promising results, with the compound being highly effective against clinical isolates from 21 European countries [29]. Zoliflodacin showed an MIC range of ≤0.002–0.25 μg/mL, considerably lower than that of most drugs currently being used for treatment but, most importantly, it did not present any cross-resistance to these antimicrobials.

Similarly, Farrell et al. studied the antigonococcal activity of Gepotidacin, a novel triazaacenaphthylene antibacterial which inhibits bacterial DNA gyrase and topoisomerase IV via a unique mechanism [30,42]. The compound had an MIC_{50} and MIC_{90} of 0.12 and 0.25 mg/L, respectively, against 25 *N. gonorrhoeae* strains, including five ciprofloxacin non-susceptible strains. Moreover, synergism studies showed that no antagonism occurred when gepotidacin was combined with levofloxacin, azithromycin, tetracycline, and ceftriaxone; while the combination of gepotidacin with moxifloxacin had a synergistic effect. This drug candidate underwent a Phase II evaluation, showing that oral doses of gepotidacin were ≥95% effective in treating uncomplicated urogenital gonorrhea [31].

Along with these three drugs in clinical trials, other compounds being developed to treat gonorrhea are still in early experimental phases. This is the case of Lefamulin, a novel semi-synthetic pleuromutilin, recently evaluated against 251 gonococcal clinical isolates, including multidrug-resistant and extensively-drug resistant samples [32]. The compound showed potent activity, an MIC range of 0.004–2 mg/L, against gonococcal isolates and no significant cross-resistance to other antimicrobials. Furthermore, this compound has also been proven to be active against the other most relevant bacterial pathogens causing sexually transmitted infections (STIs), *Chlamydia trachomatis* and *Mycoplasma genitalium*, proving to be a good candidate first-line antibiotic for the treatment of STIs [33]. However promising, further studies are required in order to consider the introduction of Lefamulin as a first-line treatment option.

For that matter, Butler et al. studied aminoethyl spectinomycins, a new class of semisynthetic analogs of the antibiotic spectinomycin, for the treatment of drug-resistant gonococci [34]. The studied compounds presented increased potency against *N. gonorrhoeae* compared to spectinomycin. Furthermore, these compounds also demonstrated activity against *C. trachomatis*, which is not observed with spectinomycin. The study concludes that aminoethyl spectinomycins are a promising alternative for spectinomycin and antibiotics such as ceftriaxone against drug-resistant gonorrhea, with the added benefit of treating chlamydial co-infections.

Furthermore, novel antibacterials in the earliest stages of drug design and screening have also been reported. Fedarovich et al. screened a 50,000 compound library for potential inhibitors of *N. gonorrhoeae* penicillin binding protein 2 (PBP 2) using fluorescence polarization [35]. The screening resulted in 32 compounds exhibiting >50% inhibition of Bocillin-FL binding to PBP 2, of which seven showed antimicrobial activity against susceptible and penicillin- or cephalosporin-resistant strains. These seven molecules remain as lead compounds for future optimization as anti-gonococcal agents.

3.3. Alternative Therapies

In addition to new antibiotics, alternative therapies to combat increasingly resistant *N. gonorrhoeae* are being developed. These alternatives are mainly focused on the prevention of recurring infections rather than on the treatment of the disease. In this regard, early in vivo studies have been performed regarding the intravaginal administration of interleukin-12 (IL-12) in mice [36]. The study concludes that intravaginally administered IL-12 promotes the Th1-driven adaptive immune response, including the production of specific anti-gonococcal antibodies which would prevent recurring infection.

On a similar note, Foschi et al. studied the efficacy of vaginal lactobacilli in reducing *N. gonorrhoeae* viability [37]. The study assessed the anti-gonococcal activity of 14 vaginal *Lactobacillus* strains belonging to *L. crispatus, L. gasseri,* and *L. vaginalis.* It was found that the acidic environment associated with lactobacilli metabolism is extremely effective in counteracting gonococcal growth, with complete abolishment of gonococci viability being observed at pH < 4.0. Furthermore, results showed that lactobacilli cells are able to reduce viability and co-aggregate with gonococci. This is achieved by released-surface components with biosurfactant properties produced by lactobacilli. The study concludes that specific *Lactobacillus* strains, mainly belonging to *L. crispatus*, are able to counteract gonococcal viability through multiple mechanisms, representing a new potential probiotic strategy for the prevention of infection in women.

Prophylaxis is especially important during pregnancy, seeing as neonatal conjunctivitis is commonly caused by *N. gonorrhoeae* [38]. The most common approach is ophthalmic prophylaxis with antibiotic ointments. However, due to the increasing appearance of resistances, these are becoming less effective. Churchward et al. studied 37 fatty acids or fatty acid derivatives for fast antigonococcal activity [39]. Two lead candidates, monocaprin and myristoleic acid, were bactericidal at 1 mM and remained active in artificial tear fluid, becoming promising alternatives to conventional antibacterial ointments. They went on to study the ability of *N. gonorrhoeae* to develop resistance when grown in sub-lethal concentrations of monocaprin [43]. Results showed that, after growing gonococci on growth media containing sub-lethal concentrations of monocaprin, the MIC showed a two-fold change, which cannot be considered as the development of resistance. Thus, the study concludes that *N. gonorrhoeae* in not capable of developing resistances against monocaprin, making it an ideal long-term alternative for neonatal conjunctivitis prophylaxis.

Another alternative treatment that has gained importance recently is bacteriophage therapy, as a therapeutic option on its own and also in combination with currently used antimicrobials [44,45]. However promising, this type of therapy is still in early stages when it comes to treating gonorrhea. Experiments with peptide inhibitors targeting gonococci identified using phage display have been reported in recent years [40,41]. Connor et al. constructed open reading frame phagemid (pHORF) oligopeptide phage display libraries of the entire *N. gonorrhoeae* genome, identifying six immunogenic proteins for the first time and verifying 13 additional proteins as immunogenic in *N. gonorrhoeae* [40]. Similarly, Sikora et al. focused on targeting the nitrite reductase AniA, a key component of gonococcal anaerobic respiration and biofilm formation [41]. One of the 29 unique peptides identified, C7-3, and its derivative (C7-3m2), demonstrated potent inhibition of AniA, with an MIC50 value of 0.6 mM against anaerobically grown *N. gonorrhoeae*. These studies show promising results towards the development of bacteriophage therapy for the treatment of gonorrhea; however, further studies are required in this field.

4. Conclusions

Neisseria gonorrhoeae is a public health threat worldwide due to the increasing number of antibiotic-resistant strains. Current treatment guidelines include first-line treatments, as well as alternative treatments which should only be prescribed in case of allergy or presence of resistance. However, most of these guidelines are already being challenged by this "Superbug". This has led the scientific community to develop new antibiotics and alternative therapies in order to control this disease. These new treatment options require not only high antigonococcal potency, but also no cross-resistance with current antibiotics in order to assure their applicability in the long-run. Alternative therapies, on the other hand, have focused on preventing infections rather than treating them and, therefore, controlling the disease before it has a chance of developing further resistances.

Author Contributions: B.S.-G. conceived and wrote the paper and M.T.P.-G. conceived and wrote the paper.

Funding: This research received no external funding.

References

1. World Health Organization (WHO). *Global Action Plan to Control the Spread and Impact of Antimicrobial Resistance in Neisseria gonorrhoeae*; WHO: Geneva, Switzerland, 2012; Available online: http://apps.who.int/iris/bitstream/10665/44863/1/9789241503501_eng.pdf (accessed on 15 May 2018).
2. Bolan, G.A.; Sparling, P.F.; Wasserheit, J.N. The emerging threat of untreatable gonococcal infection. *N. Engl. J. Med.* **2012**, *366*, 485–487. [CrossRef] [PubMed]
3. Hook, E.W., 3rd; Kirkcaldy, R.D. A Brief History of Evolving Diagnostics and Therapy for Gonorrhea: Lessons Learned. *Clin. Infect. Dis.* **2018**. [CrossRef] [PubMed]
4. Unemo, M.; Del Rio, C.; Shafer, W.M. *Emerging Infections 10*; Scheld, W.M., Hughes, J.M., Whitley, R.J., Eds.; American Society for Microbiology: Washington, DC, USA, 2016; Chapter 12.
5. Centers for Disease Control and Prevention (CDC). *Cephalosporin-Resistant Neisseria gonorrhoeae Public Health Response Plan*; CDC: Atlanta, GA, USA, 2012; pp. 1–43.
6. World Health Organization (WHO). *Global Priority List of Antibiotic-Resistant Bacteria to Guide Research, Discovery, and Development of New Antibiotics*; WHO: Geneva, Switzerland, 2017; Available online: http://www.who.int/medicines/publications/WHO-PPL-Short_Summary_25Feb-ET_NM_WHO.pdf (accessed on 15 May 2018).
7. Public Health England. *UK Case of Neisseria gonorrhoeae with High-Level Resistance to Azithromycin and Resistance to Ceftriaxone Acquired Abroad*; Health Protection Report; Public Health England: London, UK, 2018; Volume 12.
8. Australian Government. Department of Health. Multi-Drug Resistant Gonorrhoea. 2018. Available online: http://www.health.gov.au/internet/main/publishing.nsf/Content/mr-yr18-dept-dept004.htm (accessed on 15 May 2018).
9. Suay-Garcia, B.; Pérez-Gracia, M.T. Drug-Resistant *Neisseria gonorrhoeae*: Latest developments. *Eur. J. Clin. Microbiol. Infect. Dis.* **2017**, *36*, 1065–1071. [CrossRef] [PubMed]
10. World Health Organization (WHO). Strategies and Laboratory Methods for Strengthening Surveillance of Sexually Transmitted Infections. Available online: http://www.who.int/reproductivehealth/publications/rtis/9789241504478/en/ (accessed on 22 April 2018).
11. World Health Organization (WHO). Guidelines for the Treatment of Neisseria gonorrhoeae. Available online: http://www.who.int/reproductivehealth/publications/rtis/gonorrhoea-treatment-guidelines/en/ (accessed on 22 April 2018).
12. Australasia Sexual Health Alliance. Australian STI Management Guidelines for Use in Primary Care. Available online: http://www.sti.guidelines.org.au/sexually-transmissible-infections/gonorrhoea (accessed on 22 April 2018).
13. Public Health Agency of Canada. Canadian Guidelines on Sexually Transmitted Infections. Available online: https://www.canada.ca/en/public-health/services/infectious-diseases/sexual-health-sexually-transmitted-infections/canadian-guidelines/sexually-transmitted-infections/canadian-guidelines-sexually-transmitted-infections-34.html (accessed on 22 April 2018).
14. Bignell, C.; Unemo, M.; European STI Guidelines Editorial Board. European Guideline on the Diagnosis and Treatment of Gonorrhea in Adults. *Int. J. STD AIDS* **2013**, *24*, 85–92. [CrossRef] [PubMed]
15. Centers for Disease Control and Prevention (CDC). Sexually Transmitted Diseases Treatment Guidelines. Available online: https://www.cdc.gov/std/tg2015/gonorrhea.htm (accessed on 22 April 2018).

16. Bignell, C.; Fitzgerald, M.; Guideline Development Group; British Association for Sexual Health and HIV UK. UK national guideline for the management of gonorrhea in adults. *Int. J. STD AIDS* **2011**, *22*, 541–547. [CrossRef] [PubMed]
17. The New Zealand Sexual Health Society. New Zealand Guideline for the Management of Gonorrhea, 2014, and Response to the Threat of Antimicrobial Resistance. Available online: http://www.nzshs.org/docman/guidelines/best-practice-guidelines/142-new-zealand-guideline-for-the-management-of-gonorrhoea-2014-and-response-to-the-threat-of-antimicrobial-resistance/file (accessed on 22 April 2018).
18. Fifer, H.; Natarajan, U.; Jones, L.; Alexander, S.; Hughes, G.; Golparian, D.; Unemo, M. Failure of Dual Antimicrobial Therapy in Treatment of Gonorrhea. *N. Engl. J. Med.* **2016**, *734*, 2504–2506. [CrossRef] [PubMed]
19. Lee, H.; Lee, K.; Chong, Y. New treatment options for infections caused by increasingly antimicrobial-resistant *Neisseria gonorrhoeae*. *Exp. Rev. Anti-Infect. Ther.* **2016**, *14*, 243–256. [CrossRef] [PubMed]
20. Jönsson, A.; Sunniva, F.; Golparian, D.; Hamasuna, R.; Jacobsson, S.; Lindberg, M.; Jensen, J.S.; Ohnishi, M.; Unemo, M. In vitro activity and time-kill curve analysis of sitafloxacin against a global panel of antimicrobial-resistant and multidrug-resistant *Neisseria gonorrhoeae* isolates. *APMIS* **2018**, *126*, 29–37. [CrossRef] [PubMed]
21. Hamasuna, R.; Ohnishi, M.; Matsumoto, M.; Okumura, R.; Unemo, M.; Matsumoto, T. In vitro activity of sitafloxacin and additional newer generation Fluoroquinolones against ciprofloxacin-resistant *Neisseria gonorrhoeae* isolates. *Microb. Drug Resist.* **2018**, *24*, 30–34. [CrossRef] [PubMed]
22. Soge, O.O.; Salipante, S.J.; No, D.; Duffy, E.; Roberts, M.C. In Vitro Activity of Delafloxacin against Clinical *Neisseria gonorrhoeae* Isolates and Selection of Gonococcal Delafloxacin Resistance. *Antimicrob. Agents Chemother.* **2016**, *60*, 3106–3111. [CrossRef] [PubMed]
23. Singh, V.; Bala, M.; Bhargava, A.; Kakran, M.; Bhatnagar, R. In vitro efficacy of 21 dual antimicrobial combinations comprising novel and currently recommended combinations for treatment of drug resistant gonorrhoea in future era. *PLoS ONE* **2018**, *13*, e0193678. [CrossRef] [PubMed]
24. Singh, V.; Bala, M.; Bhargava, A.; Kakran, M.; Bhatnagar, R. In vitro synergy testing of gentamicin, an old drug suggested as future treatment option for gonorrhoea, in combination with six other antimicrobials against multidrug-resistant *Neisseria gonorrhoeae* strains. *Sex. Transm. Dis.* **2018**, *45*, 127–131. [CrossRef] [PubMed]
25. Alirol, E.; Wi, T.E.; Bala, M.; Bazzo, M.L.; Chen, X.S.; Deal, C.; Dillon, J.R.; Kularatne, R.; Heim, J.; Hooft van Huijsduijnen, R.; et al. Multidrug-resistant gonorrhea: A research and development roadmap to discover new medicines. *PLoS Med.* **2017**, *14*, e1002366. [CrossRef] [PubMed]
26. Golparian, D.; Fernandes, P.; Ohnishi, M.; Jensen, J.S.; Unemo, M. In vitro activity of the new fluoroketolide solithromycin (CEM-101) against a large collection of clinical *Neisseria gonorrhoeae* isolates and international reference strains, including those with high-level antimicrobial resistance: Potential treatment option for gonorrhea? *Antimicrob. Agents Chemother.* **2012**, *56*, 2739–2742. [PubMed]
27. Hook, E.W., 3rd; Golden, M.; Jamieson, B.D.; Dixon, P.B.; Harbison, H.S.; Lowens, S.; Fernandes, P. A Phase 2 Trial of Oral Solithromycin 1200 mg or 1000 mg as Single-Dose Oral Therapy for Uncomplicated Gonorrhea. *Clin. Infect. Dis.* **2015**, *61*, 1043–1048. [CrossRef] [PubMed]
28. Huband, M.D.; Bradford, P.A.; Otterson, L.G.; Basarab, G.S.; Kutschke, A.C.; Giacobbe, R.A.; Patey, S.A.; Alm, R.A.; Johnstone, M.R.; Potter, M.E.; et al. In vitro antibacterial activity of AZD0914, a new spiropyrimidinetrione DNA gyrase/topoisomerase inhibitor with potent activity against Gram-positive, fastidious Gram-Negative, and atypical bacteria. *Antimicrob. Agents Chemother.* **2015**, *59*, 467–474. [CrossRef] [PubMed]
29. Unemo, M.; Ringlander, J.; Wiggins, C.; Fredlund, H.; Jacobsson, S.; Cole, M. High in vitro susceptibility to the novel spiropyrimidinetrione ETX0914 (AZD0914) among 873 contemporary clinical *Neisseria gonorrhoeae* isolates from 21 European countries from 2012 to 2014. *Antimicrob. Agents Chemother.* **2015**, *59*, 5220–5225. [CrossRef] [PubMed]
30. Farrell, D.J.; Sader, H.S.; Rhomberg, P.R.; Scangarella-Oman, N.E.; Flamm, R.K. In vitro Activity of Gepotidacin (GSK2140944) against *Neisseria gonorrhoeae*. *Antimicrob. Agents Chemother.* **2017**, *61*, e02047-16. [CrossRef] [PubMed]

31. Taylor, S.N.; Morris, D.H.; Avery, A.K.; Workowski, K.A.; Batteiger, B.E.; Tiffany, C.A.; Perry, C.R.; Raychaudhuri, A.; Scangarella-Oman, N.E.; Hossain, M.; et al. Gepotidacin for the Treatment of Uncomplicated Urogenital Gonorrhea: A Phase 2, Randomized, Dose-Ranging, Single-Oral Dose Evaluation. *Clin. Infect. Dis.* **2018**. [CrossRef] [PubMed]
32. Jacobsson, S.; Paukner, S.; Golparian, D.; Jensen, J.S.; Unemo, M. In vitro activity of the novel pleuromutilin lefamulin (BC-3781) and effect of efflux pump inactivation on multidrug-resistant and extensively-drug resistant *Neisseria gonorrhoeae*. *Antimicrob. Agents Chemother.* **2017**, *61*, e01497. [CrossRef] [PubMed]
33. Paukner, S.; Gruss, A.; Jensen, J.S. In Vitro Activity of Lefamulin against Sexually Transmitted Bacterial Pathogens. *Antimicrob. Agents Chemother.* **2018**, *62*, e02380-17. [CrossRef] [PubMed]
34. Butler, M.M.; Waidyarachchi, S.L.; Connolly, K.L.; Jerse, A.E.; Chai, W.; Lee, R.E.; Kohlhoff, S.A.; Shinabarger, D.L.; Bowlin, T.L. Aminoethyl spectinomycins as therapeutics for drug-resistant gonorrhea and chlamydial co-infections. *Antimicrob. Agents Chemother.* **2018**, *65*. [CrossRef]
35. Fedarovich, A.; Djordjevic, K.A.; Swanson, S.M.; Peterson, Y.K.; Nicholas, R.A.; Davies, C. High-Throughput Screening for Novel Inhibitors of *Neisseria gonorrhoeae* Penicillin-Binding Protein 2. *PLoS ONE* **2012**, *7*, e44918. [CrossRef] [PubMed]
36. Liu, Y.; Perez, J.; Hammer, L.A.; Gallagher, H.C.; de Jesus, M.; Egilmez, N.K.; Russell, M.W. Intravaginal Administration of Interleukin 12 during Genital Gonococcal Infection in Mice Induces Immunity to Heterologous Strains of *Neisseria gonorrhoeae*. *mSphere* **2018**, *3*, e00421. [CrossRef] [PubMed]
37. Foschi, C.; Salvo, M.; Cevenini, R.; Parolin, C.; Vitali, B.; Marangoni, A. Vaginal Lactobacilli Reduce *Neisseria gonorrhoeae* Viability through Multiple Strategies: An in vitro Study. *Front. Cell Infect. Microbiol.* **2017**, *7*, 502. [CrossRef] [PubMed]
38. Darling, E.K.; McDonald, H. A meta-analysis of the efficacy of ocular prophylactic agents used for the prevention of gonococcal and chlamydial ophtalmia neonatorum. *J. Midwif. Womens Health* **2010**, *55*, 319–327. [CrossRef] [PubMed]
39. Churchward, C.P.; Alany, R.G.; Kirk, R.S.; Walker, A.J.; Snyder, L.A.S. Prevention of Ophthalmia Neonatorum Caused by *Neisseria gonorrhoeae* Using a Fatty Acid-Based Formulation. *MBio* **2017**, *8*, e00534-17. [CrossRef] [PubMed]
40. Connor, D.O.; Zantow, J.; Hust, M.; Bier, F.F.; von Nickisch-Rosenegk, M. Identification of Novel Immunogenic Proteins of *Neisseria gonorrhoeae* by Phage Display. *PLoS ONE* **2016**, *11*, e0148986. [CrossRef] [PubMed]
41. Sikora, A.E.; Mills, R.H.; Weber, J.V.; Hamza, A.; Passow, B.W.; Romaine, A.; Williamson, Z.A.; Reed, R.W.; Zielke, R.A.; Korotkov, K.V. Peptide Inhibitors Targeting the *Neisseria gonorrhoeae* Pivotal Anaerobic Respiration Factor AniA. *Antimicrob. Agents Chemother.* **2017**, *61*, e00186-17. [CrossRef] [PubMed]
42. Biedenbach, D.J.; Bouchillon, S.K.; Hackel, M.; Miller, L.A.; Scangarella-Oman, N.E.; Jakielaszek, C.; Sahm, D.F. In Vitro Activity of Gepotidacin, a Novel Triazaacenaphthylene Bacterial Topoisomerase Inhibitor, against a Broad Spectrum of Bacterial Pathogens. *Antimicrob. Agents Chemother.* **2016**, *60*, 1918–1923. [CrossRef] [PubMed]
43. Churchward, C.P.; Calder, A.; Snyder, L.A.S. Mutations in *Neisseria gonorrhoeae* grown in sub-lethal concentrations of monocaprin do not confer resistance. *PLoS ONE* **2018**, *13*, e0195453. [CrossRef] [PubMed]
44. Golkar, K.; Bagasra, O.; Pace, D.G. Bacteriophage therapy: A potential solution for the antibiotic resistance crisis. *J. Infect. Dev. Ctries.* **2014**, *8*, 129–136. [CrossRef] [PubMed]
45. Lin, D.M.; Koskella, B.; Lin, H.C. Phage therapy: An alternative to antibiotics in the age of multi-drug resistance. *World J. Gastrointest. Pharmacol. Ther.* **2017**, *8*, 162–173. [CrossRef] [PubMed]

10

Decreasing Inappropriate Use of Antibiotics in Primary Care in Four Countries in South America—Cluster Randomized Controlled Trial

Inés Urbiztondo [1], Lars Bjerrum [1], Lidia Caballero [2], Miguel Angel Suarez [3], Monica Olinisky [4] and Gloria Córdoba [1,*]

1 The Research Unit for General Practice and Section of General Practice, Department of Public Health, University of Copenhagen, 1353 Copenhagen, Denmark; inesurbiztondo@gmail.com (I.U.); lbjerrum@sund.ku.dk (L.B.)
2 Dr. Pedro Baliña Hospital, Public Health Ministry, Posadas 3300, Misiones, Argentina; lidia.gladis@gmail.com
3 Policlínica Central de la Caja Nacional de Salud, La Paz 15000, Bolivia; sucumian@gmail.com
4 Department of Family and Community Medicine, Faculty of Medicine, University of the Republic, Montevideo 11600, Uruguay; molinisky@gmail.com
* Correspondence: gloriac@sund.ku.dk

Academic Editor: Jeffrey Lipman

Abstract: High antibiotic prescribing and antimicrobial resistance in patients attending primary care have been reported in South America. Very few interventions targeting general practitioners (GPs) to decrease inappropriate antibiotic prescribing have been investigated in this region. This study assessed the effectiveness of online feedback on reducing antibiotic prescribing in patients with suspected respiratory tract infections (RTIs) attending primary care. The aim was to reduce antibiotic prescribing in patients with acute bronchitis and acute otitis media. Both are RTIs for which antibiotics have a very limited effect. A cluster randomized two-arm control trial was implemented. Healthcare centres from Bolivia, Argentina, Paraguay and Uruguay participating in the quality improvement program HAPPY AUDIT were randomly allocated to either intervention or control group. During ten consecutive weeks, GPs in the intervention group received evidence-based online feedback on the management of suspected RTIs. In patients with acute bronchitis, the intervention reduced the antibiotic prescribing rate from 71.6% to 56% (control group from 61.2% to 52%). In patients with acute otitis media, the intervention reduced the antibiotic prescribing from 94.8% to 86.2% (no change in the control group). In all RTIs, the intervention reduced antibiotic prescribing rate from 37.4% to 28.1% (control group from 29% to 27.2%). Online evidence-based feedback is effective for reducing antibiotic prescribing in patients with RTIs attending primary care in South America.

Keywords: antibiotics; educational intervention; general practice

---

1. Introduction

Inappropriate use of antibiotics generates Antimicrobial Resistance (AMR), which represents a serious threat for societal development due to its health and economic impact [1,2].

Antimicrobial resistance (AMR) is an increasing global problem. Studies have found a high prevalence of AMR in several countries in Latin America, particularly for pathogens involved in community acquired respiratory tract infections (RTIs) [3–5] such as *Streptococcus pneumoniae, Haemophilus influenza*, and *Moraxella catarrhalis*. For example, the latest report from the World Health

Organization on antimicrobial resistance found a prevalence of *Streptococcus pneumoniae* resistant to penicillin of 65% in Bolivia and 30% in Argentina [1].

There is a lack of data on the use of antibiotics in South America. In a previous study [6], we found that general practitioners (GPs) from Argentina prescribed antibiotics on average to 41% of the patients consulting with respiratory tract symptoms. Population-based data have shown an increase in antibiotic consumption [7]. This study analyzed consumption of antibiotics between 1997 and 2007 in eight Latin American countries. In general, there was an increase in consumption of antibiotics and great variation across countries. For example, in Uruguay, during this period, the consumption of antibiotics increased from 5.43 Defined Daily Dosis per 1000 inhabitants per day (DID) in 1997 to 8.90 DID in 2007. Argentina maintained high levels of consumption 16.64 DID. In all countries, there was a significant increase in the consumption of broad-spectrum antibiotics. These types of antibiotics are those with the highest probability of triggering AMR. Due to the high prevalence of AMR and high use of antibiotics in South America, effective interventions should be implemented to reduce antibiotic overprescription.

The implementation of effective interventions to reduce inappropriate prescription of antibiotics in primary care in Latin America is challenging. Not only is it important to take into consideration the fragmented health care systems (e.g., differing populations between general practitioners depending on the type of health insurance the patient belong to), but also the problem of poor compliance with regulations to prohibit the sale of antibiotics over the counter [8].

RTIs are the most common reasons for antibiotic prescribing in primary care [9]. Most RTIs are caused by a virus, and in the majority of patients, antibiotics have no beneficial effect [10,11]. In a previous observational study [6], high antibiotic prescribing rates for acute bronchitis and otitis media were found. Acute bronchitis is mainly a viral infection [11], while the prescription of antibiotics in patients with Acute Otitis media requires the fulfillment of specific criteria [10].

Several strategies have been developed to reduce inappropriate prescribing of antibiotics in primary care. A systematic review comparing different interventions in primary care found that interventions aimed at reducing overall antibiotic prescribing were more effective than interventions focusing on the right choice of antibiotics [12]. A more recent review concluded that antibiotic use could be improved by educational interventions such as dissemination of printed/audiovisual educational materials, group education, personal or group feed-back, individual outreach visits, reminders at the time of prescribing, computer-assisted decision-making systems, among others. Both reviews agree on pointing out that a greater effect is achieved with multi-faceted interventions [12,13].

It is difficult to assess which element of a multifaceted program is the one driving behaviour change. Hence, as part of the quality improvement program: HAPPY AUDIT (Health Alliance for Prudent Prescribing, Yield and Use of Anti-microbial Drugs in the Treatment of Respiratory Tract Infections), we sought to assess the added effect of online evidence-based feedback.

HAPPY AUDIT South America was launched in 2013. GPs from Argentina, Bolivia, Uruguay, and Paraguay were invited to participate in a quality improvement cycle to decrease the inappropriate prescription of antibiotics in patients with suspected RTI. As part of the quality improvement cycle, all GPs collected data about their prescribing decision between June–August 2014. In March 2015, GPs in every country were invited to a two-day meeting to talk about the personal prescribing report in comparison to the general report at country and the South American level. Furthermore, GPs discussed about the challenges for the diagnosis process, as there is no national guidelines and availability of point-of-care-tests (POCTs). Afterwards, they were given educational material for their patients about the most common respiratory tract infections. Between June–August 2015 GPs registered again their prescribing decisions. During this second data collection, some GPs were randomly exposed to the evidence-based online feedback intervention.

This analysis aimed at assessing the effectiveness of online evidence-based feedback on reducing antibiotic prescribing in patients with suspected respiratory tract infection, especially in patients with the diagnoses of acute bronchitis and acute otitis media in four South-American countries.

2. Results

Table 1 shows baseline characteristics of participating GPs. There were no statistically significant differences in baseline characteristics between GPs in the intervention and control group. In 2014, 110 health care centres were randomized to intervention or control group. There were completed data from 73 health care centres; 36 (50 GPs) in the intervention arm and 37 (67 GPs) in the control arm—see Figure 1.

Table 1. Baseline characteristics of participating general practitioners (GPs).

Characteristics	Intervention Group (36 Groups; 50 GPs)	Control Group (37 Groups; 67 GPs)	*p*
Women	33 (66%)	45 (67%)	0.8
Age *	40 (8)	38 (8)	0.1
Specialization in general practice	28 (56%)	35 (52%)	0.6
>10 years work experience	17 (34%)	24 (36%)	0.8
Urban practice	29 (58%)	37 (55%)	0.7
Number of consultations per day *	24 (8)	21 (11)	0.1
High prescribers ¥	16 (32%)	14 (21%)	0.1

* Mean (SD), ¥ GPs prescribing antibiotics to more than 75% of their patients.

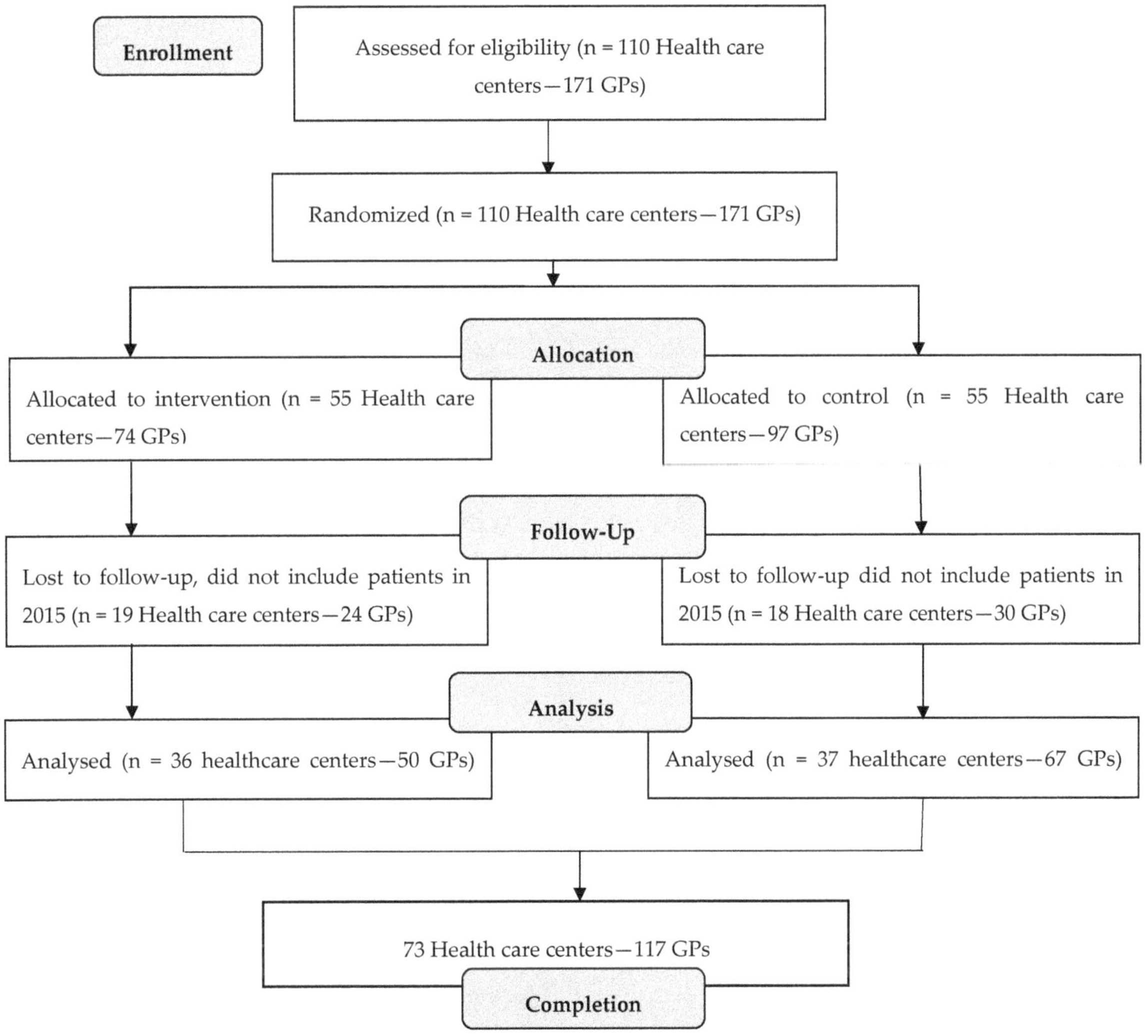

Figure 1. Flow chart of the study population.

In 2014 (before intervention), 8482 patients were registered. 2805 (33%) patients received an antibiotic prescription. In 2015 (after intervention), 8052 patients were registered; 2225 (28%) received an antibiotic prescription.

Adherence and use of the online feedback intervention were tracked in the program surveyexact. Participation was above 90% for each of the clinical cases.

Table 2 shows the antibiotic prescribing rates for acute bronchitis and acute otitis media before and after the intervention. For acute bronchitis, the intervention group reduced the antibiotic prescribing rate from 71.6% to 56% (difference 15.6%, 95%Confidence Interval (CI) 8.3; 22.7), and the control group reduced the antibiotic prescribing rate from 61.2% to 52.1% (difference 9.1%, 95%CI 2; 16). For acute otitis media, the intervention group reduced the antibiotic prescribing rate from 94.8% to 86.2% (difference 8.6%, 95%CI 0.5; 18). There was no change in antibiotic prescribing in the control group. For all RTIs, the intervention group reduced the antibiotic prescribing rate from 37.4% to 28.1% (difference 9.3%, 95%CI 7.1; 11), and the control group reduced the antibiotic prescribing rate from 29% to 27.2% (difference 1.8%, 95%CI 0.08; 3.6).

Table 2. Prescription of antibiotics in 2014 and 2015.

Outcomes	2014		2015		Difference in Proportions
	Patients	Prescribed Antibiotics (%)	Patients	Prescribed Antibiotics (%)	
Acute bronchitis					
Intervention	381	71.6	327	56	15.6 (CI 8.3; 22.7)
Control	431	61.2	378	52.1	9.1 (CI 2; 16)
Total	812	66	705	54	12 (CI 6.9; 16)
Otitis media					
Intervention	155	94.8	87	86.2	8.6 (CI 0.5; 18)
Control	138	79	134	82	3 (CI −6; 12)
Total	293	87	221	83.7	3 (CI −3; 9.9)
All RTI					
Intervention	4050	37.4	3644	28.1	9.3 (CI 7.1; 11)
Control	4433	29	4408	27.2	1.8 (CI −0.08; 3.6)
Total	8483	33	8052	28	5 (CI 3.9; 6.8)

Table 3 shows the results of the hierarchical logistic models. There was a significant reduction in antibiotic prescribing for acute bronchitis in both the intervention and the control group. The reduction in antibiotic prescribing in patients with acute bronchitis was higher in the intervention group (OR 0.25 95%CI 0.15; 0.42) than in the control group (OR 0.60 95%CI 0.38; 0.94), ($p = 0.001$).

Table 3. Reduction in prescription of antibiotics in patients with suspected RTI within and across randomization groups.

Outcomes	OR	95%CI	*p* Value ¥
Acute bronchitis			
Intervention	0.25	0.15; 0.42	0.001
Control	0.60	0.38; 0.94	
Acute Otitis			
Intervention	0.32	0.10; 1.01	0.05
Control	1.06	0.49; 2.28	
All RTI			
Intervention	0.59	0.53; 0.65	<0.001
Control	0.82	0.74; 0.91	

¥ *p* value of the interaction term: intervention * year—added value of the intervention.

3. Discussion

3.1. Summary of Main Findings

Overall, there was a decrease in antibiotic prescribing for patients with acute bronchitis, acute otitis media and in all patients with a suspected RTI. The reduction was significantly higher in the intervention group compared to the control group. A possible explanation for the reduction in antibiotic prescribing in both groups can be the participation in the HAPPY AUDIT cycle alongside the cluster randomized control trial. This could have made all participants more aware of their antibiotic prescribing. Nonetheless, a larger effect in the intervention group indicates that exposure to online feedback on evidence-based management of RTI can bring about a larger effect in the reduction of unnecessary prescriptions.

3.2. Strengths and Weaknesses of the Study

The results are based on data from 117 GPs and 16,535 patients across four countries in South America. The large sample size allowed accurate assessment of the decrease in antibiotic prescribing for the selected diagnoses: acute bronchitis, acute otitis media, and overall.

The online feedback intervention was assessed as an added feature of the quality improvement program HAPPY AUDIT. This program is based on the methodology of a medical audit developed by the Audit Project Odense group [14]. This methodology relies on voluntary participation and a bottom-up approach in which GPs themselves set their own improvement goals.

On the one hand, the voluntary participation of GPs affects the external validity of these findings. Previous research has shown that GPs participating in quality improvement programs or research tend to prescribe fewer antibiotics [15,16]. Part of the reduction may have been caused by the desire to improve their prescribing behaviour. Nonetheless, the intervention group had a larger decrease in comparison to the control group (also motivated to decrease their prescribing).

On the other hand, the voluntary participation guarantee that the recording of the data did not suffer from observation bias (i.e., change in prescribing behaviour due to participation in a research program). All participants were interested in knowing their prescribing pattern to set their own quality improvement goals. Hence, they were very interested in recording data as requested to obtain an accurate assessment of the change in their prescribing pattern. Regarding the second registration, GPs were not informed that the primary success outcome for the assessment of the online feedback intervention was a decrease in prescriptions for acute bronchitis. This ensured that they were not focusing on this diagnosis or changing the label from acute bronchitis to Pneumonia to justify the prescription of antibiotics (see Supplementary Materials Table S1).

There were no differences in the exposure to the intervention among the participating practices. All practices in the intervention group received the same information through the same channel (e-mail/surveyxact program). This is an important characteristic of the intervention because it overcomes the limitations of different peer academic detailers, who might influence the results of the intervention depending on their pedagogical skills [17].

Allocation bias at the practice level was reduced by using a computer-based allocation process. The allocation was performed before the first data collection, so there was no information about the prescribing pattern of the GPs. Furthermore, the person running the allocation did not know the GPs or have any contact with the GPs during the whole study.

Cross-contamination was minimised by allocation at the practice level. This ensured that GPs working in the same health care center were in the same randomization groups. Furthermore, the allocation was stratified by solo (one GP per health care center) or group (two or more GPs per health care center) practices. It was done to achieve a balance in the number of GPs in both randomization groups. Due to the large variation in the number of GPs per health care centre, there were more GPs in the control group.

We sought to reduce diagnostic misclassification by using the same data collection instruments before and after the intervention. The data collection instrument was designed based on the APO methodology [18], so GPs used a very small amount of time during the consultation to record the main characteristics of the patient and the treatment decision.

The cluster-randomized trial was carried out alongside the HAPPY AUDIT quality improvement program. This methodology relies on data collection under daily practice conditions. Hence, we cannot rule out diagnostic misclassification. There are no national guidelines, and the lack of POCTs makes it difficult to standardized diagnostic criteria in everyday practice. However, the similar distribution of diagnoses between 2014 and 2015 may indicate that there was no a differential misclassification during the two periods of data collection (Supplementary Materials Table S1).

There was a one-year difference between the two data collection periods. During this period, GPs could have been exposed to other types of interventions like public health campaigns or courses about appropriate use of antibiotics, which would have contributed to the decrease in the prescription of antibiotics. Unfortunately, for the GPs working within the South American context, there is a worrisome lack of engagement by the public health authorities and other scientific bodies to decrease the unnecessary prescription of antibiotics in primary care. The only source of information about appropriate use of antibiotics the GPs were exposed to during 2014 and 2015 was the material provided by HAPPY AUDIT.

At baseline, there was a higher proportion of high prescribers in the intervention group (32%) in comparison to the control group (21%). It may explain the difference in the prescription of antibiotics between the intervention and control group. A hierarchical model to assess whether prescribing style was a confounder of the effect of the intervention between the two groups was tested. The strength and direction of the results did not change (Supplementary Materials Table S2).

Finally, prescribing data were only compared before and after the intervention without multiple follow-up data points; hence, we cannot completely rule out that part of the decrease may have been caused by the regression-to-the-mean effect [19].

3.3. Comparison with Other Similar Studies

There are very few studies assessing the effectiveness of online feedback interventions on physicians' performance. Generally, online feedback programs target patients to change their lifestyle. One study [20] performed in Canada aiming to increase awareness and use of evidence-based research in clinical practice and to increase use of Internet-based resources for continuing medical education concluded that on-line case-based discussion is a promising strategy for encouraging family physicians to access current research. This study provides just a general conclusion that online feedback may be effective, but it does not assess the effects within a specific area.

There is a lack of studies on evidence-based feedback interventions aimed at decreasing inappropriate prescribing of antibiotics in the South American context. A small study performed in a hospital in Bogota-Colombia used online learning targeting general practitioners and reduced the prescribing rate of antibiotics in patients with suspected RTI [21]. Nonetheless, the results cannot be extrapolated to primary care due to different working conditions and different patient populations.

A study performed in the USA [22] targeting antibiotic prescribing for non-complicated acute bronchitis in adults also showed a substantial decline in antibiotic prescribing rates in the intervention group (from 74% to 48%; $p < 0.003$) and not in the control group (78% to 76%; $p = 0.81$). The reduction in prescribing rates in this study was larger than in our study. A plausible explanation for that difference is that their intervention targeted specifically acute bronchitis while the intervention in our study targeted all patients with suspected RTIs and GPs did not know that the primary outcome was a reduction in the proportion of prescriptions in patients with suspected acute bronchitis.

A multinational study [23] performed in Europe assessed the effects of internet-based training on antibiotic prescribing for acute respiratory tract infections. The European study included four arms: usual care; internet-based training to use a point-of-care CRP test; internet-based training in enhanced communication skills; or combined training in CRP testing and enhanced communication skills. Similar to our study, they focused on interactive interventions rather than just providing educational information. In line with our study, there was a reduction in prescription of antibiotics. Interactive methods are better than those that present information without requiring feedback from the recipient [24]. The larger effect of their intervention in comparison to our intervention can be explained by the following differences in the content of the intervention. First, our intervention did not include the use of any POCT. The use of the CRP test has demonstrated to be effective without additional interventions for decreasing prescription of antibiotics as it helps the GP to rule out a bacterial infection and helps the GP to establish a dialogue with the patient about the need for antibiotics [25,26]. Second, Little et al. intervention required more "study time" for each of the modules. Our intervention sought to use very little time from the GP to encourage them to read the clinical case, answer back and read the key literature using maximum one hour per week.

3.4. Relevance of the Findings

There are very few studies assessing the effectiveness of interventions to improve antibiotic use performed in Latin American countries [12,13]. Hence, more trials testing the same intervention or comparing online feedback with use of diagnostic test are required to get a robust assessment of the effect of these interventions within the Latin American context.

Our study proved that an online-based interactive intervention could reduce the prescribing of antibiotic for RTIs among GPs in the Latin American context, but we do not know if that leads to a reduction in antibiotic use or on the contrary leads to a higher use of antibiotic or other medications without prescriptions [8]. This can be particularly important in the South American context due to the non-negligible amount of antibiotic sales without prescription. Further research should focus on this problem and future studies should include inter-sectoral interventions.

Finally, Internet training has proved to be helpful and has the advantage that it can be disseminated widely at low cost and does not require highly trained outreach facilitators to be on site, which is especially important in low-income countries and rural areas.

4. Materials and Methods

4.1. Design

A cluster randomized two-arm controlled trial was carried out alongside the quality improvement program HAPPY AUDIT (Health Alliance for Prudent use and yield of antibiotics in patients with suspected RTI). Health care centres were the unit of allocation and intervention. Individual data at patient and GP level were collected and analysed.

4.2. Setting and Participants

GPs from the medical associations in Bolivia, Argentina, Paraguay, and Uruguay were invited to participate in the quality improvement program HAPPY AUDIT. All GPs who voluntarily accepted toparticipate in HAPPY AUDIT were randomized for participation in the cluster randomized trial (Figure 1).

4.3. Ethics

Ethics approval was granted in each country by the following authorities. Bioethics Committee, Posadas, Misiones—Argentina (File No. 022014). Department of Quality, Education and Research at "Caja Nacional de Salud" La Paz—Bolivia (File No. 29/05/2014) and the Ethics Committee of "Arco Iris" Hospital. Ministry of Health and Welfare, Seventh Health Zone, Encarnación—Paraguay (File No 116/2014). Ethics Committee for research projects at the Faculty of Medicine, University of the Republic, Montevideo—Uruguay (File No. 070153-000309-14).

4.4. Sample Size Calculation

Power calculation was based on the results of an earlier study of RTIs in Argentina [6]. According to HAPPY AUDIT, the antibiotic prescribing rate for acute bronchitis was about 60%. Thus, in order to demonstrate a 20% reduction of prescribing rate, with a power of 80%, a statistical significance level of 5% and an intra-class correlation of 0.02, we estimated to include 110 practices, 55 in the intervention group and 55 in the control group, and each practice should include at least 40 patients.

4.5. Data Collection and Outcomes

In each country, GPs registered patients with suspected RTI according to the HAPPY AUDIT procedures. It means, before the first data collection, all the GPs attended a course about the use of the data collection form and diagnosis of the most common respiratory tract infections. In South America, there is not access to point-of-care tests (POCTs), and there are no national guidelines about the diagnosis and management of RTIs. The diagnoses were only based on clinical information. For example, acute bronchitis was diagnosed on clinical basis, as C-reactive protein is not available. The secondary outcomes were: (a) reduction in prescription of antibiotics in patients with acute otitis media; (b) overall reduction in prescription of antibiotics in patients with suspected RTI. GPs registered the following information in a standardized form: age, sex, symptoms, signs, anticipated focus of infection, suspected etiology, and treatment (antibiotic prescribing).

4.6. Random Assignment

To avoid cross-contamination, the randomization procedure was done at the practice level. Practices were stratified solo practices (only one GP per health care centre) or group practices (two or more GPs per health care centre), and for each strata, the intervention was randomly assigned with half of practices in the intervention group and half in the control group. The person in charge of running the computer-based random assignment did not know the participants and had not information about their prescribing pattern.

4.7. Intervention

All GPs participating in the HAPPY AUDIT quality cycle were randomized either to intervention (evidence-based online feedback) or control (no exposure to the evidence-based online feedback). GPs in the intervention group received an e-mail with a link to an on-line intervention program that included the following three modules:

(a) Presentation of a clinical case: a patient with a RTI;
(b) Multiple choice questions focusing on evidence-based decision rules and treatment proposals (three questions per clinical case);
(c) Overall feedback with correct answers and references to key literature.

In total, GPs received ten clinical cases with questions during June–August 2015. GPs had one week to send the answer back. After one week, the GPs received the right answer from the previous clinical case with key literature and a new clinical case.

The online feedback was sent through the surveyexact program. The program registered the number of respondents per clinical case.

4.8. Statistical Analysis

Two hierarchical logistic regression models were developed for each of the following outcomes: (a) prescription of antibiotics in patients with acute bronchitis; (b) prescription of antibiotics in patients with acute otitis media and (c) prescription of antibiotics in all patients with suspected RTI. The first model tested differences in antibiotic prescribing rates before-after intervention for each group (intervention and control). The second model tested the added effect of the evidence-based online intervention. It tested the interaction between randomization group and year. The structure of the data was maintained by including two random intercepts: (a) One at the practice level and; (b) one at the GP level. All analyses were performed in the R programming language and environment v3.3.2 using the lme4 and nnet package [27].

5. Conclusions

Online evidence-based feedback is effective for reducing antibiotic prescribing in patients with suspected respiratory tract infection attending primary care in South America and it is a tool that can be widely disseminated at low cost without requiring highly trained facilitators, which is especially important in low-income countries and rural areas.

Author Contributions: The study was designed by G.C. and L.B. G.C., L.B., L.C., M.A.S., and M.O. contributed to the management of the study and implementation of the intervention. G.C. coordinated randomization and analyzed the data. G.C. and I.U. contributed to the interpretation of the data and the writing of the paper. All authors contributed to review the paper.

References

1. World Health Organization. Antimicrobial Resistance: Global Report on Surveillance 2014. Available online: http://www.who.int/drugresistance/documents/surveillancereport/en/ (accessed on 7 July 2017).
2. World Economic Forum. Global Risks 2013. Available online: http://www3.weforum.org/docs/WEF_GlobalRisks_Report_2013.pdf (accessed on 7 July 2017).
3. Mendes, C.; Marin, M.E.; Quinones, F.; Sifuentes-Osornio, J.; Siller, C.C.; Castanheira, M.; Zoccoli, C.M.; Lopez, H.; Sucari, A.; Rossi, F.; et al. Antibacterial resistance of community-acquired respiratory tract pathogens recovered from patients in Latin America: Results from the PROTEKT surveillance study (1999–2000). *Braz. J. Infect. Dis.* **2003**, *7*, 44–61. [CrossRef] [PubMed]
4. Villegas, M.V.; Guzmán Blanco, M.; Sifuentes-Osornio, J.; Rossi, F. Increasing prevalence of extended-spectrum-beta- lactamase among Gram-negative bacilli in Latin America—2008 update from the Study for Monitoring Antimicrobial Resistance Trends (SMART). *Braz. J. Infect. Dis.* **2011**, *15*, 34–39. [PubMed]
5. Garza-González, E.; Dowzicky, M.J. Changes in Staphylococcus aureus susceptibility across Latin America between 2004 and 2010. *Braz. J. Infect. Dis.* **2013**, *17*, 13–19. [CrossRef] [PubMed]
6. Bjerrum, A.; Gahrn-Hansen, B.; Hansen, M.P.; Jarbol, D.E.; Cordoba, G.; Llor, C.; Cots, J.M.; Hernandez, S.; Lopez-Valcarcel, B.G.; Perez, A.; et al. Health Alliance for prudent antibiotic prescribing in patients with Respiratory Tract Infections (HAPPY AUDIT) impact of a non-randomised multifaceted intervention programme. *BMC. Fam. Pract.* **2011**, *12*, 52. [CrossRef] [PubMed]
7. Wirtz, V.J.; Dreser, A.; Gonzales, R. Trends in antibiotic utilization in eight Latin American countries, 1997–2007. *Rev. Panam. Salud Publica* **2010**, *27*, 219–225. [CrossRef] [PubMed]
8. Santa-Ana-Tellez, Y.; Mantel-Teeuwisse, A.K.; Dreser, A.; Leufkens, H.G.M.; Wirtz, V.J. Impact of Over-the-Counter Restrictions on Antibiotic Consumption in Brazil and Mexico. *PLoS ONE* **2013**, *8*. [CrossRef] [PubMed]
9. Costelloe, C.; Lovering, A.; Mant, D.; Hay, A.D.; Metcalfe, C. Effect of antibiotic prescribing in primary care on antimicrobial resistance in individual patients: Systematic review and meta-analysis. *BMJ* **2010**, *340*, c2096. [CrossRef] [PubMed]
10. Arroll, B. Antibiotics for upper respiratory tract infections: An overview of Cochrane reviews. *Respir. Med.* **2005**, *99*, 255–261. [CrossRef] [PubMed]
11. Smith, S.M.; Fahey, T.; Smucny, J.; Becker, L.A. Antibiotics for acute bronchitis. *Cochrane Database Syst. Rev.* **2014**, *3*, CD000245. [CrossRef]

12. Van Der Velden, A.W.; Pijpers, E.J.; Kuyvenhoven, M.M.; Tonkin-Crine, S.K.G.; Little, P.; Verheij, T.J.M. Effectiveness of physician-targeted interventions to improve antibiotic use for respiratory tract infections. *Br. J. Gen. Pract.* **2012**, *62*. [CrossRef] [PubMed]
13. Roque, F.; Herdeiro, M.T.; Soares, S.; Teixeira Rodrigues, A.; Breitenfeld, L.; Figueiras, A. Educational interventions to improve prescription and dispensing of antibiotics: A systematic review. *BMC Public Health* **2014**, *14*. [CrossRef] [PubMed]
14. Munck, A.; Damsgaard, J.; Hansen, D.; Bjerrum, L.; Søndergaard, J. The Nordic method for quality improvement in general practice. *Qual. Prim. Care* **2003**, *11*, 73–78.
15. Strandberg, I.; Ovhed, I.; Troein, M.; Hakansson, A. Influence of self-registration on audit participants and their non-participating colleagues. A retrospective study of medical records concerning prescription patterns. *Scand. J. Prim. Health Care* **2005**, *23*, 42–46. [CrossRef] [PubMed]
16. Akkerman, A.E.; Kuyvenhoven, M.M.; Verheij, T.J.M.; van Dijk, L. Antibiotics in Dutch general practice: Nationwide electronic GP database and national reimbursement rates. *Pharmacoepidemiol. Drug Saf.* **2008**, *17*, 378–383. [CrossRef] [PubMed]
17. Wensing, M.; Van Der Weijden, T.; Grol, R. Implementing guidelines and innovations in general practice: Which interventions are effective? *Br. J. Gen. Pract.* **1998**, *48*, 991–997. [CrossRef] [PubMed]
18. Bentzen, N. Medical Audit—The APO-Method in General Practice. *Scand. J. Prim. Health Care* **1993**, *11*, 13–18. [CrossRef]
19. Bacchieri, A.; Della Cioppa, G. Experimental design: Fallacy of "before-after" comparisons in uncontrolled studies. In *Fundamentals of Clinical Research Bridging Medicine, Statistics and Operations*; Springer: Mailand, Italy, 2007.
20. Marshall, J.N.; Stewart, M.; Østbye, T. Small-group CME using e-mail discussions: Can it work? *Can. Fam. Physician* **2001**, *47*, 557–563. [PubMed]
21. Ospina, J.E.; Orozco, J.G. Impacto de una intervencion educativa virtual sobre la prescripcion de antibioticos en infeccion respiratoria alta aguda, Bogota, 2007. *Univ. Med. Bogota* **2008**, *49*, 293–316.
22. Gonzales, R.; Steiner, J.F.; Lum, A.; Barrett, P.H. Decreasing antibiotic use in Ambulatory Practice: Impact of a multidimensional intervenition on the treatment of uncomplicated acute bronchitis in adults. *J. Am. Med. Assoc.* **1999**, *281*, 1512–1519. [CrossRef]
23. Little, P.; Stuart, B.; Francis, N.; Douglas, E.; Tonkin-Crine, S.; Anthierens, S.; Cals, J.W.L.; Melbye, H.; Santer, M.; Moore, M.; et al. Effects of internet-based training on antibiotic prescribing rates for acute respiratory-tract infections: A multinational, cluster, randomised, factorial, controlled trial. *Lancet* **2013**, *382*, 1175–1182. [CrossRef]
24. Arnold, S.R.; Straus, S.E. Interventions to Improve Antibiotic Prescribing Practices in Ambulatory Care. *Cochrane Database Syst. Rev.* **2005**, *4*, CD003539. [CrossRef]
25. Cals, J.W.; Butler, C.C.; Hopstaken, R.M.; Hood, K.; Dinant, G.J. Effect of point of care testing for C reactive protein and training in communication skills on antibiotic use in lower respiratory tract infections: Cluster randomised trial. *Br. Med. J.* **2009**, *338*. [CrossRef] [PubMed]
26. Cals, J.W.L.; Schot, M.J.C.; de Jong, S.A.M.; Dinant, G.-J.; Hopstaken, R.M. Protein Testing and Antibiotic Prescribing for Respiratory Tract Infections: A Randomized Controlled Trial. *Ann. Fam. Med.* **2010**, *8*, 124–133. [CrossRef] [PubMed]
27. Bates, D.; Mächler, M.; Bolker, B.; Walker, S. Fitting Linear Mixed-Effects Models Using lme4. *J. Stat. Softw.* **2015**, *67*, 48. [CrossRef]

11

Conformational Response of 30S-bound IF3 to A-Site Binders Streptomycin and Kanamycin

Roberto Chulluncuy [1,†], Carlos Espiche [1,†], Jose Alberto Nakamoto [1,2,†], Attilio Fabbretti [3] and Pohl Milón [1,*]

1 Centro de Investigación e Innovación, Faculty of Health Sciences, Universidad Peruana de Ciencias Aplicadas—UPC, Lima L-33, Peru; robertochulluncuy1@gmail.com (R.C.); carlosespiche852@gmail.com (C.E.); jose.nakamoto@upch.pe (J.A.N.)

2 Facultad de Ciencias y Filosofía Alberto Cazorla Talleri, Universidad Peruana Cayetano Heredia—UPCH, Lima L-31, Peru

3 Laboratory of Genetics, Department of Biosciences and Veterinary Medicine, University of Camerino, 62032 Camerino, Italy; attilio.fabbretti@unicam.it

* Correspondence: pmilon@upc.pe

† These authors contributed equally to this work.

Academic Editor: Claudio O. Gualerzi

Abstract: Aminoglycoside antibiotics are widely used to treat infectious diseases. Among them, streptomycin and kanamycin (and derivatives) are of importance to battle multidrug-resistant (MDR) *Mycobacterium tuberculosis*. Both drugs bind the small ribosomal subunit (30S) and inhibit protein synthesis. Genetic, structural, and biochemical studies indicate that local and long-range conformational rearrangements of the 30S subunit account for this inhibition. Here, we use intramolecular FRET between the C- and N-terminus domains of the flexible IF3 to monitor real-time perturbations of their binding sites on the 30S platform. Steady and pre-steady state binding experiments show that both aminoglycosides bring IF3 domains apart, promoting an elongated state of the factor. Binding of Initiation Factor IF1 triggers closure of IF3 bound to the 30S complex, while both aminoglycosides revert the IF1-dependent conformation. Our results uncover dynamic perturbations across the 30S subunit, from the A-site to the platform, and suggest that both aminoglycosides could interfere with prokaryotic translation initiation by modulating the interaction between IF3 domains with the 30S platform.

Keywords: streptomycin; kanamycin; translation initiation; 30S subunit; IF3; tuberculosis; FRET

---

1. Introduction

Bacterial pathogens account for 38% of human infections [1] and, because of their potential to develop antibiotic resistance, represent a severe threat to human health. The problem is of particular importance in underdeveloped countries, where the incidence of multidrug-resistant (MDR) and extensively drug-resistant (XDR) mycobacteria and bacteria is rapidly increasing (World Health Organization, WHO). Tuberculosis (TB), caused by *Mycobacterium tuberculosis*, is a devastating disease with higher incidence in underdeveloped countries than in their developed counterparts ([2] and references therein). Antibiotics are the only option to treat TB efficiently. Streptomycin along with kanamycin and its derivative Amikacin are used as second-line drugs for the treatment of MDR tuberculosis [3,4].

Kanamycin and Streptomycin bind the decoding site (A-site) of the minor ribosomal subunit (30S) and inhibit protein synthesis mainly by causing misreading of the mRNA [5] or translocation inhibition (Kanamycin) [6,7]. The streptomycin-resistant strains contain hyper-accurate ribosomes [8].

During decoding the 30S subunit samples various conformations (Figure 1a) and the accuracy of the process can be affected by favoring a particular 30S state [9]; it can be surmised that streptomycin increases the misreading insofar as it promotes a ribosomal conformation that decreases the decoding accuracy.

Due to streptomycin's effects, it was proposed that this drug could trigger an "error catastrophe" during protein elongation [10]. However, this model is in conflict with bot, the observation that ribosomes isolated from streptomycin-treated cells do not differ in speed and accuracy from those isolated from untreated *E. coli* cells [11], and that streptomycin causes 70S monomer accumulation and polysome depletion in vivo [12].

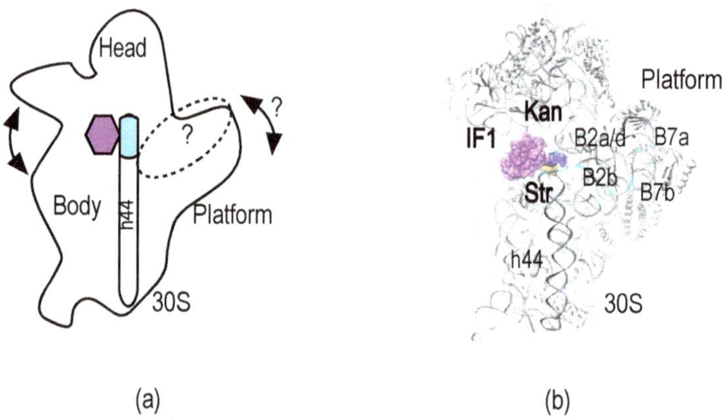

Figure 1. 30S subunit, dynamic domains, and inter-subunit bridges. (**a**) Representation of the 30S subunit as seen from the 50S-interacting side. The main dynamic domains of the small subunit are indicated. Arrows represent the known and potential movements involved in mistranslation of the mRNA. The purple hexagon indicates the decoding center and binding site of IF1, streptomycin and kanamycin. The dotted oval indicates the overall binding surface of IF3 on the 30S platform; (**b**) Crystal structure of the IF1-30S subunit complex (Purple surface, PDB: 1HR0) [13]. Streptomycin (orange) and kanamycin (blue) were aligned from PDB: 4DR3 and PDB: 2ESI, respectively [14,15]. Cyan ribbons highlight residues involved in inter-subunit bridges of the 30S platform that overlap with IF3 binding sites.

Streptomycin, kanamycin and initiation factor IF1 bind nearby within the decoding center of the 30S subunit and promote diverse local and long range conformational perturbations [13–17]. IF3 binds to the 30S platform, making contacts with h45, h23, and h24 of the 16S rRNA and ribosomal proteins uS7 and uS11 [18–22]. IF3 is a basic protein constituted by two globular domains of similar masses, N-terminal (NTD) and C-terminal (CTD), connected by a flexible linker [23,24]. The two domains are separated by a hydrophilic, lysine-rich flexible linker. Results of NMR spectroscopy, neutron scattering, mutagenesis, and accessibility to proteolysis indicate that IF3 NTD and CTD move independently [25–27]. Furthermore, real-time probing experiments [19] have demonstrated that IF3 CTD is the first to contact the 30S platform, immediately followed by the IF3 NTD. Interestingly, streptomycin binding was found to increase the dissociation rate of IF3 from non-canonical 30S initiation complexes (IC) [28].

The 30S platform greatly contributes to the association of the small subunit with the major ribosomal subunit (50S) through the formation of several inter-subunit bridges (Figure 1). The interaction of IF3 with the 30S subunit lays across the platform and regulates the progression of the 30S IC towards elongation of protein synthesis [19,20]. Here, we specifically labeled each domain of IF3 with fluorescent dyes ($IF3_{DL}$) to develop an intramolecular Förster resonance energy transfer (FRET) system capable of sensing rapid conformational changes of the factor and/or its binding sites at the 30S platform. In combination with pre-steady state kinetics, the FRET signal of $IF3_{DL}$ responds to the interaction of streptomycin, kanamycin, and IF1 with the A-site of the 30S subunit.

Our data, in combination with recent structural studies, suggest a novel molecular mechanism for the aminoglycosides as capable of perturbing IF3 binding sites on the 30S platform.

2. Results

2.1. Experimental Outline

IF3 binds across the 30S platform, interacts with several intersubunit bridges, and responds to conformational states of the small subunit (Figure 1) [17,19,20,28,29]. Therefore, IF3 could be used as sensor of structural changes occurring in the 30S platform. The structure of IF3 NTD consists of a globular α/β fold, constituted by a four-stranded b-sheet onto which an α-helix is packed [30]. IF3 CTD is composed by a two-layered α/β sandwich fold with a $\beta\alpha\beta\alpha\beta\beta$ topology with two parallel α-helices packed against a four-stranded β-sheet [23] (Figure 2a,c). Naturally, IF3 contains a sterically buried single cysteine at position 65 of the NTD which reacts slowly with maleimide moieties [31,32]. We introduced a second cysteine at a solvent-exposed position of the CTD (E166C) to kinetically enhance the fluorescent modification of the CTD over the NTD. Aiming to obtain a very sensitive intramolecular FRET system, Atto-488 and Atto-540Q were chosen as the fluorescence donor and non-emitting acceptor (quencher), respectively.

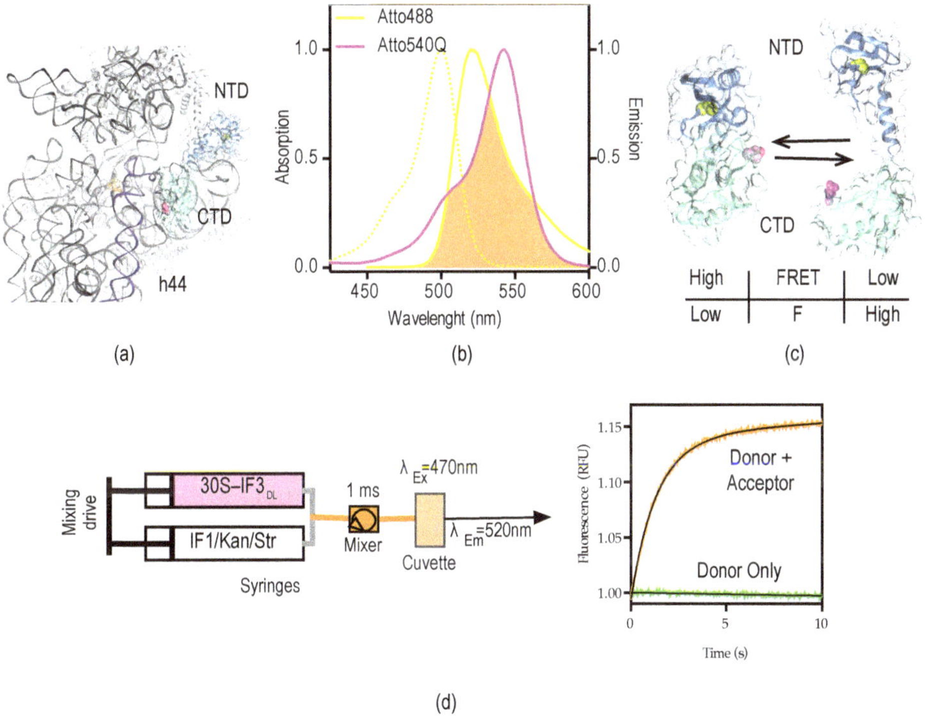

Figure 2. $IF3_{DL}$ intramolecular FRET for dynamic measurements of the 30S platform. (**a**) Crystal structure of the 30S subunit, depicting a possible orientation of IF3 across the platform, CTD (turquoise), and NTD (steel blue); (**b**) absorption and emission spectra of Atto-488 fluorescent dye (yellow) and Atto-540Q quencher (purple). The overlap area between donor emission fluorescence (Atto-488) and acceptor absorption of quencher (Atto-540Q) is indicated in orange. R_0 distance for the FRET couple is 64 Å according to the producer (Atto-tec, Siegen, Germany); (**c**) Potential arrangements of IF3 domains with respect to each other. Colors are as in (**a**); cysteine residues for donor (C65, yellow) and acceptor (E166C, purple) dyes are shown as spheres. The bottom table indicates the possible readouts of fluorescence and FRET for the corresponding states of $IF3_{DL}$; (**d**) Scheme of stopped-flow experimental set-up and the typical signal read out upon mixing 30S–$IF3_{DL}$ with a 30S binder (orange trace). In order to assign the signal as FRET, the same experiment is performed in the absence of the acceptor, in this case $IF3_{NAtto488}$, IF3 labeled at the natural cysteine in the NTD (green trace).

The R_0 between the dyes is Å 64, providing a wide range of distances to be monitored by changes of FRET efficiencies (Figure 2b). Under native buffer conditions $IF3_{E166C}$ reacted efficiently with Atto-540Q maleimide (Figure S1c). In order to enhance the poor reactivity of C65 at the NTD, $IF3_{E166C}$–Atto540Q was subsequently modified with Atto-488 maleimide under denaturing conditions. Finally, the resulting doubly labeled protein ($IF3_{DL}$) contained a non-emitting acceptor (quencher) at the CTD and a fluorescent dye at the NTD (Figure S1c) (see Materials and Methods for details). Therefore, the vicinity of the dyes (domains) would result in donor fluorescence quenching, while the opposite would increase the observed fluorescence. A high FRET state corresponds to low fluorescence read-outs, indicating the vicinity of IF3 domains with respect to each other (Figure 2c).

2.2. *Probing the Sensing Limits of $IF3_{DL}$*

IF3 and IF1 cooperatively increase their affinity for the 30S subunit [21,33]. Along the pathway of translation initiation, both factors rapidly join the 30S subunit concomitantly with IF2. The whole process of 30S pre-Initiation Complex (pre-IC) formation takes around 100 ms and precedes fMet-$tRNA^{fMet}$ (initiator tRNA) recruitment [33,34]. This multi-component process can follow multiple pathways, as shown by single molecule measurements [35]. The cooperation between IF1 and IF3 is suggested to maintain the fidelity of translation initiation; however, its molecular dynamics remain elusive [28,36].

Here, we measure the binding kinetics of $IF3_{DL}$ to the 30S subunit and the influence of IF1 in the resulting 30S–$IF3_{DL}$ complex (Figure 2d). NMR measurements of full-length IF3 indicated that its domains can freely move in solution, adopting almost random orientations [25]. However, molecular modeling and site-directed mutagenesis proposed that IF3 can transiently establish inter-domain contacts [27]. In any case, the transition from unbound to bound to the 30S subunit would result in IF3 adopting an elongated conformation on the 30S platform [19,20,37] (Figure 3a).

Indeed, fluorescence equilibrium measurements of $IF3_{DL}$ titrations at increasing concentrations of 30S subunits (0.2–2.5 μM) resulted in proportional increased emission fluorescence (Figure 3b), indicating that IF3 transits towards an extended open state in the 30S platform. Fitting of the measurements with a quadratic function for binding kinetics yielded a dissociation constant K_D for the 30S–IF3 complex in the low nanomolar range, consistent with previous pre-steady state measurements [33]. Binding of IFs to the 30S subunit and their subsequent conformational rearrangements are rapid, taking place in few seconds. Therefore, to measure the pre-steady state binding of $IF3_{DL}$ to the 30S subunit we rapidly mixed 30S subunits with $IF3_{DL}$ in a stopped-flow apparatus (KintekCorp, Snow Shoe, PA, USA) and measured fluorescence emission after passing a 515 nm long-pass optical filter.

Upon mixing of $IF3_{DL}$ with 30S subunits, the fluorescence increased with time with a biphasic behavior (Figure 3c). In contrast, a control where the factor was mixed with buffer or lacked the acceptor at the CTD did not show a change of fluorescence (Figure S3). Non-linear regression fitting of the recorded measurements with an equation containing two exponential terms yielded two apparent rate constants, k_{app1} and k_{app2}, and two associated fluorescence amplitudes, F_1 and F_2 (Equation (2)). Analysis is consistent with an initial bimolecular encounter between $IF3_{DL}$ and the 30S subunit, $k_{app1} = 16 \pm 1\ s^{-1}$, followed by a conformational rearrangement of the factor, $k_{app2} = 2 \pm 0.05\ s^{-1}$. These measurements are in agreement with previous rapid kinetic studies, although different fluorescent reporters, 30S subunits, and IFs purification methods were used [33,38].

Then we investigated whether $IF3_{DL}$ pre-bound to the 30S subunit could monitor IF1 interactions with the ribosome. Equilibrium titrations of $IF3_{DL}$–30S with increasing concentrations of IF1 resulted in a decrease of emitted fluorescence, indicating that IF3 domains reach closer distances, consistent with previous single-molecule studies [37] (Figure 3d). Fitting of the measurements for one-site binding yielded a K_D of about 100 nM, consistent with measurements by pre-steady state methods [33].

Equilibrium measurements of the interaction of IF1 with the 30S–$IF3_{DL}$ complex indicated a decrease in distance between the domains of IF3. We then explored whether the kinetics of the interaction would reflect a bimolecular encounter of IF1 with the complex or a later conformational rearrangement. Preformed 30S–$IF3_{DL}$ complexes were rapidly mixed with a 10-fold molar excess of IF1 in a stopped-flow apparatus and fluorescence was measured with time as described above. Upon mixing, the fluorescence of $IF3_{DL}$ decreased exponentially and was best described by a single exponential term equation (Equation (4)) (Figure 3e). Fitting of the measurements yielded an apparent rate constant k_{app} = 0.26 ± 0.01 s^{-1}. Previous studies reported an association constant for the bimolecular encounter of IF1 with the 30S–IF3 complex of 20 $\mu M^{-1} \cdot s^{-1}$ [33], thus we expected an apparent rate for IF1 of ≈20 s^{-1} (IF1 = 1 μM). Then, $IF3_{DL}$ reports an IF1-dependent FRET change that is ≥75-fold slower than the initial binding, suggesting that $IF3_{DL}$ is monitoring a successive step, i.e., a conformational rearrangement of IF3 on the platform resulting in the accommodation of one of IF3 domains.

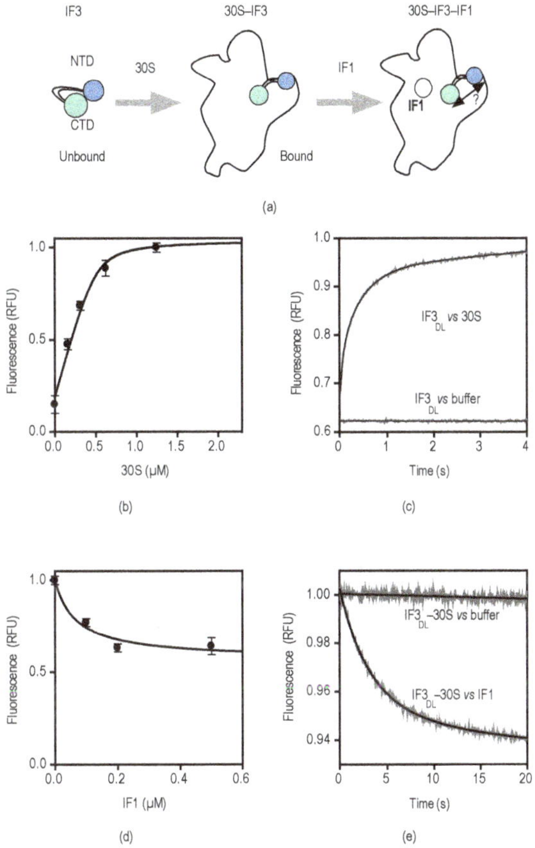

Figure 3. Steady and pre-steady binding of $IF3_{DL}$ and IF1 to the 30S subunit. (**a**) Experimental scheme depicting the binding reactions of IF3 and IF1; (**b**) $IF3_{DL}$ titration with increasing concentrations of 30S subunits. $IF3_{DL}$ (0.5 μM) was incubated with the indicated concentrations of 30S subunits for 10 min. 5 replicates of 2 μL were measured in a NanoDrop 3000 fluorimeter (Thermo Fisher Scientific, Waltham, MA, USA). Error bars indicate standard deviations (SD). Continuous line shows fitting with a quadratic equation for binding (see Materials and Methods); (**c**) Time courses of $IF3_{DL}$ binding to 30S subunits and a buffer control to assign the specific amplitude change. 30S subunits (0.1 μM) were mixed with equimolar $IF3_{DL}$ in a stopped-flow apparatus. Ten to 12 individual traces were recorded and averaged. Smooth lines indicate fits by non-linear regression with two exponential terms; (**d**) 30S–$IF3_{DL}$ (0.5 μM) titration with IF1 at the indicated concentrations. Five replicates of 2 μL were measured as above. Error bars indicate standard deviations (SD); (**e**) Time courses of 30S–$IF3_{DL}$ binding to IF1 and a buffer control to assign the specific amplitude change. See Figure S3 for no acceptor controls. 30S–$IF3_{DL}$ complexes (0.1 μM) were mixed with a 10-fold molar excess of IF1 (1 μM) in a stopped-flow apparatus. Twelve individual traces were recorded and averaged. Smooth lines indicate fits by non-linear regression with a single exponential term.

IF3$_{DL}$ allows monitoring equilibrium and real-time kinetics of factor binding, dissociation, as well as conformational changes induced by IF1. The intramolecular FRET sensibility and versatility of IF3$_{DL}$ provide solid bases to test 30S subunit binders, with a special emphasis for those targeting the A-site. Among them, streptomycin and kanamycin stood out because of their medical importance as second-line drugs to treat MDR TB.

2.3. Counter Effects between IF1 and Streptomycin/Kanamycin

The conformational cooperation between IF1 and IF3 observed above has been suggested to maintain the fidelity of translation initiation [28,36]. On the other hand, streptomycin was shown to disrupt the cooperation between the factors, and possibly overall fidelity, by increasing the velocity of formation of 70S IC programmed with non-canonical mRNAs [28]. Here, we use 30S–IF3$_{DL}$ complexes to monitor real-time conformational perturbations of IF3 on the platform upon the binding of streptomycin and kanamycin to the A-site (Figure 4a).

Rapid mixing of either aminoglycoside with 30S–IF3$_{DL}$ complexes in a stopped-flow apparatus results in an exponential increase of fluorescence over time, indicating that IF3 domains get further apart (Figure 4b). The measurements were best described by a single exponential term yielding an apparent rate (k_{app}) and an associated fluorescent amplitude (F) (Equation (4)). Analysis by non-linear regression fitting returned apparent rates for streptomycin and kanamycin ${k_{app}}^{Str} = 4.6 \pm 0.1\ s^{-1}$ and ${k_{app}}^{Kan} = 1.4 \pm 0.1\ s^{-1}$ (Figure 4d).

Streptomycin and kanamycin have opposite effects on the 30S platform if compared to IF1 as observed by IF3$_{DL}$. While IF1 closes up IF3 domains, the aminoglycosides bring them apart. Each A-site binder is also characterized by different extents of FRET change with IF1 promoting an opposite and greater (≈3-fold) perturbation if compared to the aminoglycosides. Consequently, we probed whether the interaction of streptomycin and kanamycin with the 30S subunit could revert IF1-dependent closing up of IF3$_{DL}$ (Figure 4c).

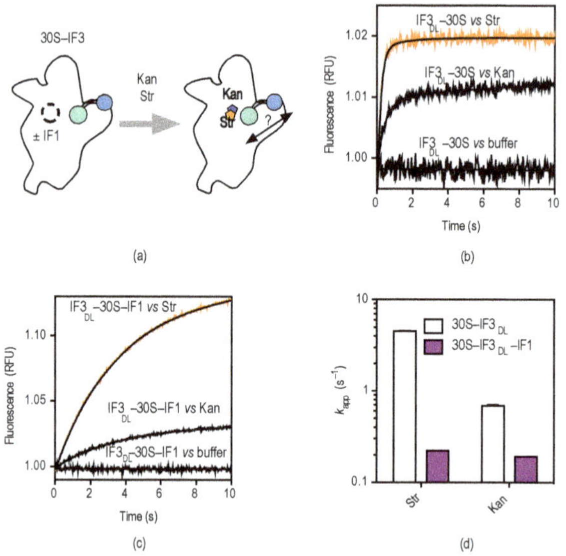

Figure 4. Pre-steady state kinetics of streptomycin and kanamycin binding to 30S–IF3$_{DL}$ complexes. (**a**) Scheme depicting the experimental approach to monitoring conformational effects as a function of streptomycin (orange) and kanamycin (blue); (**b**) time courses of 30S–IF3$_{DL}$ (0.1 μM) interacting with each aminoglycoside; colors are as in (**a**). The trace for buffer control indicates no dissociation of IF3$_{DL}$ during rapid mixing in the stopped-flow apparatus. See Figure S3 for controls in the absence of fluorescence acceptor; (**c**) Time courses of streptomycin and kanamycin binding to 30S–IF3$_{DL}$–IF1 (0.1 μM). Smooth lines indicate fits by non-linear regression (Equation (4)); (**d**) Influence of IF1 over the kinetics of IF3$_{DL}$ conformational changes caused by streptomycin and kanamycin.

Rapid mixing of 30S–IF3$_{DL}$–IF1 complexes with either streptomycin or kanamycin in a stopped-flow apparatus resulted in an exponential increase of fluorescence (Figure 4c). Comparisons of the drugs binding to 30S–IF3$_{DL}$ complexes (without IF1) showed an increased amplitude of fluorescence change and slower apparent rates (Figure 4d). Nonlinear fitting of the time dependencies with a single exponential function (Equation (4)) indicated a 20-fold and 7-fold decrease of the k_{app} for streptomycin and kanamycin in the presence of IF1, respectively (Figure 4d). On the contrary, the amplitudes of FRET changes were increased in the presence of IF1. Thus, kanamycin and streptomycin seem to compete with IF1, imposing an IF3 layout on the platform similar to that in 30S complexes lacking IF1 (Figure 5). In addition, reversion of the IF1-dependent conformation shows similar apparent rates for both aminoglycosides (${k_{app}}^{Str} = 0.2 \pm 0.01\ s^{-1}$ and ${k_{app}}^{Kan} = 0.22 \pm 0.01\ s^{-1}$), suggesting they are rate-limited by a similar reaction.

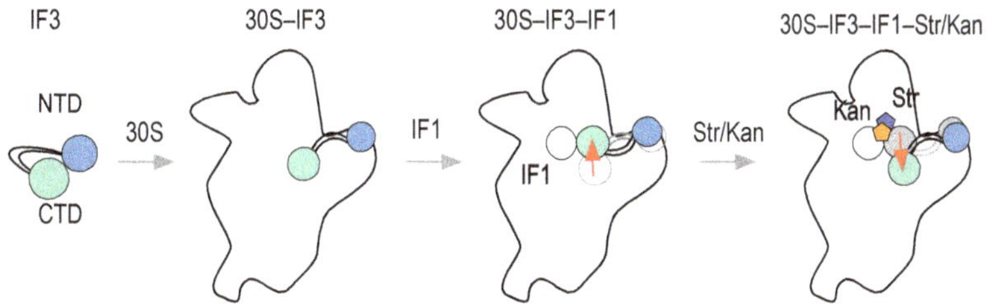

Figure 5. Scheme of IF3 movements during early stages of translation initiation and response to antibiotics streptomycin and kanamycin. IF3 binding to the 30S subunit results in opening of the factor and adopting an overall elongated state. The interaction of IF1 (purple) results in repositioning of IF3, probably shifting the CTD (magenta) towards the P-site and possibly interacting with IF1. Streptomycin (orange) and kanamycin (blue) would perturb the equilibrium between binding sites of IF3, promoting a displacement of the factor. Red arrows indicate possible movements of IF3. Gray shadows indicate IF3 states prior to the interaction of the binder with the 30S subunit.

The intrinsic flexibility and dynamics of IF3 seem to sample different conformational states of the 30S subunit, at the 30S platform where the factor binds. With opposing directions, IF1 together with streptomycin and kanamycin alter the relative disposition of IF3 domains, revealing molecular mechanisms of antibiotic action at an unexpected site but with potential functional implications. Perturbing IF3 binding sites by streptomycin, even in the presence of IF1, provides a rationale to previous reports where the absence of IF1 or the addition of streptomycin increased the rates of non-canonical translation initiation [28].

3. Discussion

Both, streptomycin and kanamycin, disturb the positioning of IF3 at the 30S platform, possibly affecting translation initiation (Figure 4) in addition to later steps of translation. It is generally accepted that streptomycin and kanamycin inhibit cell growth by increasing mRNA misreading during elongation of protein synthesis (reviewed in [39]). This notion is derived from polyU directed poly-Phe synthesis experiments where the drugs induced mis-incorporation of other amino acids into the peptide chain [40]. In support, streptomycin caused phenotypic suppression of nonsense mutations in vivo [41]. More recent biochemical, structural, and single-molecule studies strengthen the notion of streptomycin and kanamycin (and other aminoglycosides) affecting decoding, elongation, and translocation [39,42,43]. On the initiation side, streptomycin increased the velocity of 70S IC formation if programmed with non-canonical mRNAs, suggesting that the aminoglycoside could cause loss of translation initiation fidelity [28]. The effect was associated with an increase of IF3 dissociation rate through a conformational switch at the 30S subunit. Streptomycin would weaken the binding sites of IF3 at the platform, therefore increasing premature 50S joining. Thus, streptomycin would result in *in vivo* formation of unproductive 70S complexes. This postulation is supported by experiments from the late 1960s which indeed showed streptomycin to cause an accumulation of 70S monomers concomitantly to a reduction of polysomes, consistent with streptomycin preferentially inhibiting early steps of translation [12,44].

We observe that IF1 binding decreases the donor fluorescence of $IF3_{DL}$ (increased FRET), interpreted as a closing up of IF3 domains (Figure 3). IF1 was shown to bind away (>50 Å) from either domain of IF3, suggesting that the closing up of IF3 is rather indirect, through an allosteric effect of IF1 across the 30S subunit [21]. However, recent structural studies show that each domain of IF3 can occupy at least two positions on the 30S subunit as a function of ligands bound to the initiation complex [18]. The CTD seem to contact IF1 in complexes lacking initiator tRNA. In full 30S ICs the CTD positions under the tRNA, moving away from its initial position. Also the NTD of IF3 was shown to interact nearby uS11, at the tip of the platform, or to initiator tRNA in full complexes. In a lesser extent, single molecule approaches observed similar dynamics of IF3. Specifically, the effect of IF1 on IF3 layout was shown to transit away from an extended conformation towards a more closed state [37].

Functionally, rapid kinetic and biochemical assays showed a close relationship between IF3 and the mRNA in an IF1-dependent manner. IF3 can promote mRNA shift and can indirectly discriminate unfit mRNAs, i.e., non-canonical codons [28,45–47]. The crosstalk between IF3 and IF1 is also supported by several isolated mutations, which increased translation initiation from non-canonical codons, clustered in the 790 loop (interacting with IF3) and h44 (at residues known to be distorted by IF1).A cooperation between IF1 and IF3 enhances the fidelity of translation initiation [36].

Consistently, IF1 increases IF3 affinity for the 30S subunit in a cooperative manner [33]. Omission of IF1 resulted in an increased premature 70S IC formation, a similar effect obtained in the presence of streptomycin [28]. Thus, streptomycin and IF1 would favor opposite states of IF3 on the 30S subunit. The closer distances between IF3 domains observed in this study would represent a 30S subunit with the most 50S anti-association property. On the other hand, a more open state of the factor would facilitate the arrival of the major subunit. Streptomycin and kanamycin promote the opening of the factor (this study, Figure 4) and streptomycin increases the speed of IF3 dissociation and subunit association [28].

Streptomycin would perturb initiation of protein synthesis by reverting a high-fidelity IF3 layout on the 30S subunit that is induced by IF1. Consequently, the overall initiation fidelity threshold is lowered by the aminoglycoside, allowing premature joining of the major subunit. Our results expand the range of reactions that aminoglycosides may affect and provide insights into the dynamic molecular network that they exploit. Streptomycin stabilizes the pairing of A1413-G1487 as it hinders G1487 from kethoxal modification [48] (Figure S4). Additionally, streptomycin is proposed to cause conformational changes in the h45 tetraloop. This loop was shown to adopt two different states, called "engaged and disengaged", with respect to h44 (nucleotide C1496), with streptomycin favoring the disengaged state [14]. In this state the h45 tetraloop moves away from the h44, with G1517 swinging counter-clockwise about 5 Å away (Table S1 and Figure S4). Streptomycin interacts with G1491, not affecting A1492 and A1493. On the contrary, IF1 flips out both residues (1492–1493), promotes the engaged state between h44 and h45 (C1496-G1517), and unpairs A1413 and U1414 from G1487 and G1486, respectively [13] (Figure S4). Altogether, streptomycin promotes opposite to IF1 structural changes across three directions, towards the tip of h44, downstream h44, and towards the platform, through the h44/h45 interaction (Table S2 and Figure S4).

Thus, IF1 and streptomycin seem to exploit the same structural network, yet in opposite directions (Figure 5). Our results indicate that IF1 and streptomycin/kanamycin also display opposite effects for the inter-domain distance of IF3, with the antibiotics increasing the distance while IF1 decreases it. These counter effects may find a rationale in the structural network described above, where different residues of the 30S subunit may be exposed for preferential binding of IF3. As observed by cryoEM, IF3 domains can bind to different sites on the 30S platform [18]. Our results may indicate that IF1, streptomycin, and kanamycin perturb the equilibrium of the CTD between its two binding sites.

A direct interaction of IF1 with the CTD of IF3 may contribute to enhance the close state of IF3 observed here.

Structural and kinetic analysis show that the engaged/disengaged state of the 30S subunit is also affected by the novel antibiotic GE81112, resulting in a blockade of the 30S IC progression by preventing initiation codon decoding [49]. Whether GE81112 perturbs the IF3 layout of the 30S subunit remains elusive; however, our model would suggest that the drug promotes a close distance conformation between domains. Conformational changes that are sensed by IF3 in the platform area may also affect the association of the 30S with the 50S through differential exposure of intersubunit bridges (Figure 1b). Besides B2b, which is collocating with the IF3 binding site, B7a–b may be regulated as in different rotate states of the ribosome. Altogether, the dynamic platform could provide a rationale for the tight regulation of the anti-association function of IF3 as modulating the accessibility of each domain for their binding sites.

Finally, the biophysical system depicted in this work can be used as a novel platform to identify and characterize compounds targeting initiation of translation [50]. Indeed, screening systems to identify compounds that preferentially inhibit the initiation phase have proved successful [51–53]. In addition, our $IF3_{DL}$-30S reporter assay can provide novel aspects of the inhibiting mechanism of known 30S-binding drugs. Similar approaches have allowed detailed descriptions for other inhibitors of the ribosome [54,55].

4. Materials and Methods

4.1. *Escherichia coli Strains, Expression Vectors, Cell Growth, and Protein Expression Induction*

Competent *E. coli* $BL21_{DE3}$ cells were $CaCl_2$ transformed (Mix & Go, Zymo Research, Irvine, CA, USA) with either expression vector pET24c *Inf*A, pET24c *Inf*C *wt*, or pET24c *Inf*C E166C, coding for IF1, IF3 *wt*, or $IF3_{E166C}$, respectively. pET24c vectors containing *wt* and mutant genes were commercially acquired (GenScript, Piscataway, NJ, USA). Typically, 2 L of Luria–Bertoni (LB) medium were used to grow $BL21_{DE3}$ pET24c *Inf*A or pET24c *Inf*C to an OD_{600nm} of 0.5. Protein expression was induced by adding 1 mM Isopropyl β-D-1-thiogalactopyranoside (IPTG, Thermo Fisher Scientific). Cells were allowed to express IF1 or IF3 for 3 h prior to harvesting by centrifugation at 5000× *g* at 4 °C. Cells were lysed in Lysis Buffer (50 mM Hepes pH: 7, 100 mM NH_4Cl, 10 mM $MgCl_2$, 10% Glycerol, 6 mM 2-mercaptoetanol) supplemented with 0.1 mg/mL of Lysozyme (Merck, Darmstadt, Germany). After five cycles of freezing and thawing, 1 U/mL DNAse I was added to reduce the viscosity in 20 min of incubation at 4 °C. Membranes and supernatant were separated by centrifugation at 15,000× *g* for 30 min.

4.2. *IF1, IF3, and 30S Subunits Purification*

Both initiation factors were purified by Cation exchange chromatography on HiTrap SP HP (Amersham, Uppsala, Sweden). Supernatants were manually loaded to the column (1 mL column volume) and subsequently subjected to a linear NH_4Cl gradient (0.05–1 M) in a Jasco HPLC system (Jasco, Tokyo, Japan). The gradient was prepared in $Buffer_A$ (50 mM Hepes pH 7.1, 10% Glycerol, 6 mM 2-Mercaptoethanol). IF3 and IF1 were eluted at 700 mM and 400 mM of NH_4Cl, respectively, in (Figures S1a and S2a). The best separation conditions were 1 mL/min flow rate and 20 Column Volumes (CV) long gradient, collecting fractions of 1 mL each. Protein elution was followed by absorbance at 290 nm and SDS-Polyacrylamide Gel Electrophoresis (SDS-PAGE, 15%) (Figures S1 and S2). While IF3 was eluted with an elevated degree of purity, IF1 fractions contained high molecular weight contaminates (Figure S2b). Full elimination of the contaminants was obtained by subjecting the combined IF1 fractions to Amicon® Ultra 30K Da centrifugal filters (Merck) followed by concentration on a HiTrap SP HP (Amersham), single step eluted with 1 M NH_4CL $Buffer_A$ (Figure S2c).

30S subunits purification methods are described in detail in [38].

4.3. Double Labeling of IF3 with Atto-Tec Dyes

$IF3_{E166C}$ was subjected to extensive dialysis in labeling buffer (50 mM Hepes pH: 7.1, 100 mM NH_4Cl, 10% glycerol, 0.5 mM TCEP) in a D-Tube™ Dialyzer Maxi (Merck) to remove traces of 2-mercaptoethanol as the reducing agent strongly inhibits the coupling of maleimide-linked dyes to cysteines. First, the C-terminal was labeled at the recombinant cysteine (166) as it is exposed and efficiently reacts with maleimide derivatives [38]. A 10-fold excess of Atto-540Q maleimide (Atto-Tec) over $IF3_{E166C}$ was incubated in labeling buffer for 20 min. The reaction was stopped by the addition of 6 mM 2-mercaptoethanol. The modified $IF3_{CTD}{}^{540Q}$ was purified from unreacted dyes on a HiTrap SP HP column. After 10 CV washes with $Buffer_A$ containing 100 mM NH_4Cl, a single step elution was applied using 3 mL of 1 M NH_4Cl in $Buffer_A$. Typically, full protein recovery is achieved in 0.5 mL and elution of the labeled protein is readily visible. IF3 $_{CTD}{}^{540Q}$ was subsequently dialyzed as mentioned above in a labeling buffer containing 2 M UREA.

Denaturation of IF3 results in the exposure of the otherwise buried cysteine at position 65 of the NTD. The denatured protein was incubated with a 10-fold molar excess of Atto-488 maleimide for 1 h at RT, mild shacking was applied. $IF3_{CTD}{}^{540Q}{}_{-NTD}{}^{488}$ ($IF3_{DL}$) was purified from the unreacted dye as described above using HiTrap SP HP column (Merck). Eluted proteins were dialyzed against storage buffer (Hepes pH: 7.1, 100 mM NH_4Cl, 10% Glycerol, 6 mM 2-mercaptoethanol) and small aliquots were stored at −80 °C. Purity and efficiency of labeling was assayed by 15% SDS-PAGE, where fluorescence was observed under a UV trans-illuminator and total protein by blue Coomassie staining (Figure S1c).

4.4. Equilibrium Binding Measurements

All reactions were performed in $HAKM_{10}$ buffer (50 mM HEPES 70mM, NH_4Cl, 30 mM KCl, 10 mM $MgCl_2$, 6 mM 2-Mercaptoethanol). 30S titrations of $IF3_{DL}$ (0.5 μM) were incubated with varying concentrations of 30S subunits (0.16, 0.3125, 0.625, 1.25, 2.5 μM). Reactions were incubated for 10 min at 37 °C. Fluorescence was measured in a NanoDrop 3000 fluorimeter (Thermo) using blue LED excitation and emission at maximum for Atto-488 (518 nm) at room temperature. Typically, five independent measurements were performed for each reaction to calculate mean and standard deviation values. Binding of IF1 to 30S–IF3DL complexes was performed as above after pre-incubating $IF3_{DL}$ with 30S subunits for 10 min at 37 °C. IF1 influence was measured at varying concentration of the factor (0.1, 0.2, 0.5, 1, 2 μM). 30S subunits were $MgCl_2$ (20 mM) activated for 30 min at 42 °C prior to being used.

4.5. Stopped-Flow Measurements and Analysis

Fluorescence stopped-flow measurements were performed using a SF-300X stopped-flow apparatus (KintekCorp) by rapidly mixing equal volumes (30 μL each) of reacting solutions (Figure 2a). Excitation wavelength for Atto-488 was 470 nm and emission was measured after a long-pass optical filter with a 515 nm cut-off. One thousand points were acquired in 20–30 s of each measurement. Ten to 15 replicates were recorded for each reaction and subsequently averaged. All stopped flow reactions were performed in $TAKM_{10}$ buffer (50 mM Tris (pH: 7.5), 70 mM NH_4Cl, 30 mM KCl, 10 mM $MgCl_2$, 6 mM 2-Mercaptoethanol) at 25 °C; 30S and IFs concentrations are given in the figure legends.

4.6. Data Analysis

Non-linear regressions by Prism 6.0 (Graphpad Software, La Jolla, CA, USA) were performed using the following equations:

$$[C] = \frac{([A] + [B] + K_D) - \sqrt{([A] + [B] + K_D)^2 - 4[A][B]}}{2}, \quad (1)$$

with A = 30S; B = $IF3_{DL}$; C = 30S–$IF3_{DL}$ and K_D is the dissociation constant.

$$F = F_0 + F_1 e^{kapp1 \times t} + F_2 e^{kapp2 \times t} \quad (2)$$

$$[C] = \frac{[A][B]}{K_D + [B]}; \quad (3)$$

A = 30S–$IF3_{DL}$; B = IF1; C = 30S–$IF3_{DL}$–IF1.

$$F = F_0 + F_1 e^{kapp1 \times t} \quad (4)$$

4.7. Structural Models

Molecular models were derived from the structures of 30S–bound IF1 of *Thermus thermophiles* (PDB 1HR0; [13]), streptomycin bound to the 30S (PDB 4DR3; [14]), kanamycin bound to the site-A section of h44 (PDB 2ESI; [15]) and the apo-30S subunit (PDB 4DR1; [14]) (Table S3). The structural models showing the binding site of IF1, streptomycin and kanamycin where generated by aligning the structures through the backbone atoms of the 16S rRNA (Full sequence for 30S/IF1 and 30S/streptomycin and partial sequence for the A-site with kanamycin) using Chimera and Swiss PDB viewer [56,57]. Molecular graphics and analyses were performed with the UCSF Chimera package. Chimera is developed by the Resource for Biocomputing, Visualization, and Informatics at the University of California, San Francisco (supported by NIGMS P41-GM103311). Through this work the new nomenclature for ribosomal proteins has been used [58].

Acknowledgments: We especially thank Annamaria Giuliodori for critically reading the manuscript, Pablo Soriano for his technical support, and Alon Gregory Rutigliano for helping during his laboratory training. **Funding:** Programa Nacional de Innovación para la Competitividad y Productividad (382-PNICP-PIBA-2014 (to Pohl Mil6n and Attilio Fabbretti)); Fondo Nacional de Desarrollo Científico, Tecnol6gico y de Innovación Tecnol6gica (FONDECYT–084–2015 (to Pohl Mil6n)). FIRB Futuro in Ricerca from the Italian Ministero dell'Istruzione, dell'Universitá e della Ricerca (RBFR130VS5 001 to Attilio Fabbretti).

Author Contributions: Attilio Fabbretti and Pohl Mil6n conceived the project; Attilio Fabbretti, Roberto Chulluncuy, Carlos Espiche and Jose Alberto Nakamoto designed, performed, and analyzed the experiments; Attilio Fabbretti and Pohl Mil6n wrote the article with the input of Jose Alberto Nakamoto, Roberto Chulluncuy and Carlos Espiche.

Abbreviations

The following abbreviations are used in this manuscript:

MDR	Multidrug-resistant
XDR	Extensively drug-resistant
TB	Tuberculosis
IF3	Initiation factor 3
IF1	Initiation factor 1
CDC	Centers for Disease Control and Prevention
30S	Minor ribosomal subunit
IC	Initiation complexes
SD	Shine–Dalgarno sequence
NTD	N-terminal domain
CTD	C-terminal domain
FRET	Fluorescence Resonance Energy Transfer
$IF3_{DL}$	Double-labeled IF3
Pre-IC	Pre-initiation complex
Initiatior tRNA	fMet-$tRNA^{fMet}$

K_D	Dissociation constant
k_{app}	Apparent rate constant
SEM	Standard error of the mean
F	fluorescent amplitude
LB	Luria–Bertoni medium
IPTG	Isopropyl β-D-1-thiogalactopyranoside
SDS-PAGE	Sodium-dodecyl-sulfate-Polyacrylamide Gel Electrophoresis
HEPES	4-(2-hydroxyethyl)-1-piperazineethanesulfonic acid
TCEP	tris(2-carboxyethyl)phosphine

References

1. Taylor, L.H.; Latham, S.M.; Woolhouse, M.E.J. Risk factors for human disease emergence. *Philos. Trans. R. Soc. B Biol. Sci.* **2001**, *356*, 983–989. [CrossRef] [PubMed]
2. Zumla, A.; Raviglione, M.; Hafner, R.; von Reyn, C.F. Tuberculosis. *N. Engl. J. Med.* **2013**, *368*, 745–755. [CrossRef] [PubMed]
3. Blumberg, H.M.; Burman, W.J.; Chaisson, R.E.; Daley, C.L.; Etkind, S.C.; Friedman, L.N.; Fujiwara, P.; Grzemska, M.; Hopewell, P.C.; Iseman, M.D.; et al. Centers for Disease Control and Prevention/Infectious Diseases Society of America: Treatment of tuberculosis. *Am. J. Respir. Crit. Care Med.* **2003**, *167*, 603–662. [PubMed]
4. Horsburgh, C.R.; Feldman, S.; Ridzon, R. Infectious Diseases Society of America Practice guidelines for the treatment of tuberculosis. *Clin. Infect. Dis.* **2000**, *31*, 633–639. [CrossRef] [PubMed]
5. Mingeot-Leclercq, M.P.; Glupczynski, Y.; Tulkens, P.M. Aminoglycosides: Activity and resistance. *Antimicrob. Agents Chemother.* **1999**, *43*, 727–737. [PubMed]
6. Pestka, S. [28] The use of inhibitors in studies of protein synthesis. *Methods Enzymol.* **1974**, *30*, 261–282. [PubMed]
7. Misumi, M.; Tanaka, N. Mechanism of inhibition of translocation by kanamycin and viomycin: A comparative study with fusidic acid. *Biochem. Biophys. Res. Commun.* **1980**, *92*, 647–654. [CrossRef]
8. Gorini, L.; Jacoby, G.A.; Breckenridge, L. Ribosomal ambiguity. *Cold Spring Harb. Symp. Quant. Biol.* **1966**, *31*, 657–664. [CrossRef] [PubMed]
9. Lodmell, J.S.; Dahlberg, A.E. A conformational switch in *Escherichia coli* 16S ribosomal RNA during decoding of messenger RNA. *Science* **1997**, *277*, 1262–1267. [CrossRef] [PubMed]
10. Blomberg, C.; Johansson, J.; Liljenström, H. Error propagation in *E. coli* protein synthesis. *J. Theor. Biol.* **1985**, *113*, 407–423. [CrossRef]
11. Fast, R.; Eberhard, T.H.; Ruusala, T.; Kurland, C.G. Does streptomycin cause an error catastrophe? *Biochimie* **1987**, *69*, 131–136. [CrossRef]
12. Luzzatto, L.; Apirion, D.; Schlessinger, D. Streptomycin action: Greater inhibition of *Escherichia coli* ribosome function with exogenous than with endogenous messenger ribonucleic acid. *J. Bacteriol.* **1969**, *99*, 206–209. [PubMed]
13. Carter, A.P.; Clemons, W.M.; Brodersen, D.E.; Morgan-Warren, R.J.; Hartsch, T.; Wimberly, B.T.; Ramakrishnan, V. Crystal structure of an initiation factor bound to the 30S ribosomal subunit. *Science* **2001**, *291*, 498–501. [CrossRef] [PubMed]
14. Demirci, H.; Murphy, F.; Murphy, E.; Gregory, S.T.; Dahlberg, A.E.; Jogl, G. A structural basis for streptomycin-induced misreading of the genetic code. *Nat. Commun.* **2013**, *4*. [CrossRef] [PubMed]
15. François, B.; Russell, R.J.M.; Murray, J.B.; Aboul-ela, F.; Masquida, B.; Vicens, Q.; Westhof, E. Crystal structures of complexes between aminoglycosides and decoding A site oligonucleotides: Role of the number of rings and positive charges in the specific binding leading to miscoding. *Nucleic Acids Res.* **2005**, *33*, 5677–5690. [CrossRef] [PubMed]
16. Carter, A.P.; Clemons, W.M.; Brodersen, D.E.; Morgan-Warren, R.J.; Wimberly, B.T.; Ramakrishnan, V. Functional insights from the structure of the 30S ribosomal subunit and its interactions with antibiotics. *Nature* **2000**, *407*, 340–348. [PubMed]
17. Moazed, D.; Samaha, R.R.; Gualerzi, C.O.; Noller, H.F. Specific protection of 16S rRNA by translational initiation factors. *J. Mol. Biol.* **1995**, *248*, 207–210. [CrossRef]
18. Hussain, T.; Llácer, J.L.; Wimberly, B.T.; Kieft, J.S.; Ramakrishnan, V. Large-scale movements of IF3 and tRNA during bacterial translation initiation. *Cell* **2016**, *167*, 133–144. [CrossRef] [PubMed]

19. Fabbretti, A.; Pon, C.L.; Hennelly, S.P.; Hill, W.E.; Lodmell, J.S.; Gualerzi, C.O. The real-time path of translation factor IF3 onto and off the ribosome. *Mol. Cell* **2007**, *25*, 285–296. [CrossRef] [PubMed]
20. Dallas, A.; Noller, H.F. Interaction of translation initiation factor 3 with the 30S ribosomal subunit. *Mol. Cell* **2001**, *8*, 855–864. [CrossRef]
21. Julián, P.; Milon, P.; Agirrezabala, X.; Lasso, G.; Gil, D.; Rodnina, M.V.; Valle, M. The Cryo-EM structure of a complete 30S translation initiation complex from *Escherichia coli*. *PLoS Biol.* **2011**, *9*, e1001095. [CrossRef] [PubMed]
22. Pon, C.L.; Pawlik, R.T.; Gualerzi, C. The topographical localization of IF3 on *Escherichia coli* 30S ribosomal subunits as a clue to its way of functioning. *FEBS Lett.* **1982**, *137*, 163–167. [CrossRef]
23. Biou, V.; Shu, F.; Ramakrishnan, V. X-ray crystallography shows that translational initiation factor IF3 consists of two compact alpha/beta domains linked by an alpha-helix. *EMBO J.* **1995**, *14*, 4056–4064. [PubMed]
24. Garcia, C.; Fortier, P.L.; Blanquet, S.; Lallemand, J.Y.; Dardel, F. Solution structure of the ribosome-binding domain of *E. coli* translation initiation factor IF3. Homology with the U1A protein of the eukaryotic spliceosome. *J. Mol. Biol.* **1995**, *254*, 247–259. [CrossRef] [PubMed]
25. Moreau, M.; de Cock, E.; Fortier, P.L.; Garcia, C.; Albaret, C.; Blanquet, S.; Lallemand, J.Y.; Dardel, F. Heteronuclear NMR studies of *E. coli* translation initiation factor IF3. Evidence that the inter-domain region is disordered in solution. *J. Mol. Biol.* **1997**, *266*, 15–22. [CrossRef] [PubMed]
26. Gualerzi, C.O.; Pon, C.L. Initiation of mRNA translation in bacteria: Structural and dynamic aspects. *Cell. Mol. Life Sci.* **2015**, *72*, 4341–4367. [CrossRef] [PubMed]
27. De Cock, E.; Springer, M.; Dardel, F. The interdomain linker of *Escherichia coli* initiation factor IF3: A possible trigger of translation initiation specificity. *Mol. Microbiol.* **1999**, *32*, 193–202. [CrossRef] [PubMed]
28. Milon, P.; Konevega, A.L.; Gualerzi, C.O.; Rodnina, M.V. Kinetic checkpoint at a late step in translation initiation. *Mol. Cell* **2008**, *30*, 712–720. [CrossRef] [PubMed]
29. Hennelly, S.P.; Antoun, A.; Ehrenberg, M.; Gualerzi, C.O.; Knight, W.; Lodmell, J.S.; Hill, W.E. A time-resolved investigation of ribosomal subunit association. *J. Mol. Biol.* **2005**, *346*, 1243–1258. [CrossRef] [PubMed]
30. Garcia, C.; Fortier, P.L.; Blanquet, S.; Lallemand, J.Y.; Dardel, F. 1H and 15N resonance assignments and structure of the N-terminal domain of *Escherichia coli* initiation factor 3. *Eur. J. Biochem.* **1995**, *228*, 395–402. [CrossRef] [PubMed]
31. Pon, C.; Cannistraro, S.; Giovane, A.; Gualerzi, C.O. Structure-function relationship in *Escherichia coli* initiation factors. Environment of the Cys residue and evidence for a hydrophobic region in initiation factor IF3 by fluorescence and ESR spectroscopy. *Arch. Biochem. Biophys.* **1982**, *217*, 47–57. [CrossRef]
32. Pon, C.L.; Gualerzi, C.O. Effect of initiation factor 3 binding on the 30S ribosomal subunits of *Escherichia coli*. *Proc. Natl. Acad. Sci. USA* **1974**, *71*, 4950–4954. [CrossRef] [PubMed]
33. Milon, P.; Maracci, C.; Filonava, L.; Gualerzi, C.O.; Rodnina, M.V. Real-time assembly landscape of bacterial 30S translation initiation complex. *Nat. Struct. Mol. Biol.* **2012**, *19*, 609–615. [CrossRef] [PubMed]
34. Milon, P.; Carotti, M.; Konevega, A.L.; Wintermeyer, W.; Rodnina, M.V.; Gualerzi, C.O. The ribosome-bound initiation factor 2 recruits initiator tRNA to the 30S initiation complex. *EMBO Rep.* **2010**, *11*, 312–316. [CrossRef] [PubMed]
35. Tsai, A.; Petrov, A.; Marshall, R.A.; Korlach, J.; Uemura, S.; Puglisi, J.D. Heterogeneous pathways and timing of factor departure during translation initiation. *Nature* **2012**, *487*, 390–393. [CrossRef] [PubMed]
36. Qin, D.; Fredrick, K. Control of translation initiation involves a factor-induced rearrangement of helix 44 of 16S ribosomal RNA. *Mol. Microbiol.* **2009**, *71*, 1239–1249. [CrossRef] [PubMed]
37. Elvekrog, M.M.; Gonzalez, R.L. Conformational selection of translation initiation factor 3 signals proper substrate selection. *Nat. Struct. Mol. Biol.* **2013**, *20*, 628–633. [CrossRef] [PubMed]
38. Milon, P.; Konevega, A.L.; Peske, F.; Fabbretti, A.; Gualerzi, C.O.; Rodnina, M.V. Transient kinetics, fluorescence, and FRET in studies of initiation of translation in bacteria. *Methods Enzymol.* **2007**, *430*, 1–30. [PubMed]
39. Wilson, D.N. The A-Z of bacterial translation inhibitors. *Crit. Rev. Biochem. Mol. Biol.* **2009**, *44*, 393–433. [CrossRef] [PubMed]
40. Davies, J.; GILBERT, W.; Gorini, L. Streptomycin, suppression, and the code. *Proc. Natl. Acad. Sci. USA* **1964**, *51*, 883–890. [CrossRef] [PubMed]
41. Gorini, L.; Gundersen, W.; Burger, M. Genetics of regulation of enzyme synthesis in the arginine biosynthetic pathway of *Escherichia coli*. *Cold Spring Harb. Symp. Quant. Biol.* **1961**, *26*, 173–182. [CrossRef] [PubMed]

42. Tsai, A.; Uemura, S.; Johansson, M.; Puglisi, E.V.; Marshall, R.A.; Aitken, C.E.; Korlach, J.; Ehrenberg, M.; Puglisi, J.D. The impact of aminoglycosides on the dynamics of translation elongation. *Cell Rep.* **2013**, *3*, 497–508. [CrossRef] [PubMed]
43. Gromadski, K.B.; Rodnina, M.V. Streptomycin interferes with conformational coupling between codon recognition and GTPase activation on the ribosome. *Nat. Struct. Mol. Biol.* **2004**, *11*, 316–322. [CrossRef] [PubMed]
44. Luzzatto, L.; Apirion, D.; Schlessinger, D. Mechanism of action of streptomycin in *E. coli*: Interruption of the ribosome cycle at the initiation of protein synthesis. *Proc. Natl. Acad. Sci. USA* **1968**, *60*, 873–880. [CrossRef] [PubMed]
45. La Teana, A.; Gualerzi, C.O.; Brimacombe, R. From stand-by to decoding site. Adjustment of the mRNA on the 30S ribosomal subunit under the influence of the initiation factors. *RNA* **1995**, *1*, 772–782. [PubMed]
46. La Teana, A.; Pon, C.L.; Gualerzi, C.O. Translation of mRNAs with degenerate initiation triplet AUU displays high initiation factor 2 dependence and is subject to initiation factor 3 repression. *Proc. Natl. Acad. Sci. USA* **1993**, *90*, 4161–4165. [CrossRef] [PubMed]
47. Grigoriadou, C.; Marzi, S.; Pan, D.; Gualerzi, C.O.; Cooperman, B.S. The translational fidelity function of IF3 during transition from the 30 S initiation complex to the 70 S initiation complex. *J. Mol. Biol.* **2007**, *373*, 551–561. [CrossRef] [PubMed]
48. Moazed, D.; Noller, H.F. Interaction of antibiotics with functional sites in 16S ribosomal RNA. *Nature* **1987**, *327*, 389–394. [CrossRef] [PubMed]
49. Fabbretti, A.; Schedlbauer, A.; Brandi, L.; Kaminishi, T.; Giuliodori, A.M.; Garofalo, R.; Ochoa-Lizarralde, B.; Takemoto, C.; Yokoyama, S.; Connell, S.R.; et al. Inhibition of translation initiation complex formation by GE81112 unravels a 16S rRNA structural switch involved in P-site decoding. *Proc. Natl. Acad. Sci. USA* **2016**, *113*, E2286–E2295. [CrossRef] [PubMed]
50. Fabbretti, A.; Gualerzi, C.O.; Brandi, L. How to cope with the quest for new antibiotics. *FEBS Lett.* **2011**, *585*, 1673–1681. [CrossRef] [PubMed]
51. Brandi, L.; Fabbretti, A.; Milon, P.; Carotti, M.; Pon, C.L.; Gualerzi, C.O. Methods for identifying compounds that specifically target translation. *Methods Enzymol.* **2007**, *431*, 229–267. [PubMed]
52. Fabbretti, A.; He, C.-G.; Gaspari, E.; Maffioli, S.; Brandi, L.; Spurio, R.; Sosio, M.; Jabes, D.; Donadio, S. A derivative of the thiopeptide GE2270A highly selective against *Propionibacterium acnes*. *Antimicrob. Agents Chemother.* **2015**, *59*, 4560–4568. [CrossRef] [PubMed]
53. Brandi, L.; Maffioli, S.; Donadio, S.; Quaglia, F.; Sette, M.; Milon, P.; Gualerzi, C.O.; Fabbretti, A. Structural and functional characterization of the bacterial translocation inhibitor GE82832. *FEBS Lett.* **2012**, *586*, 3373–3378. [CrossRef] [PubMed]
54. Fabbretti, A.; Brandi, L.; Petrelli, D.; Pon, C.L.; Castanedo, N.R.; Medina, R.; Gualerzi, C.O. The antibiotic Furvina(R) targets the P-site of 30S ribosomal subunits and inhibits translation initiation displaying start codon bias. *Nucleic Acids Res.* **2012**, *40*, 10366–10374. [CrossRef] [PubMed]
55. Kaminishi, T.; Schedlbauer, A.; Fabbretti, A.; Brandi, L.; Ochoa-Lizarralde, B.; He, C.-G.; Milon, P.; Connell, S.R.; Gualerzi, C.O.; Fucini, P. Crystallographic characterization of the ribosomal binding site and molecular mechanism of action of Hygromycin A. *Nucleic Acids Res.* **2015**, *43*, 10015–10025. [CrossRef] [PubMed]
56. Guex, N.; Peitsch, M.C. SWISS-MODEL and the Swiss-PdbViewer: An environment for comparative protein modeling. *Electrophoresis* **1997**, *18*, 2714–2723. [CrossRef] [PubMed]
57. Pettersen, E.F.; Goddard, T.D.; Huang, C.C.; Couch, G.S.; Greenblatt, D.M.; Meng, E.C.; Ferrin, T.E. UCSF Chimera—A visualization system for exploratory research and analysis. *J. Comput. Chem.* **2004**, *25*, 1605–1612. [CrossRef] [PubMed]
58. Ban, N.; Beckmann, R.; Cate, J.H.D.; Dinman, J.D.; Dragon, F.; Ellis, S.R.; Lafontaine, D.L.J.; Lindahl, L.; Liljas, A.; Lipton, J.M.; et al. A new system for naming ribosomal proteins. *Curr. Opin. Struct. Biol.* **2014**, *24*, 165–169. [CrossRef] [PubMed]

12

In Vitro Synergism of Silver Nanoparticles with Antibiotics as an Alternative Treatment in Multiresistant Uropathogens

Montserrat Lopez-Carrizales [1], Karla Itzel Velasco [1], Claudia Castillo [2], Andrés Flores [3], Martín Magaña [3], Gabriel Alejandro Martinez-Castanon [4] and Fidel Martinez-Gutierrez [1,*]

1 Laboratorio de Microbiología, Universidad Autónoma de San Luis Potosí, San Luis Potosí, CP 78210, Mexico; montsecarrizales@icloud.com (M.L.-C.); kivg56@hotmail.com (K.I.V.)
2 Laboratorio de Células Neurales Troncales, CIACYT-Facultad de Medicina, Universidad Autónoma de San Luis Potosí, San Luis Potosí, CP 78210, Mexico; claudiacastillo@gmail.com
3 Hospital Central Dr. Ignacio Morones Prieto, San Luis Potosí, CP 78290, Mexico; santosf2000@yahoo.com (A.F.); mmaganaa@hotmail.com (M.M.)
4 Facultad de Estomatología, Universidad Autónoma de San Luis Potosí, San Luis Potosí, CP 78290, Mexico; mtzcastanon@fciencias.uaslp.mx
* Correspondence: fidel@uaslp.mx

Abstract: The increase in the prevalence of bacterial resistance to antibiotics has become one of the main health problems worldwide, thus threatening the era of antibiotics most frequently used in the treatment of infections. The need to develop new therapeutic strategies against multidrug resistant microorganisms, such as the combination of selected antimicrobials, can be considered as a suitable alternative. The in vitro activities of two groups of conventional antimicrobial agents alone and in combination with silver nanoparticles (AgNPs) were investigated against a set of ten multidrug resistant clinical isolate and two references strains by MIC assays and checkerboard testing, as well as their cytotoxicity, which was evaluated on human fibroblasts by MTT assay at the same concentration of the antimicrobial agents alone and in combination. Interesting results were achieved when the AgNPs and their combinations were characterized by Dynamic Light Scattering (DLS), Zeta Potential, Transmission Electron Microscopy (TEM), UV–visible spectroscopy and Fourier Transforms Infrared (FTIR) spectroscopy. The in vitro activities of ampicillin, in combination with AgNPs, against the 12 microorganisms showed one Synergy, seven Partial Synergy and four Additive effects, while the results with amikacin and AgNPs showed three Synergy, eight Partial Synergy and one Additive effects. The cytotoxic effect at these concentrations presented a statistically significant decrease of their cytotoxicity ($p < 0.05$). These results indicate that infections caused by multidrug resistant microorganisms could be treated using a synergistic combination of antimicrobial drugs and AgNPs. Further studies are necessary to evaluate the specific mechanisms of action, which could help predict undesirable off-target interactions, suggest ways of regulating a drug's activity, and identify novel therapeutic agents in this health problem.

Keywords: antimicrobial activity; biofilm; urinary infection; silver nanoparticles; bacterial resistance

---

1. Introduction

Urinary tract infections (UTIs) are defined as inflammatory processes related to the invasion and multiplication of microorganisms that occur at any level of the urinary tract, including urethral (urethritis), bladder (cystitis), ureters (ureteritis) and kidney infections (pyelonephritis) [1].

Approximately between 150 and 250 million cases of UTIs occur each year worldwide [2]. In 2011, more than 8 million cases were reported in the U.S. [1], of which 93,300 were acquired in intensive care units [3]. Recently, the epidemiological bulletin of the Ministry of Health reported in 2016 a total of 4,023,432 cases of UTIs in Mexico, of which 76.68% were in women and only 23.31% in men.

Gram-negative intestinal bacteria are the most common etiology agents of UTIs, where uropathogenic *Escherichia coli* (UPEC) is the major microorganism isolate, which is a member of the Enterobacteriacea family [4]. Other commonly associated pathogens include *Klebsiella* sp. and *Proteus mirabilis*, both of which are characterized by their urease enzyme and Gram-positive bacteria such as *Staphylococcus saprophyticus* and *Enterococcus faecalis* [5].

Urinary Tract Infections Associated with Catheters (CAUTI) are one of the most frequent explanations of nosocomial infections [6]. Patients with urinary catheters show an increment of bacteriuria in relation to duration of catheterization [7], however, the most important factor is the biofilm formation along the catheter surface [7,8]. A biofilm is a resistance mechanism that consists in a self-organized community of microorganisms embedded in a matrix of extracellular polymeric substances synthesized by themselves [9]. Many bacterial species show growth in the form of biofilms, which gives them various advantages [10]. Some of the benefits are metabolic cooperation (nutrients) [11], horizontal gene transfer [12], protection against environmental stresses, lower susceptibility to antimicrobial agents [13,14] and prevention of host defense mechanisms (immune system) [15]. The most common organisms that contaminate the urinary catheter and develop biofilms are strains of *Escherichia coli, Pseudomonas aeruginosa, Enterococcus, Proteus mirabilis, Klebsiella pneumoniae* and coagulase-negative staphylococci [10,16].

The antibiotic resistance of bacteria is a global health problem that is continually expanding, and is recognized as a medical problem that increases morbidity and mortality rates, which implies length of hospital stays as well as cost and bad prognosis [17,18]. In fact, the speed at which bacteria are establishing resistance to current antibiotics is faster than the development of new molecules with antimicrobial features. Unfortunately, it is very difficult to identify new bacterial targets that can be used to develop new classes of antimicrobial agents that are safe and effective.

In this context, nanotechnology opens new possibilities, allowing new solutions with old resources. Nanoscale materials such as silver nanoparticles (AgNPs) have emerged as novel agents due to their unique physicochemical properties and remarkable antimicrobial activities that confer a great advantage for the development of alternative products against, for example, multi-drug resistant microorganisms [19,20]. Due to the above, it has been proposed to implement the use of AgNPs on different devices for medical use. One of the strategies is the modification of surfaces of the devices to inhibit the formation of bacterial biofilms [21].

Recently, several studies have indicated that AgNPs can enhance the effect of antibiotics against susceptible and resistant bacteria, [22] as a well as decrease bacterial adhesion in the early stages of biofilm formation. In 2016, Rajendran and et al., impregnated urinary catheters with antibiotics (amikacin and nitrofurantoin) and a synergistic combination of antibiotics and AgNPs (synthesized by a biological method) in order to evaluate antibiofilm activity. The authors reported that the synergistic combination showed a 90% inhibition of bacterial adhesion, whereas functionalization with antibiotics showed only 25% inhibition [23].

Some authors have reported that AgNPs have toxic effects on mammalian cells; for example, impairment of normal mitochondrial function, increased membrane permeability and generation of reactive oxygen species [24,25].

In this study, the synergistic activity of AgNPs was evaluated with conventional antibiotics against Gram-positive and Gram-negative multi-drug resistant isolates from clinical samples. Results presented here show that AgNPs, in combination with antibiotics, increase the antimicrobial effect in an additive or synergistic manner. Furthermore, MTT assays suggest that at low concentrations the AgNPs and their combinations do not present cytotoxic effects in eukaryotic cells.

2. Results and Discussion

2.1. Synthesis and Characterization of AgNPs

TEM micrograph revealed that the AgNPs were of spherical and pseudospherical shapes (Figure 1). Based on the particle size distribution histogram evaluated from the corresponding TEM micrograph (n = 100), the mean (±SD) size of AgNPs 8.57 ± 1.17 nm was calculated. The mean size for the combination of AgNPs with ampicillin (AgNPs + AMP) was 4.01 ± 0.80 nm and for the combination of AgNPs with amikacin (AgNPs + AMK) was 6.03 ± 0.87 nm (Table 1).

The particle size distributions of AgNPs + AMP and AgNPs + AMK were also evaluated in Dulbecco's Modified Eagle Medium (DMEM).

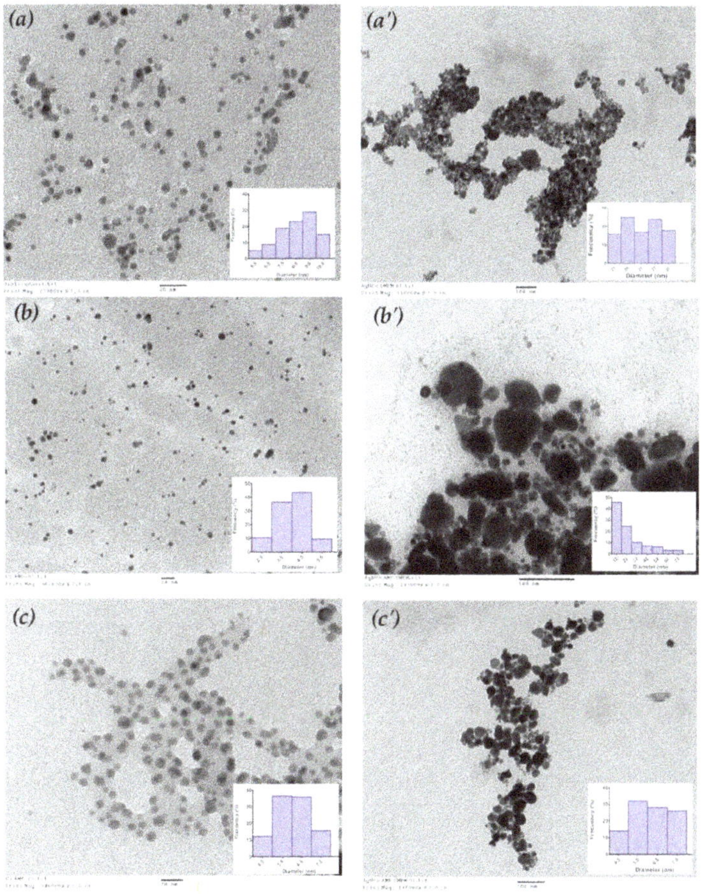

Figure 1. Morphological characterization of silver nanoparticles and their combinations with antibiotics. Transmission electron micrographs showing the formation of spherical and pseudospherical nanoparticles. (**a**) AgNPs; (**a'**) AgNPs in DMEM; (**b**) AgNPs + AMP; (**b'**) AgNPs + AMP in DMEM; (**c**) AgNPs + AMK; (**c'**) AgNPs + AMK in DMEM. Insets: Particle size distribution histogram. DMEM: Dulbecco's Modified Eagle Medium. AMP: Ampicillin. AMK: Amikacin.

AgNPs synthesized in aqueous solution and their combinations with antibiotics were characterized by DLS (Table 1). The results of the dialyzed AgNPs showed a narrow size distribution with a hydrodynamic diameter of (±SD) 8.23 nm ± 0.91 nm and a zeta potential value of −40.80 mV ± 9.54 mV. The combination of AgNPs + AMP also showed a narrow size distribution with a hydrodynamic diameter of 4.69 nm ± 0.51 nm. This decrease in size was attributed to the fact that ampicillin favors the homogeneous dispersion of the nanoparticles and gives it a greater stability when it obtains a zeta potential value of −51.00 mV ± 20.20 mV. The results of combination of AgNPs + AMK showed a narrow distribution of sizes with a hydrodynamic diameter of 947.90 nm ± 65.30 nm and a value of −21.10 mV ± 4.63 mV for zeta potential. The increase of size of the nanoparticles are attributed to the addition of amikacin, which favors agglomeration of the AgNPs and causes an increase in the zeta potential, which translates in less stable nanoparticles.

The hydrodynamic diameters and zeta potentials of AgNPs and their combinations were also evaluated in DMEM.

Table 1. Characterization of silver nanoparticles and their combinations with antibiotics by DLS and TEM.

	DLS				TEM	
	Hydrodynamic Diameter (nm)	Hydrodynamic Diameter in DMEM (nm)	Zeta Potential (mV)	Zeta Potential in DMEM (mV)	Diameter (nm)	Diameter in DMEM (nm)
AgNPs	8.23 ± 0.91	39.25 ± 6.42	−40.80 ± 9.54	−16.20 ± 0.0	8.57 ± 1.17	25.08 ± 2.74
AgNPs + AMP	4.69 ± 0.51	26.25 ± 5.55	−51.00 ± 20.20	−15.60 ± 0.0	4.01 ± 0.80	24.17 ± 16.29
AgNPs + AMK	947.90 ± 65.30	222.50 ± 47.10	−21.10 ± 4.63	−18.10 ± 7.56	6.03 ± 0.87	6.14 ± 0.99

Data are expressed as mean and standard deviation. DLS: Dynamic Light Scattering. TEM: Transmission Electron Microscopy. DMEM: Dulbecco's Modified Eagle Medium. AMP: Ampicillin. AMK: Amikacin.

The UV–visible spectrum revealed a peak at a wavelength of 412 nm for AgNPs whereas in the combination AgNPs + AMP, the peak was observed at 410 nm and in the combination AgNPs + AMK, the peak appeared at a wavelength of 450 nm (Figure 2). These peaks correspond to the excitation of the surface plasmon of AgNPs. The plasmonic resonance depends on several parameters, like the nature, size and geometry of the nanoparticles and the physical properties of the medium in which the nanoparticles are dispersed. In the case of AgNPs, the plasmon peak appears at a wavelength around 400 nm [26].

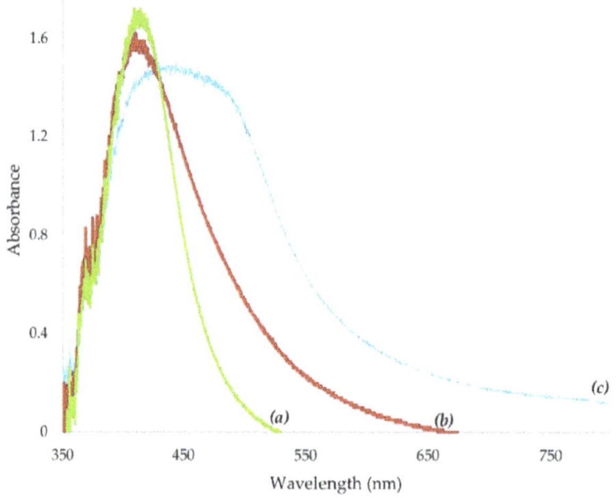

Figure 2. UV–visible absorption spectra of silver nanoparticles and their combinations with antibiotics. UV–visible spectrum showed the maximum absorbance at (**a**) 412 nm for AgNPs, (**b**) 410 nm for AgNPs + AMP and (**c**) 450 nm for AgNPs + AMK. AMP: Ampicillin. AMK: Amikacin.

In this study, gallic acid was used as a reducing and stabilizing agent, a molecule with a carboxylic group and rich in hydroxyl functional groups. Yoosaf et al. proposed that AgNPs are stabilized by gallic acid through electrostatic interactions through their oxidized carboxylic group and the afore-cited hydroxyl groups were capable of forming hydrogen bonds [27].

To study the possible interactions between antibiotics and the surface of the AgNPs, FTIR was performed (Figure 3). FTIR is useful for determining the chemical composition of antibiotics involved in the coating of AgNPs. The observed intense bands were compared with standard values to identify the functional groups. The FTIR spectra of the antibiotics (Figure 3a,b) changed greatly upon the combination with AgNPs (AgNPs + AMP and AgNPs + AMK), as displayed in Figure 3a′,b′. Ampicillin is a molecule that has carbonyl and amine functional groups, while amikacin is a molecule rich in hydroxyl and amine groups. In the case of ampicillin, the band at 1759 cm^{-1} disappeared completely (Figure 3a′), which suggests that the antibiotic interacts with the AgNPs through its carbonyl group (C=O). Furthermore, the peak of the primary amine at 3380 cm^{-1} (Figure 3a) shifted to 3130 cm^{-1} (Figure 3a′) after the combination with nanoparticles, indicating that the amine functional group was involved in the interaction with the surface of the AgNPs. Therefore, the spectrum of the amikacin showed that the bands at 1626 cm^{-1} corresponding to a carbonyl group and 3400 cm^{-1} for a primary amine disappeared completely (Figure 3b′) after being combined with the nanoparticles. Those results of the FTIR suggest that the functional groups of the antibiotics could be involved in the interaction by hydrogen bonds with gallic acid [28,29]. The results showed in Figure 3 are in concordance with the previous results of the Hua Deng et al., 2016, who carried out UV–Vis and Raman spectroscopy studies reveal that amikacin can form complexes with AgNPs, while ampicillin do not [30]. The authors reported that no Raman enhancement is observed when AgNPs are combined with ampicillin at any test concentrations. This implies that the antibiotics do not strongly interact with AgNPs to replace the stabilizer molecules on the surface of AgNPs. Moreover, they infer that the combinations of antibiotics and AgNPs have different ways to develop antimicrobial activities.

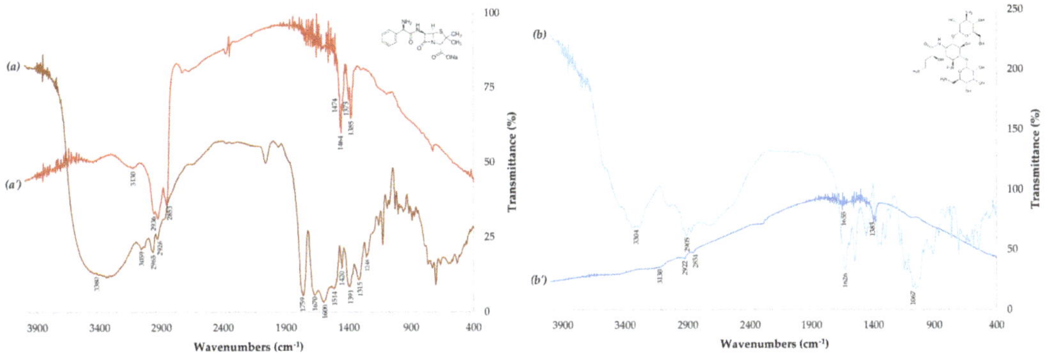

Figure 3. FTIR spectra of the antibiotics and their combinations with silver nanoparticles. (**a**) AMP: Ampicillin; (**a′**) AgNPs + AMP; (**b**) AMK: Amikacin; (**b′**) AgNPs + AMK. Insets: AMP and AMK structure.

2.2. Samples and Bacterial Strains

The multidrug resistance clinical strains used for this experiment were isolated from the urine of patients with CAUTI; microbiological analysis showed that the clinical pathogenic strains isolated were in accordance with the main etiologic agents causing CAUTI; these results are in accordance with previously results reported when the UTI were evaluated on hospitalized patients in Kolkata, an eastern region of India, as well as in studies where complicate and non-complicate UTI were studied [4,31].

2.3. Antimicrobial Test

A set of ten clinical pathogenic strains resistant to antibiotics associated with CAUTI were evaluated, of which two corresponded to Gram-positive strains and the rest to Gram-negative strains. The results showed that all clinical isolates (*E. faecium*, *S. aureus*, *A. baumannii*, *E. cloacae*, three different isolates of *E. coli*, *K. pneumoniae*, *M. morgannii* and *P. aeruginosa*) showed a MIC to AgNPs between 4 and 16 μg/mL. The bacterial strains showed MIC values of 4–128 μg/mL for amikacin and all Gram-negative strains were resistant to ampicillin.

2.4. Checkerboard Synergy

Table 2 shows the MIC archived with the ten multidrug resistance clinical strains grown in Mueller Hinton Broth with amikacin and ampicillin, both in the absence of AgNPs and when present; when the bacteria were incubated with the combination of AgNPs and antibiotic (AgNPs + AMK and AgNPs + AMP), the ampicillin and amikacin MICs decreased drastically for all strains. The combination of AgNPs + AMK reduce the MIC by 2 to 32-fold. By contrast, with the combination of AgNPs + AMP reduce the MIC just with *S. aureus* and *E. cloacae* by 1- and 4-fold respectively; with the other microorganisms, the MICs were reduced by 16- and 32-fold. These results show a better antimicrobial activity of the combination of AgNPs + AMP, which could be explained by the interaction between the AgNPs and ampicillin and, therefore, arrangement of the molecules in a new compound, which could work in both ways, like independent chemical entities or a new compound; more experiments are needed to explain the role and proportion of each one of them.

Table 2. Efficacy of silver nanoparticles, antibiotics and their combinations against clinical strains.

Clinical Strains	MIC (μg/mL)			Fold Change	MIC (μg/mL)		Fold Change
	AgNPs	AMK	AgNPs + AMK *		AMP	AgNPs + AMP *	
Gram-positive							
Enterococcus faecium	8	128	4	32	128	8	16
Staphylococcus aureus	8	4	2	2	4	4	1
Gram-negative							
Acinetobacter baumannii	16	128	4	32	128	8	16
Enterobacter cloacae	16	16	8	2	128	32	4
Escherichia coli (501) **	8	64	4	16	128	8	16
Escherichia coli (508) **	8	4	1	4	128	8	16
Escherichia coli (515) **	8	32	8	4	128	8	16
Klebsiella pneumoniae	4	4	2	2	128	4	32
Morganella morganii	8	8	4	2	128	8	16
Pseudomonas aeruginosa	4	32	4	8	128	4	32

* Minimum Inhibitory Concentration (MIC) represents the concentration of antibiotic (amikacin or ampicillin) present in the combination. AMK: Amikacin. AMP: Ampicillin. ** The numbers in parentheses indicate that *E. coli* corresponds to a different clinical sample.

The synergistic effects of AgNPs and conventional antibiotics were evaluated by determination of the Fractional Inhibitory Concentration (FIC) index (Figure 4). Synergistic interactions of AgNPs and amikacin were observed against *Acinetobacter baumannii*, *Escherichia coli* (508) and *E. coli* (ATCC 25922). Synergistic interactions of AgNPs and ampicillin were found only against *Acinetobacter baumannii*. Other combinational activities of AgNPs and antibiotics were considered as partially synergistic interactions. These synergistic activities of AgNPs in combination with conventional antibiotics suggest that it may be possible to reduce the viability of bacterial strains at lower antibiotic concentrations (Table 3).

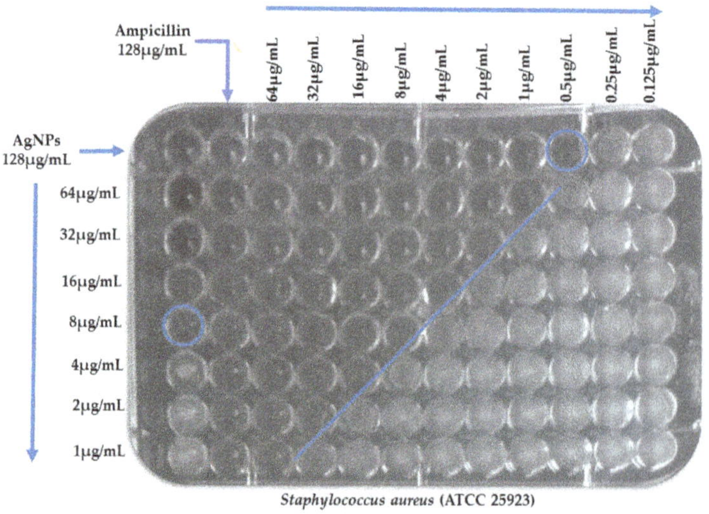

Figure 4. Example of checkerboard testing. Blue circles denote the MIC of antimicrobial agents (alone) and blue line denote the FIC (combination of both). MIC: Minimum Inhibitory Concentration. FIC: Fractional Inhibitory Concentration.

Table 3. FIC index of combinations among silver nanoparticles and antibiotics against clinical and reference strains.

Bacterial Strains	FIC Index			
	AgNPs + AMK		AgNPs + AMP	
Gram-positive				
Staphylococcus aureus (ATCC 25923)	1.06	(AD)	1.03	(AD)
Enterococcus faecium	0.53	(PS)	0.56	(PS)
Staphylococcus aureus	0.63	(PS)	1.25	(AD)
Gram-negative				
Escherichia coli (ATCC 25922)	0.31	(S)	1.50	(AD)
Acinetobacter baumannii	0.28	(S)	0.31	(S)
Enterobacter cloacae	0.75	(PS)	1.25	(AD)
Escherichia coli (501) **	0.56	(PS)	0.56	(PS)
Escherichia coli (508) **	0.31	(S)	0.56	(PS)
Escherichia coli (515) **	0.75	(PS)	0.56	(PS)
Klebsiella pneumoniae	0.75	(PS)	0.53	(PS)
Morganella morganii	0.75	(PS)	0.56	(PS)
Pseudomonas aeruginosa	0.63	(PS)	0.53	(PS)

FIC: Fractional Inhibitory Concentration. AMK: Amikacin. AMP: Ampicillin. ATCC: American Type Culture Collection. The FIC index was interpreted as follows: FIC $\leq$ 0.5, Synergy (S); 0.5 $\leq$ FIC < 1, Partial Synergy (PS); FIC = 1, Additive (AD); 2 $\leq$ FIC < 4, Indifferent (I); FIC > 4, Antagonism (AN) [32,33]. ** The numbers in parentheses indicate that *E. coli* corresponds to a different clinical sample.

2.5. Cytotoxicity of AgNPs

The cytotoxicity of AgNPs and antibiotics was evaluated separately and in combination by the MTT assay. AgNPs were tested at concentrations of 0.25, 1, 4, 16, 64 and 128 µg/mL in human fibroblasts. The percentages of living and dead cells were determined after 24 h of being exposed in contact with the AgNPs. AgNPs concentrations less than 4 µg/mL showed a cytotoxic effect that resulted in a death rate of 13.8% or less. However, concentrations greater than 64 µg/mL caused significant cell death of approximately 67%. In addition, antibiotics (ampicillin and amikacin) were tested at concentrations of 64, 32, 8, 2, 0.5 and 0.125 µg/mL in human fibroblasts. It was found that the viability percentage for each of the concentrations of ampicillin was greater than 80% and for amikacin greater than 76%. To evaluate the cytotoxic effects of the combination of AgNPs and conventional antibiotics, ten combinations of different concentrations (AgNPs µg/mL + antibiotic µg/mL: 128 + 64; 64 + 32; 32 + 16; etc.) were tested. It was found that there is no statistically significant difference between the two treatments (AgNPs + AMP and AgNPs + AMK) with respect to cell viability when the two-way ANOVA was performed ($p < 0.05$). However, combinations of 128 µgAgNPs/mL + 64 µg of antibiotic/mL and 64 µgAgNPs/mL + 32 µg of antibiotic/mL caused a statistically significant decrease in cell viability when compared with the rest of the combinations tested ($p < 0.05$) evidenced by the reduction of the mitochondrial activity. On the other hand, it is important to highlight that when AgNPs were combined with antibiotics, at concentrations equal to or less than 8 µg AgNPs/mL showed a viability percentage between 90–95% (Figure 5).

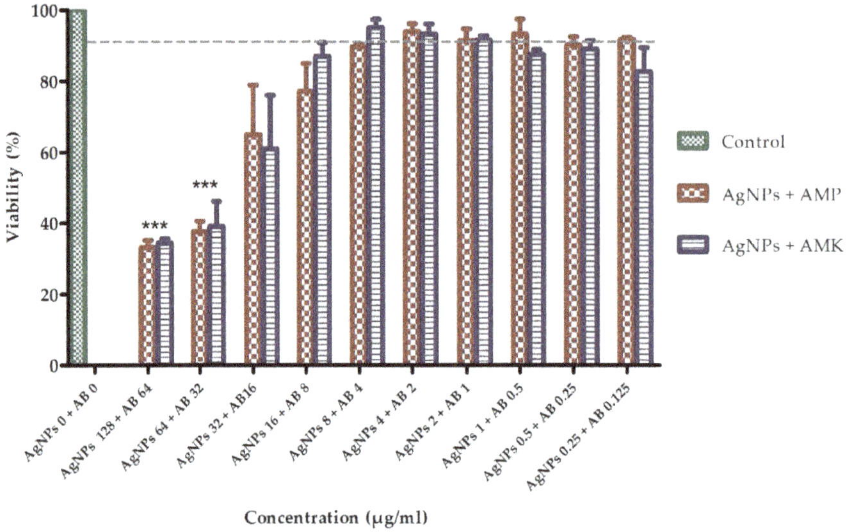

Figure 5. Viability of cells treated with combinations of silver nanoparticles and antibiotics. To measure cytotoxicity, fibroblasts were treated with increasing concentrations of AgNPs + AMP (red) or AgNPs + AMK (blue) (n = 3). Twenty-four hours after of addition of treatment cell viability was determined using MTT. Results are expressed as mean and standard deviation. * $p < 0.05$, ** $p < 0.01$, *** $p < 0.001$ by two-way ANOVA. Control: DMEM. AB: Antibiotic = Amikacin (AMK) or Ampicillin (AMP).

Interesting results were archived when two specific multi-resistant strains, *E. faecium* with resistance to vancomycin and *A. baumannii* with resistance to meropenem, were tested and both showed, with the combination of AgNPs + AMK, a reduction of the MIC by 32-fold, as well as with the combination of AgNPs + AMP of the MIC by 16-fold. In both cases, the cytotoxicity to fibroblasts, of the concentrations of AgNPs + Antibiotic which showed a reduction of MIC, showed a reduction with statistical significance (Table 4).

Table 4. Viability of fibroblasts treated with silver nanoparticles, antibiotics and their combinations using concentrations corresponding to the MIC value.

Clinical Strains	Viability of Fibroblasts (%)				
	AgNPs	AMK	AgNPs + AMK	AMP	AgNPs + AMP
E. faecium	>80	≈55	>90	>90	85–95
A. baumannii	72	≈55	>90	>90	85–95

MIC: Minimum Inhibitory Concentration. AMK: Amikacin. AMP: Ampicillin.

3. Materials and Methods

3.1. Synthesis of AgNPs

For the synthesis of nanoparticles, $AgNO_3$ (0.01 M) was used as a metallic precursor and gallic acid (0.1 g) was used as a reducer and stabilizer agent. NaOH (3 M) was used for pH regulation. AgNPs were synthesized by dissolving 0.0169 g of $AgNO_3$ in 90 mL of deionized water and this solution was placed in a 250 mL reaction vessel. A total of 0.01 g gallic acid was dissolved in 10 mL of deionized water and was added to the $AgNO_3$ solution with magnetic stirring. After the addition of gallic acid, the pH value of the solution was adjusted using a solution of NaOH 3 M. At the end of the synthesis, approximately 100 mL of nanoparticles were obtained with a pH of 12.66, of which 50 mL were dialyzed for 48 h on a 12 kDa nitrocellulose membrane.

3.2. Characterization of AgNPs

AgNPs were characterized by Dynamic Light Scattering (DLS), the hydrodynamic diameter and zeta potential were determined using a Malvern Zetasizer Nano ZS (Malvern Panalytical, Malvern, United Kingdom) operating with a He-Ne laser at a wavelength of 633 nm and a detection angle of 90°. Samples were analyzed for 60 s at 25 °C. To confirm the shape, each sample was diluted with deionized water and 50 μL of each suspension was placed on a copper wire for Transmission Electron Microscopy (TEM). All samples were analyzed by Transmission Electron Microscopy (JEOL JEM-1230, Tokyo, Japan) at an acceleration voltage of 100 kV. Afterwards, AgNPs were characterized by UV-visible spectroscopy using an S2000 UV-Vis spectrophotometer from OceanOptics Inc. (Dunedin, FL, USA). The functional groups present in the antibiotics were identified by Fourier Transform Infrared Spectroscopy (Shimadzu, IRaffinity-1, Osaka, Japan). A certain amount of nanopowder was collocated in the equipment and the spectrum was taken in the range of 400–4000 cm^{-1} with a resolution of 2 cm^{-1} and 200 times scanning using the attenuated total reflection (ATR) method.

3.3. Preparation and Characterization of Combinations of AgNPs with Antibiotics

To study the effect of ampicillin and amikacin on the size, shape and stability of the AgNPs, an aqueous solution containing a 1:1 ratio of antibiotic (128 μg/mL) and nanoparticles (128 μg/mL) was prepared for each antibiotic. These solutions were characterized by TEM, DLS, zeta potential and UV-visible spectroscopy. On the other hand, the chemical interaction between the AgNPs and antibiotics was carried out by FTIR, we prepared an aqueous solution containing higher concentrations of antimicrobials (500 μg/mL), the combinations preserved the ratio of 1:1. Subsequently, these solutions were centrifuged, keeping only the precipitate, which was left to dry for 24 h at room temperature.

3.4. Patients

The study protocol and the letter of informed consent were approved by the local Hospital's Ethics and Science Committee with the number 102-16.

The study included urine samples from patients with urinary catheters treated at the local Hospital. Patients were selected in basis to NOM-045-SSA2-2005. For the purposes of this study, only samples of patients older than 15 years, of any genus, whose culture had a bacterial count greater than or equal to 50,000 CFU/mL were selected, and also with an antimicrobial resistance profile.

3.5. Microbiological Analysis

3.5.1. Sample Collection and Bacterial Culture

Urine samples were collected in 5 mL syringes using the probe puncture technique under aseptic conditions by trained personnel. Microbiological analysis was performed according to the established criteria by the American Society for Microbiology (ASM) for urine samples. A count greater than or equal to 50 colonies (equivalent to 50,000 CFU/mL) was considered as the cutoff point for diagnosing infection. Plaques without development at 24-h incubation were discarded and indicated absence of urinary tract infection.

3.5.2. Identification and Antimicrobial Susceptibility Profile of Clinical Strains

The identification and antimicrobial susceptibility of the microorganisms isolated were determined by VITEK2 equipment. From a pure culture grown for 24 h, an inoculum was transferred to a test tube with 3 mL of solution sterile saline (0.45% to 0.5% NaCl aqueous solution, pH 4.5 to 7.0). Subsequently, the turbidity was adjusted to 0.50–0.63 units of the McFarland scale with the densitometer. The bacterial suspension was placed inside the cassette. The identification and susceptibility cards were placed in the nearby slot, inserting the transfer tube into the test tube with the corresponding suspension. The cassette was placed with the samples in the VITEK2 system. The resistance profiles are shown in Table S1.

3.5.3. Conservation of Strains

The conservation of the strains was carried out by the freeze conservation method. Glycerol was used as the cryoprotective agent. The samples were stored at −20 °C.

3.6. Antimicrobial Test

The Minimum Inhibitory Concentration (MIC) was determined by broth microdilution assay in accordance with the procedures recommended by the Clinical and Laboratory Standards Institute (CLSI) [34]. MICs were determined by incubating the microorganisms in 96-well microplates for 24 h at 37 °C. Microorganisms were exposed to serial dilutions of the antimicrobial agent (AgNPs, ampicillin and amikacin), and the end points were determined when no turbidity in the well was observed. The standardization of the method was made based on the criteria established by the CLSI. The strains used were *Staphylococcus aureus* ATCC 25923 and *Escherichia coli* ATCC 25922. The antibiotics used were oxacillin (64 μg/mL) and ceftazidime (32 μg/mL). The assay was performed in duplicate for four days. The results of the standardization of the MIC are shown in Table S2.

3.7. Checkerboard Synergy

The MIC of each antimicrobial substance alone or in combination was determined by a broth microdilution method in accordance with CLSI standards. The assay was performed in 96-well microtiter plates, a two-fold dilution of the antibiotic was distributed into each well to obtain a varying concentration of 128, 64, 32, 16, 8, 4, 2, 1, 05, 0.25 and 0.125 μg/mL in the wells of the first row, while those of the AgNPs were similarly distributed among the first column (128 to 1 μg/mL). The AgNPs dilutions were started from the columns to the right and the antibiotic dilutions were started from the first row downwards. Thus, each of the wells held a unique combination of concentrations of AgNPs and the antibiotic. The broth microdilution plates were inoculated with each test microorganism to yield the appropriate density (10^5 CFU/mL) in 100 μL Mueller–Hinton broth and incubated at the optimum temperature and time of growth conditions (37 °C/24 h). The MIC was determined as the least dilution without any turbidity. The MICs of single antimicrobial A and B (MIC_A and MIC_B) and in combination were determined. The ten multidrug resistant clinical strains were exposed to serial dilutions of the antimicrobial agents. Subsequently, we calculated the proportion: $MIC_{\text{Antibiotic alone}}/MIC_{\text{Antibiotic in combination}}$ (fold-change) to describe the number of times that MIC decreased from an initial to final value.

3.8. Cytotoxicity of AgNPs

To evaluate the toxicity of AgNPs in combination with antibiotics, human fibroblasts (baby foreskin) were used. Cells were dispensed in 96-well microplates at a density of 5000 cells per well in DMEM supplemented with 1% fetal bovine serum (FBS) for 24 h at 37 °C. After 24 h the cells were incubated with the established concentrations of AgNPs and antibiotics for 24 h at 37 °C. Treatment was withdrawn and 100 μL MTT (3-(4,5-cimethylthiazol-2-yl)-2,5-diphenyl tetrazolium bromide) (0.5 mg/mL) was added in DMEM without FBS for 4 h at 37 °C for the formation of formazan crystals. MTT was removed from the wells and 100 μL of DMSO was added to read absorbance in a Synergy H1 microplate reader with Gen 5 software (Biotek Instruments, Winooski, VT, USA) at a wavelength of 595 nm. As a positive control, cells were treated with hydrogen peroxide and as a negative control, they were only treated with medium. The assay was performed in triplicate.

3.9. Statistical Analysis

Each assay was repeated three times. Data are presented as mean $\pm$ standard deviation (SD). The comparison between the effects of the two sources of variation was made using the two-way analysis of variance (ANOVA). The analysis was performed with the statistical software SPSS 23.0 (IBM, New York, NY, USA). A value of $p < 0.05$ was considered significant.

4. Conclusions

These results indicate that infections due to multidrug resistant microorganisms could be treated by the use of a synergistic combination of antimicrobial drugs and AgNPs. Further studies are necessary to evaluate the specific mechanisms of action, which could help predict undesirable off-target interactions, suggest ways of regulating a drug's activity, and identify novel therapeutics to this health problem.

Author Contributions: F.M.-G. is the intellectual author of the project who designed the microbiological experiments. G.A.M.-C. designed the experiments related to the synthesis and characterization of silver nanoparticles and contributed to the analysis and interpretation of the data. A.F. performed the isolation of the pathogens and the sensitivity profile. M.L.-C. performed the microbiological experiments and the statistical analysis of the data. C.C. designed the experiments related to the study of the cytotoxic activity of silver nanoparticles and K.I.V. performed these experiments. M.M. oversaw the follow-up of the patients. F.M.-G. and M.L.-C. wrote this paper.

Acknowledgments: This work was supported by the Fondo de Apoyo a la Investigación (FAI) UASLP, C16-FAI-09-23.23 and Doctorado en Ciencias Odontológicas, Facultad de Estomatología, UASLP.

Appendix FIC Calculation

One strategy used to overcome the resistance mechanism of the microorganisms is the use of the combination of drugs. The way to measure their effectiveness is through the calculation of the Fractional Inhibitory Concentration (FIC) index.

The FIC index was calculated as follows:

$$\text{FIC of AgNPs} = \text{MIC}_{\text{AgNPs}} \text{ in combination}/\text{MIC}_{\text{AgNPs}} \text{ alone}$$
$$\text{FIC of Antibiotic} = \text{MIC}_{\text{Antibiotic}} \text{ in combination}/\text{MIC}_{\text{Antibiotic}} \text{ alone}$$
$$\text{FIC index} = \text{FIC of AgNPs} + \text{FIC of Antibiotic}$$

The FIC index was interpreted as follows: FIC < 0.5, Synergy (S); $0.5 \leq$ FIC <1, Partial Synergy (PS); FIC = 1, Additive (AD); $2 \leq$ FIC < 4, Indifferent (I); FIC > 4, Antagonism (AN).

References

1. Dielubanza, E.J.; Schaeffer, A.J. Urinary tract infections in women. *Med. Clin. N. Am.* **2011**, *95*, 27–41. [CrossRef] [PubMed]
2. Stamm, W.E.; Norrby, S.R. Urinary tract infections: Disease panorama and challenges. *J. Infect. Dis.* **2001**, *183* (Suppl. 1), S1–S4. [CrossRef] [PubMed]
3. Magill, S.S.; Edwards, J.R.; Bamberg, W.; Beldavs, Z.G.; Dumyati, G.; Kainer, M.A.; Lynfield, R.; Maloney, M.; McAllister-Hollod, L.; Nadle, J.; et al. Multistate point-prevalence survey of health care-associated infections. *N. Engl. J. Med.* **2014**, *370*, 1198–1208. [CrossRef] [PubMed]
4. Mukherjee, M.; Basu, S.; Mukherjee, S.K.; Majumder, M. Multidrug-Resistance and Extended Spectrum Beta-Lactamase Production in Uropathogenic *E. coli* which were Isolated from Hospitalized Patients in Kolkata, India. *J. Clin. Diagn. Res.* **2013**, *7*, 449–453. [CrossRef] [PubMed]
5. Ronald, A. The etiology of urinary tract infection: Traditional and emerging pathogens. *Am. J. Med.* **2002**, *113* (Suppl. 1A), 14S–19S. [CrossRef]

6. Iacovelli, V.; Gaziev, G.; Topazio, L.; Bove, P.; Vespasiani, G.; Finazzi Agrò, E. Nosocomial urinary tract infections: A review. *Urologia* **2014**, *81*, 222–227. [CrossRef] [PubMed]
7. Saint, S.; Lipsky, B.A.; Goold, S.D. Indwelling urinary catheters: A one-point restraint? *Ann. Intern. Med.* **2002**, *137*, 125–127. [CrossRef] [PubMed]
8. Stickler, D.J. Bacterial biofilms in patients with indwelling urinary catheters. *Nat. Clin. Pract. Urol.* **2008**, *5*, 598–608. [CrossRef] [PubMed]
9. Costerton, J.W.; Stewart, P.S.; Greenberg, E.P. Bacterial biofilms: A common cause of persistent infections. *Science* **1999**, *284*, 1318–1322. [CrossRef] [PubMed]
10. Subramanian, P.; Shanmugam, N.; Sivaraman, U.; Kumar, S.; Selvaraj, S. Antiobiotic resistance pattern of biofilm-forming uropathogens isolated from catheterised patients in Pondicherry, India. *Australas. Med. J.* **2012**, *5*, 344–348. [PubMed]
11. Goller, C.C.; Romeo, T. Environmental influences on biofilm development. *Curr. Top. Microbiol. Immunol.* **2008**, *322*, 37–66. [PubMed]
12. Mah, T.F.; O'Toole, G.A. Mechanisms of biofilm resistance to antimicrobial agents. *Trends Microbiol.* **2001**, *9*, 34–39. [CrossRef]
13. Mittal, S.; Sharma, M.; Chaudhary, U. Biofilm and multidrug resistance in uropathogenic Escherichia coli. *Pathog. Glob. Health* **2015**, *109*, 26–29. [CrossRef] [PubMed]
14. Stewart, P.S.; Costerton, J.W. Antibiotic resistance of bacteria in biofilms. *Lancet* **2001**, *358*, 135–138. [CrossRef]
15. Trautner, B.W.; Darouiche, R.O. Role of biofilm in catheter-associated urinary tract infection. *Am. J. Infect. Control* **2004**, *32*, 177–183. [CrossRef] [PubMed]
16. Stickler, D.J. Clinical complications of urinary catheters caused by crystalline biofilms: Something needs to be done. *J. Intern. Med.* **2014**, *276*, 120–129. [CrossRef] [PubMed]
17. Theuretzbacher, U. Antibiotic innovation for future public health needs. *Clin. Microbiol. Infect.* **2017**, *23*, 713–717. [CrossRef] [PubMed]
18. Walsh, T.R.; Toleman, M.A. The emergence of pan-resistant Gram-negative pathogens merits a rapid global political response. *J. Antimicrob. Chemother.* **2012**, *67*, 1–3. [CrossRef] [PubMed]
19. Martinez-Gutierrez, F.; Olive, P.L.; Banuelos, A.; Orrantia, E.; Nino, N.; Sanchez, E.M.; Ruiz, F.; Bach, H.; Av-Gay, Y. Synthesis, characterization, and evaluation of antimicrobial and cytotoxic effect of silver and titanium nanoparticles. *Nanomedicine* **2010**, *6*, 681–688. [CrossRef] [PubMed]
20. Morones, J.R.; Elechiguerra, J.L.; Camacho, A.; Holt, K.; Kouri, J.B.; Ramírez, J.T.; Yacaman, M.J. The bactericidal effect of silver nanoparticles. *Nanotechnology* **2005**, *16*, 2346–2353. [CrossRef] [PubMed]
21. Hajipour, M.J.; Fromm, K.M.; Ashkarran, A.A.; Jimenez de Aberasturi, D.; de Larramendi, I.R.; Rojo, T. Antibacterial properties of nanoparticles. *Trends Biotechnol.* **2012**, *30*, 499–511. [CrossRef] [PubMed]
22. Birla, S.S.; Tiwari, V.V.; Gade, A.K.; Ingle, A.P.; Yadav, A.P.; Rai, M.K. Fabrication of silver nanoparticles by *Phoma glomerata* and its combined effect against *Escherichia coli, Pseudomonas aeruginosa* and *Staphylococcus aureus*. *Lett. Appl. Microbiol.* **2009**, *48*, 173–179. [CrossRef] [PubMed]
23. Mala, R.; Annie Aglin, A.; Ruby Celsia, A.S.; Geerthika, S.; Kiruthika, N.; VazagaPriya, C.; Srinivasa Kumar, K. Foley catheters functionalised with a synergistic combination of antibiotics and silver nanoparticles resist biofilm formation. *IET Nanobiotechnol.* **2017**, *11*, 612–620. [CrossRef] [PubMed]
24. Braydich-Stolle, L.; Hussain, S.; Schlager, J.J.; Hofmann, M.C. In vitro cytotoxicity of nanoparticles in mammalian germline stem cells. *Toxicol. Sci.* **2005**, *88*, 412–419. [CrossRef] [PubMed]
25. Hussain, S.M.; Hess, K.L.; Gearhart, J.M.; Geiss, K.T.; Schlager, J.J. In vitro toxicity of nanoparticles in BRL 3A rat liver cells. *Toxicol. In Vitro* **2005**, *19*, 975–983. [CrossRef] [PubMed]
26. Tauran, Y.; Brioude, A.; Coleman, A.W.; Rhimi, M.; Kim, B. Molecular recognition by gold, silver and copper nanoparticles. *World J. Biol. Chem.* **2013**, *4*, 35–63. [CrossRef] [PubMed]
27. Yoosaf, K.; Ipe, B.I.; Suresh, C.H.; Thomas, K.G. In situ synthesis of metal nanoparticles and selective naked-eye detection of lead ions from aqueous media. *J. Phys. Chem. C* **2007**, *111*, 12839–12847. [CrossRef]
28. Hur, Y.E.; Kim, S.; Kim, J.-H.; Cha, S.-H.; Choi, M.-J.; Cho, S.; Park, Y. One-step functionalization of gold and silver nanoparticles by ampicillin. *Mater. Lett.* **2014**, *129*, 185–190. [CrossRef]
29. Rogowska, A.; Rafińska, K.; Pomastowski, P.; Walczak, J.; Railean-Plugaru, V.; Buszewska-Forajta, M.; Buszewski, B. Silver nanoparticles functionalized with ampicillin. *Electrophoresis* **2017**, *38*, 2757–2764. [CrossRef] [PubMed]

30. Deng, H.; McShan, D.; Zhang, Y.; Sinha, S.S.; Arslan, Z.; Ray, P.C.; Yu, H. Mechanistic Study of the Synergistic Antibacterial Activity of Combined Silver Nanoparticles and Common Antibiotics. *Environ. Sci. Technol.* **2016**, *50*, 8840–8848. [CrossRef] [PubMed]
31. Flores-Mireles, A.L.; Walker, J.N.; Caparon, M.; Hultgren, S.J. Urinary tract infections: Epidemiology, mechanisms of infection and treatment options. *Nat. Rev. Microbiol.* **2015**, *13*, 269–284. [CrossRef] [PubMed]
32. Odds, F.C. Synergy, antagonism, and what the chequerboard puts between them. *J. Antimicrob. Chemother.* **2003**, *52*. [CrossRef] [PubMed]
33. Hwang, I.S.; Hwang, J.H.; Choi, H.; Kim, K.J.; Lee, D.G. Synergistic effects between silver nanoparticles and antibiotics and the mechanisms involved. *J. Med. Microbiol.* **2012**, *61*, 1719–1726. [CrossRef] [PubMed]
34. Clinical and Laboratory Standards Institute. *Performance Standards for Antimicrobial Susceptibility Testing*; CLSI Supplement M100; CLSI: Wayne, PA, USA, 2017.

13

Sperm Quality during Storage Is Not Affected by the Presence of Antibiotics in EquiPlus Semen Extender but Is Improved by Single Layer Centrifugation

Ziyad Al-Kass [1,2], Joachim Spergser [3], Christine Aurich [4], Juliane Kuhl [4], Kathrin Schmidt [4], Anders Johannisson [1] and Jane M. Morrell [1,*]

1 Clinical Sciences, Swedish University of Agricultural Sciences (SLU), SE-75007 Uppsala, Sweden; ziyad.al.kass@slu.se or ziyadalkass@gmail.com; (Z.A.-K.); Anders.Johannisson@slu.se (A.J.)
2 Department of Surgery and Theriogenology, College of Veterinary Medicine, University of Mosul, Mosul 41002, Iraq
3 Institute of Microbiology, Vetmeduni Vienna, 1210 Vienna, Austria; joachim.spergser@vetmeduni.ac.at
4 Centre for Artificial Insemination and Embryo Transfer, Vetmeduni Vienna, 1210 Vienna, Austria; Christine.Aurich@vetmeduni.ac.at (C.A.); juliane.kuhl@vetmeduni.ac.at (J.K.); kathrin.schmidt@vetmeduni.ac.at (K.S.)
* Correspondence: jane.morrell@slu.se

Academic Editor: Leonard Amaral

Abstract: Contamination of semen with bacteria arises during semen collection and handling. This bacterial contamination is typically controlled by adding antibiotics to semen extenders but intensive usage of antibiotics can lead to the development of bacterial resistance and may be detrimental to sperm quality. The objective of this study was to determine the effects of antibiotics in a semen extender on sperm quality and to investigate the effects of removal of bacteria by modified Single Layer Centrifugation (MSLC) through a colloid. Semen was collected from six adult pony stallions (three ejaculates per male). Aliquots of extended semen were used for MSLC with Equicoll, resulting in four treatment groups: control and MSLC in extender with antibiotics (CA and SA, respectively); control and MSLC in extender without antibiotics (CW and SW, respectively). Sperm motility, membrane integrity, mitochondrial membrane potential and chromatin integrity were evaluated daily by computer-assisted sperm analysis (CASA) and flow cytometry. There were no differences in sperm quality between CA and CW, or between SA and SW, although progressive motility was negatively correlated to total bacterial counts at 0 h. However, MSLC groups showed higher mean total motility ($P < 0.001$), progressive motility ($P < 0.05$), membrane integrity ($P < 0.0001$) and mitochondrial membrane potential ($P < 0.05$), as well as better chromatin integrity ($P < 0.05$), than controls. Sperm quality remained higher in the MSLC groups than controls throughout storage. These results indicate that sperm quality was not adversely affected by the presence of antibiotics but was improved considerably by MSLC.

Keywords: pony stallions; bacteria; semen evaluation

---

1. Introduction

Semen often contains bacteria due to contamination during collection and processing. Bacteria originate from the penis and prepuce of the stallion, the environment, and from semen handling. These bacteria may cause endometritis in inseminated mares [1], contribute to decreased semen quality [2], and affect fertility [3]. To avoid such problems, antibiotics are added to semen extenders. However, excessive use of antibiotics may lead to the development of antibiotic resistance [4].

In addition, antibiotics in the semen extender may be detrimental to semen characteristics during cooled-storage [5,6]. Therefore, controlling bacteria with antibiotics may not be desirable.

No single method of sperm quality evaluation can be used on its own to predict fertility [7]. Previously, sperm number, sperm motility and morphology were used to evaluate "sperm quality", but now additional assays are available to evaluate sperm functionality. Computer Assisted Sperm Analyzers for motility (CASA) and Flow cytometry (FC) enable additional parameters of sperm quality to be tested [8]. The CASA is able to analyze sperm motility and kinematics [9]. Flow cytometry can be used to evaluate sperm plasma membrane integrity, acrosome integrity, chromatin integrity, mitochondrial status and other parameters [10]. These assays provide an objective means of analyzing several thousand spermatozoa per sample, enabling an objective assessment of the effects of the presence of bacteria, or of antibiotics, on sperm quality to be made.

An alternative method to control bacteria in semen would be to remove them physically. The technique of Single Layer Centrifugation (SLC) through a colloid was shown to improve sperm quality [11] and to separate spermatozoa from seminal plasma. It has also been reported to separate spermatozoa from bacteria in boar semen [12]. A modification of this technique, MSLC, was shown to reduce bacterial contamination in stallion semen [11,13] but did not remove all the bacteria. Therefore, it is important to investigate the effects of these residual bacteria on sperm quality after SLC and to determine whether antibiotics are needed to control such contamination.

The aims of this study were (1) to determine the effect of antibiotics on spermatozoa, by comparing sperm quality in extender with and without antibiotics; and (2) to investigate the effect of removal of bacteria on sperm quality, by monitoring sperm quality in SLC-selected samples and controls during storage for several days.

2. Materials and Methods

2.1. Animals

Semen was collected from six adult pony stallions (5–25 years old). The animals were housed according to standard husbandry practices at the Center for Artificial Insemination and Embryo Transfer, Vetmeduni Vienna, Austria. The semen collection was approved by the competent authority for animal experimentation (Austrian Federal Ministry for Science and Research, license number BMWFW-68.205/0150-WF/V/3b/2015).

2.2. Semen

2.2.1. Semen Collection

The ejaculates (3 per male) were collected using a sterilized Hannover artificial vagina after the stallion had mounted a phantom. Each ejaculate was split into two parts and extended in EquiPlus (Minitüb, Tiefenbach, Germany), either with (A) or without (W) antibiotics, to give a sperm concentration of 100×10^6/mL. The extender is a commercially available product; according to the manufacturer, it contains lincomycin 0.015 g and spectinomycin 0.025 g per 100 mL with pH 6.8 $\pm$ 0.2 and 320 $\pm$ mOs·mol/L osmotic pressure.

2.2.2. Semen Preparation with Modified Single Layer Centrifugation

Aliquots of extended semen were used for MSLC with Equicoll [11] under aseptic conditions. Briefly, the colloid (15 mL) was poured into a 50 mL sterile tube and a sterile 5 mL plastic tube (the sheath from a Cytology Brush; Minitube, Celadice, Slovakia) was inserted through the middle of the cover [13]. An aliquot (15 mL) of semen, adjusted to a sperm concentration of 100×10^6/mL, was pipetted on top of the colloid through a small hole that had previously been made at the edge of the lid. The tube was centrifuged at $300 \times g$ for 20 min using a swing-out rotor. The sperm pellet was then recovered using a long Pasteur pipette passed through the tube insert and was resuspended in the appropriate extender (Figure 1). Four treatment groups were formed: control and MSLC in EquiPlus with antibiotics (CA and SA, respectively); control and MSLC in EquiPlus without antibiotics (CW and SW, respectively). The sperm concentration was adjusted to 50×10^6/mL in all samples, which were then stored at 6 °C for 96 h.

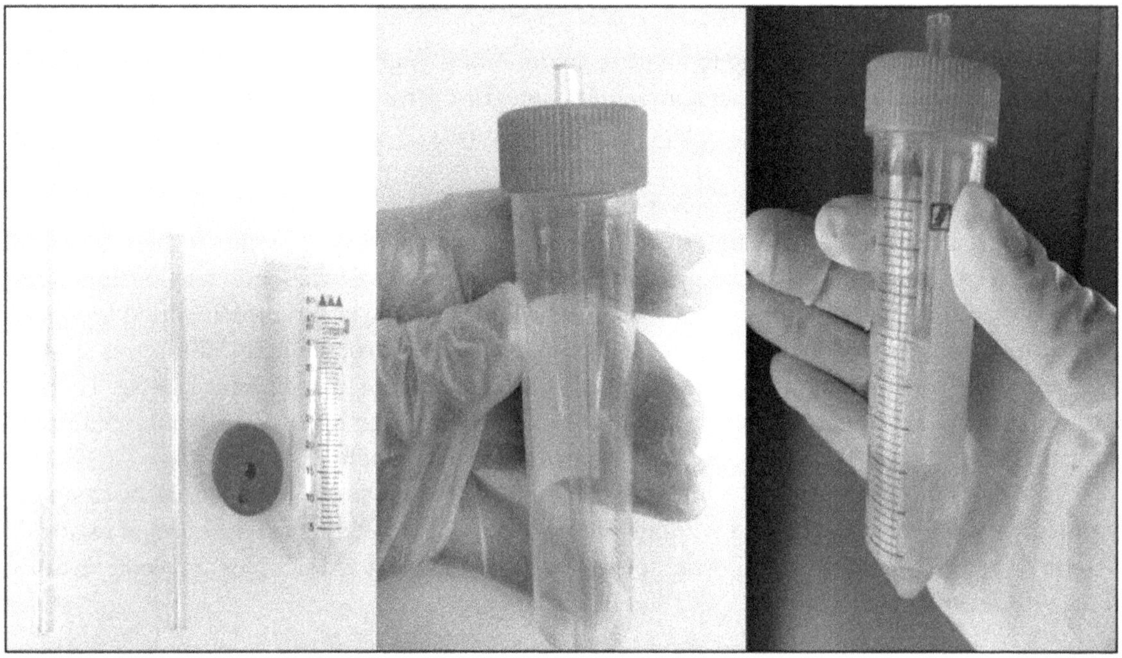

Figure 1. Modified Single Layer Centrifugation (MSLC). A 50 mL sterile tube with a sterile 5 mL plastic inner tube inserted through the middle of the cover, and a small hole that had previously been made at the edge of the lid. The colloid is poured into the 50 mL tube, the lid containing the insert is screwed on, and the semen samples are added through the small hole near the edge of the lid. After centrifugation, the sperm pellet can be retrieved easily by passing a long Pasteur pipette through the plastic insert.

2.3. Evaluation

2.3.1. Sperm Concentration

Sperm concentration was measured using a Nucleocounter-SP 100 (Chemometec, Allerød, Denmark) as follows: 50 µL semen sample were mixed with 5 mL reagent S100 (Chemometic, Allerød, Denmark) and this mixture was loaded into a cassette containing the fluorescent dye propidium iodide (PI). The cassette was inserted into the fluorescence meter, which displayed the sperm concentration after 30 s.

2.3.2. Computer-Assisted Sperm Analysis (CASA)

Motility evaluation was performed using a SpermVision analyzer (Minitüb GmbH, Tiefenbach, Germany), connected to an Olympus BX 51 microscope (Olympus, Tokyo, Japan) with a heated stage (38 °C); samples were equilibrated to room temperature before motility analysis. Sperm motility was analyzed in eight fields (at least 1000 spermatozoa in total) using the SpermVision software program with settings adjusted for stallion spermatozoa. Spermatozoa were considered as immotile if VAP < 20; locally motile if VAP > 20 and < 30, STR < 0.5, VCL < 9. The following kinematics were assessed at 0, 24, 48, 72 and 96 h: total motility (TM, %), progressive motility (PM, %), velocity of the average path (VAP, µm/s), curvilinear velocity (VCL, µm/s), straight line velocity (VSL, µm/s), straightness (STR, %), linearity (LIN, %), wobble (WOB, %) lateral head displacement (ALH, µm), beat cross frequency (BCF, Hz).

2.3.3. Membrane Integrity

Aliquots of each sample were adjusted to a sperm concentration of approximately 2×10^6 spermatozoa/mL with CellWASH (Becton Dickinson, San José, CA, USA). Assessment of plasma membrane integrity was made in 300 μL of the diluted sample after staining with 0.6 μL of 0.02 μM SYBR14 and 3 μL of 12 μM PI (Live-Dead Sperm Viability Kit L-7011; Invitrogen, Eugene, OR, USA) and incubating for 10 min at 37 °C [14]. The green and red fluorescence, as well as forward and side scatter, were measured using a FACSVerse™ flow cytometer (BD Biosciences). Membrane integrity was assessed at 24, 48, 72 and 96 h, using the classification intact membranes (SYBR14 positive, PI negative) and damaged membranes (SYBR14 positive or negative/PI positive). For the purposes of this study, only the proportion of spermatozoa with intact membranes was reported.

2.3.4. Assessment of Mitochondrial Membrane Potential (MMP)

Aliquots of the diluted sperm samples (1000 μL) were stained with 0.5 μL of 3 mM JC-1, followed by incubation at 37 °C for 30 min and evaluation by FC [15]. The green and orange fluorescence, as well as forward and side scatter were measured using a FACSVerse™ flow cytometer. Proportions of the sperm population with JC-1 high and JC-1 low fluorescence (orange and green fluorescence, respectively, representing high and low mitochondrial activity) were determined. Samples were assessed at 24, 48, 72 and 96 h after collection.

2.3.5. Sperm Chromatin Structure Assay (SCSA)

Equal volumes (50 μL) of sperm samples and buffer containing 0.01 M Tris-HCl, 0.15 M sodium chloride and 1 mM EDTA (pH 7.4; TNE) were mixed and snap-frozen in liquid nitrogen before being transferred to a −80 °C freezer for storage. Samples were taken for SCSA at 24, 48, 72 and 96 h after collection.

For evaluation, samples were thawed on crushed ice immediately before staining; 80 μL of TNE were added to 20 μL semen, 200 μL of a low-pH detergent solution containing 0.17% Triton X-100, 0.15 M NaCl and 0.08 M HCl (pH 1.2), followed 30 s later by 600 μL acridine orange (AO) (6 μg mL^{-1} in 0.1 M citric acid, 0.2 M Na_2HPO_4, 1 mM EDTA, 0.15 M NaCl, pH 6.0) [16]. Spermatozoa with single stranded DNA fluoresce red, whereas those with normal double stranded DNA fluoresce green. The ratio of red to (green + red) provides a measure of the proportion of spermatozoa with damaged DNA in the population (%DFI). The green and red fluorescence, as well as forward and side scatter, were measured using a FACSVerse™ flow cytometer. After collection of data, the ratio for each of the cells was calculated using FCSExpress version 2 (DeNovo Software, Thornhill, ON, Canada), and a histogram of the distribution was used to calculate %DFI.

2.3.6. Bacteriology

Aliquots of the diluted samples (1 mL) on ice were sent for bacteriological culture and analysis 1 to 5 h after collection. An aliquot (1 mL) of each sample was added to 9 mL 2SP medium (0.2 mol/L sucrose in 0.02 mol/L phosphate buffer, supplemented with 10% fetal calf serum), vortexed, and serially diluted up to 1×10^{-8}. Appropriate dilutions (0.1 mL) were plated in triplicate on Columbia Agar with 5% sheep blood, Schaedler Agar with vitamin K1 and 5% sheep blood (both BBL™, BD Diagnostics, Schwechat, Austria), and PPLO (Pleuropneumonia-Like-Organism) Agar (Difco™, BD Diagnostics, Schwechat, Austria) supplemented with 20% horse serum (Gibco™, Thermo Fisher Scientific, Vienna, Austria). Columbia Agar plates were incubated in ambient air at 33 °C, PPLO Agar at 37 °C under microaerobic conditions and Schaedler Agar at 37 °C in an anaerobic jar with gas packs (BD Diagnostics, Schwechat, Austria). Culture plates were examined daily for growth up to 96 h of incubation. Bacterial colonies were counted and mean total colony counts per sample were calculated from triplicates. The counts in each treatment were normalized to CA (i.e., expressed in relation to CA) since CA (control with antibiotics) was considered to be the industry standard.

2.3.7. Statistics

Data were analyzed using PROC MIXED (repeated measures data) with stallions and ejaculates as random factors, and treatments and time as variables in the SAS software (ver. 9.4, SAS Inst. Inc., Cary, NC, USA) [17]. To test normality, diagnostic plots were used. The results are presented as Least Squares Means ± Standard Error; the differences were considered significant at level $P < 0.05$. Pearson correlations were made between the various parameters of sperm quality and bacterial count.

3. Results

3.1. Sperm Motility

There were significant differences between treatments in TM e.g., between control and MSLC from 48 h onwards, and also with and without antibiotics (Figure 2). At each time point, TM was higher for MSLC than for control and higher for the treatments without antibiotics than with antibiotics. There was a significant decrease in TM with time for all samples.

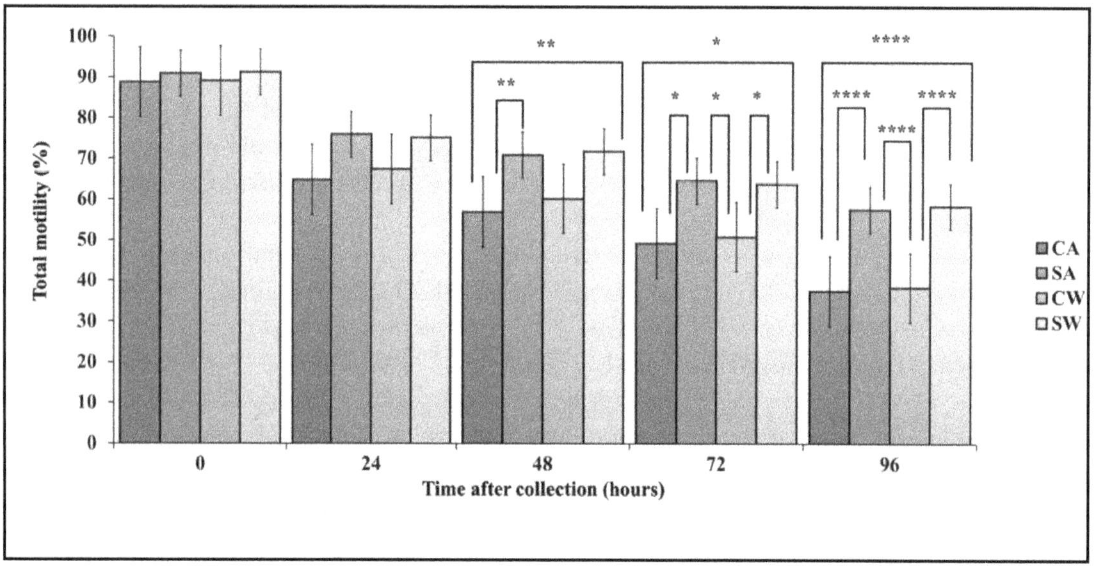

Figure 2. Total motility in control and MSLC samples, with and without antibiotics, during storage for 96 h at 6 °C. Values are Least Squares Means ± SE ($n = 18$). Note: * $P < 0.05$, ** $P < 0.01$, **** $P < 0.0001$. Abbreviations: CA, control with antibiotics; SA, modified single layer centrifugation with antibiotics; CW, control without antibiotics; SW, modified single layer centrifugation without antibiotics.

There were significant differences between treatments for some other kinematics (Table 1): between CA and SA for, VAP and VSL at 0 h, for VCL and ALH at 24 h, for STR and LIN at 96 h; between CA and SW for VSL at 24 h, for VAP at 72 h; for VCL and ALH at 48 h; between CW and SW for VSL at 0 h and at 24 h; for VAP and VSL at 48 h, for VCL at 72 h, for STR at 96 h ($P < 0.05$); and between CA and SA for VCL at 0 h and for ALH at 72 h; between CA and SW for VAP, VCL, VSL, ALH at 48 h and for ALH at 72 h; between CW and SA for VAP, VCL, VSL at 0 h and for STR at 96 h; between CW and SW for VCL and ALH at 48 h ($P < 0.01$). Lower values for SLC were observed for VAP, VCL, VSL, ALH and STR than controls.

Table 1. Sperm kinematics for control and treatment groups, with and without antibiotics at 0 to 96 h (Least Squares Means ± Standard Error; n = 18).

Time		CA	SA	CW	SW
0 h	PM%	80.83 ± 4.62	83.60 ± 4.62	81.27 ± 4.62	84.29 ± 4.62
	VAP (μm/s)	93.97 ± 3.20 ^{a}	79.02 ± 3.20 ^{a,c}	95.30 ± 3.20 ^{c}	82.13 ± 3.20
	VCL (μm/s)	166.14 ± 5.44 ^{c}	137.84 ± 5.44 ^{c,d}	163.80 ± 5.44 ^{d}	143.15 ± 5.44
	VSL (μm/s)	83.75 ± 2.86 ^{a}	70.76 ± 2.86 ^{a,c}	85.46 ± 2.86 ^{b,c}	73.29 ± 2.86 ^{b}
	STR%	0.89 ± 0.01	0.89 ± 0.01	0.89 ± 0.01	0.89 ± 0.01
	LIN%	0.50 ± 0.01	0.50 ± 0.01	0.51 ± 0.01	0.50 ± 0.01
	WOB%	0.56 ± 0.01	0.56 ± 0.01	0.57 ± 0.01	0.57 ± 0.01
	ALH (μm)	3.68 ± 0.14	3.18 ± 0.14	3.74 ± 0.14	3.19 ± 0.14
	BCF(Hz)	33.90 ± 0.63	33.14 ± 0.63	34.40 ± 0.63	32.68 ± 0.63
24 h	PM%	49.74 ± 4.62	59.41 ± 4.62	52.61 ± 4.62	57.97 ± 4.62
	VAP (μm/s)	78.60 ± 3.20	68.40 ± 3.20	78.71 ± 3.20	65.59 ± 3.20
	VCL (μm/s)	144.83 ± 5.44	129.60 ± 5.44	145.28 ± 5.44	124.82 ± 5.44
	VSL (μm/s)	61.38 ± 2.86 ^{a}	52.31 ± 2.86	61.91 ± 2.86 ^{b}	49.32 ± 2.86 ^{a,b}
	STR%	0.78 ± 0.01	0.76 ± 0.01	0.78 ± 0.01	0.75 ± 0.01
	LIN%	0.42 ± 0.01	0.40 ± 0.01	0.42 ± 0.01	0.39 ± 0.01
	WOB%	0.54 ± 0.01	0.52 ± 0.01	0.54 ± 0.01	0.52 ± 0.01
	ALH (μm)	3.91 ± 0.14	3.62 ± 0.14	3.84 ± 0.14	3.45 ± 0.14
	BCF (Hz)	31.30 ± 0.63	29.79 ± 0.63	31.27 ± 0.63	29.41 ± 0.63
48 h	PM%	44.20 ± 4.62	52.28 ± 4.62	44.92 ± 4.62	50.94 ± 4.64
	VAP (μm/s)	73.58 ± 3.20 ^{a,c}	59.66 ± 3.20 ^{a}	72.58 ± 3.20 ^{b}	57.39 ± 3.26 ^{c,b}
	VCL (μm/s)	139.63 ± 5.44 ^{a,c}	114.81 ± 5.44 ^{a,b}	138.72 ± 5.44 ^{d,b}	111.84 ± 5.43 ^{c,d}
	VSL (μm/s)	56.01 ± 2.86 ^{c}	44.19 ± 2.86	55.07 ± 2.86 ^{a}	41.71 ± 2.91 ^{c,a}
	STR%	0.75 ± 0.01	0.73 ± 0.01	0.75 ± 0.01	0.72 ± 0.01
	LIN%	0.39 ± 0.01	0.38 ± 0.01	0.39 ± 0.01	0.37 ± 0.01
	WOB%	0.52 ± 0.01	0.52 ± 0.01	0.52 ± 0.01	0.51 ± 0.01
	ALH (μm)	3.79 ± 0.14 ^{a,c}	3.20 ± 0.14 ^{a,b}	3.82 ± 0.14 ^{b,d}	3.10 ± 0.14 ^{c,d}
	BCF (Hz)	29.11 ± 0.63	29.27 ± 0.63	29.53 ± 0.63	28.61 ± 0.63
72 h	PM%	35.13 ± 4.62	42.97 ± 4.62	37.44 ± 4.62	43.46 ± 4.62
	VAP (μm/s)	67.02 ± 3.20 ^{a}	55.49 ± 3.20	65.79 ± 3.20	53.26 ± 3.20 ^{a}
	VCL (μm/s)	129.66 ± 5.44	107.80 ± 5.44	128.44 ± 5.44 ^{a}	104.56 ± 5.44 ^{a}
	VSL (μm/s)	49.33 ± 2.86	39.17 ± 2.86	48.40 ± 2.86	37.87 ± 2.86
	STR%	0.73 ± 0.01	0.70 ± 0.01	0.73 ± 0.01	0.71 ± 0.01
	LIN%	0.38 ± 0.01	0.36 ± 0.01	0.37 ± 0.01	0.36 ± 0.01
	WOB%	0.52 ± 0.01	0.51 ± 0.01	0.51 ± 0.01	0.51 ± 0.01
	ALH (μm)	3.70 ± 0.14 ^{c,d}	3.04 ± 0.14 ^{c}	3.56 ± 0.14	3.00 ± 0.14 ^{d}
	BCF (Hz)	27.54 ± 0.63	28.21 ± 0.63	27.86 ± 0.63	28.30 ± 0.63
96 h	PM%	25.77 ± 4.62	34.97 ± 4.62	28.52 ± 4.62	35.11 ± 4.62
	VAP (μm/s)	58.22 ± 3.20	53.72 ± 3.20	60.50 ± 3.20	51.10 ± 3.20
	VCL (μm/s)	110.36 ± 5.44	104.95 ± 5.44	121.38 ± 5.44	98.54 ± 5.44
	VSL (μm/s)	42.47 ± 2.86	37.33 ± 2.86	44.71 ± 2.86	35.84 ± 2.86
	STR%	0.73 ± 0.01 ^{a}	0.69 ± 0.01 ^{a,c}	0.73 ± 0.01 ^{b,c}	0.69 ± 0.01 ^{b}
	LIN%	0.39 ± 0.01 ^{a}	0.35 ± 0.01 ^{a}	0.36 ± 0.01	0.36 ± 0.01
	WOB%	0.54 ± 0.01	0.51 ± 0.01	0.49 ± 0.01	0.52 ± 0.01
	ALH (μm)	3.56 ± 0.14	3.12 ± 0.14	3.42 ± 0.14	3.00 ± 0.14
	BCF (Hz)	25.55 ± 0.63	27.89 ± 0.63	27.38 ± 0.63	27.41 ± 0.63

Note: Similar letters within rows indicate statistical difference between columns for the same parameter, ^{a,b} $P < 0.05$, ^{c,d} $P < 0.01$. Abbreviations: CA, control with antibiotics; SA, modified single layer centrifugation with antibiotics; CW, control without antibiotics; SW, modified single layer centrifugation without antibiotics; PM, progressive motility; VAP, velocity of the average path; VCL, curvilinear velocity; VSL, straight line velocity; STR, straightness, LIN, linearity; WOB, wobble; ALH, lateral head displacement; BCF, beat cross frequency.

3.2. Membrane Integrity

There were significant differences (P < 0.05) in membrane intact spermatozoa between CA and SA, CA and SW, CW and SA, CW and SW at 24 h. There were also significant differences (P < 0.001–P < 0.0001) between treatments at 48, 72 and 96 h (Figure 3). There were no differences in membrane integrity between treatments with or without antibiotics at any time points.

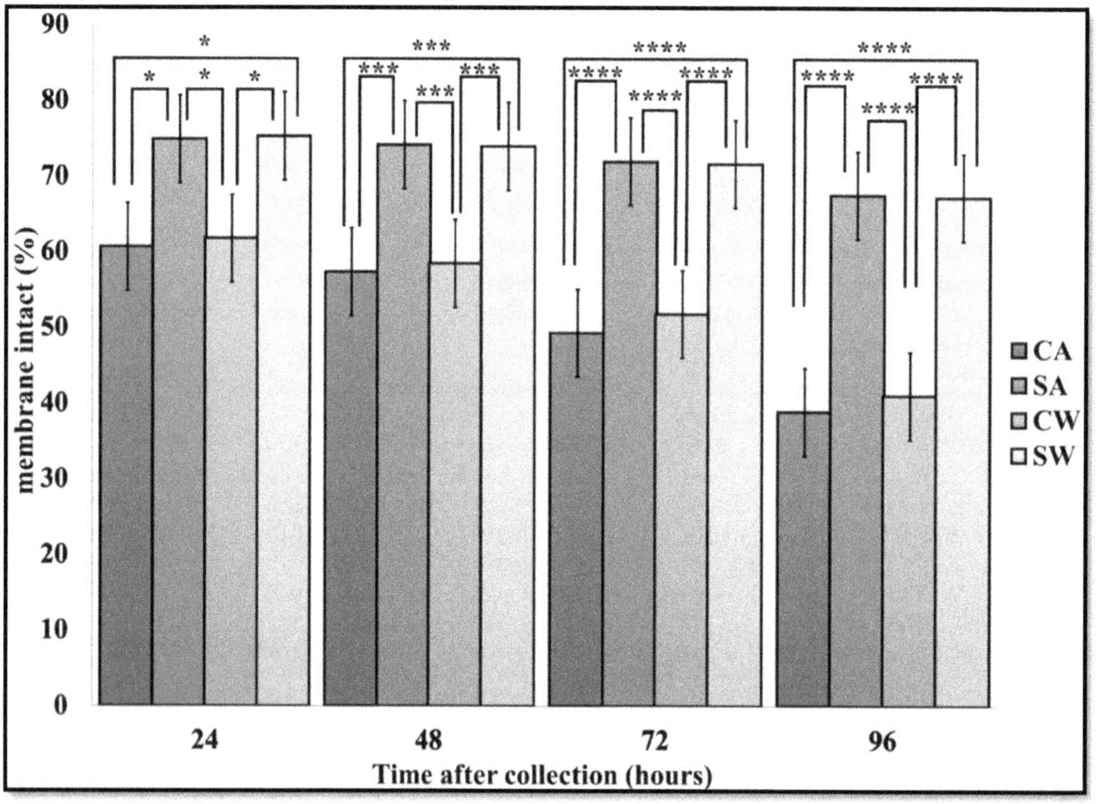

Figure 3. Membrane integrity in control and MSLC samples, with and without antibiotics, during storage for 96 h at 6 °C. Values are Least Squares Means ± SE (n = 18). Note: * P < 0.05, *** P < 0.001, **** P < 0.0001; not possible to analyze samples at 0 h. Abbreviations: CA, control with antibiotics; SA, modified single layer centrifugation with antibiotics; CW, control without antibiotics; SW, modified single layer centrifugation without antibiotics.

3.3. Mitochondrial Membrane Potential

The results for MMP are shown in (Table 2). Significant differences (P < 0.05) were found between CA and SA at 24 h in both MMP low and high; between CA and SW at 24 and 72 h for MMP low (P < 0.01), and at 24 and 72 h for MMP high. The SLC treatments had higher high MMP levels and lower low MMP levels than controls at each time point. There were no differences between extender with or without antibiotics at any time points.

Table 2. Mitochondrial membrane potential for control and treatment groups, with and without antibiotics (Least Squares Means ± Standard Error; $n = 18$).

JC-1 Low %	CA	SA	CW	SW
24 h	48.97 ± 6.63 ^{a,b}	34.60 ± 6.63 ^{a}	46.83 ± 6.63	33.61 ± 6.66 ^{b}
48 h	55.96 ± 6.63	51.70 ± 6.63	56.03 ± 6.63	48.74 ± 6.63
72 h	69.64 ± 6.63 ^{a}	59.11 ± 6.63	64.93 ± 6.63	55.37 ± 6.63 ^{a}
96 h	77.23 ± 6.63	66.14 ± 6.63	73.11 ± 6.63	66.88 ± 6.63
JC-1 high %				
24 h	48.92 ± 6.63 ^{a,b}	62.96 ± 6.63 ^{a}	50.87 ± 6.63	64.05 ± 6.63 ^{b}
48 h	41.85 ± 6.63	46.65 ± 6.63	42.22 ± 6.63	49.36 ± 6.66
72 h	29.15 ± 6.63 ^{b}	39.83 ± 6.63	34.14 ± 6.63	43.59 ± 6.63 ^{b}
96 h	21.83 ± 6.63	33.16 ± 6.63	26.27 ± 6.63	32.40 ± 6.63

Note: Similar letters indicate statistical difference between columns at the same time point, ^{a} $P < 0.05$, ^{b} $P < 0.01$. Abbreviations: JC-1 low, low Mitochondrial Membrane Potential; JC-1 high, high Mitochondrial Membrane Potential. It was not possible to analyze samples at 0 h.

3.4. SCSA

Controls had significantly ($P < 0.05$) higher levels of %DFI than MSLC at all time points (Figure 4). There was also a significant increase in %DFI with time for control groups, whereas there was no change in chromatin damage in the MSLC groups. There were no differences between the groups with and without antibiotics.

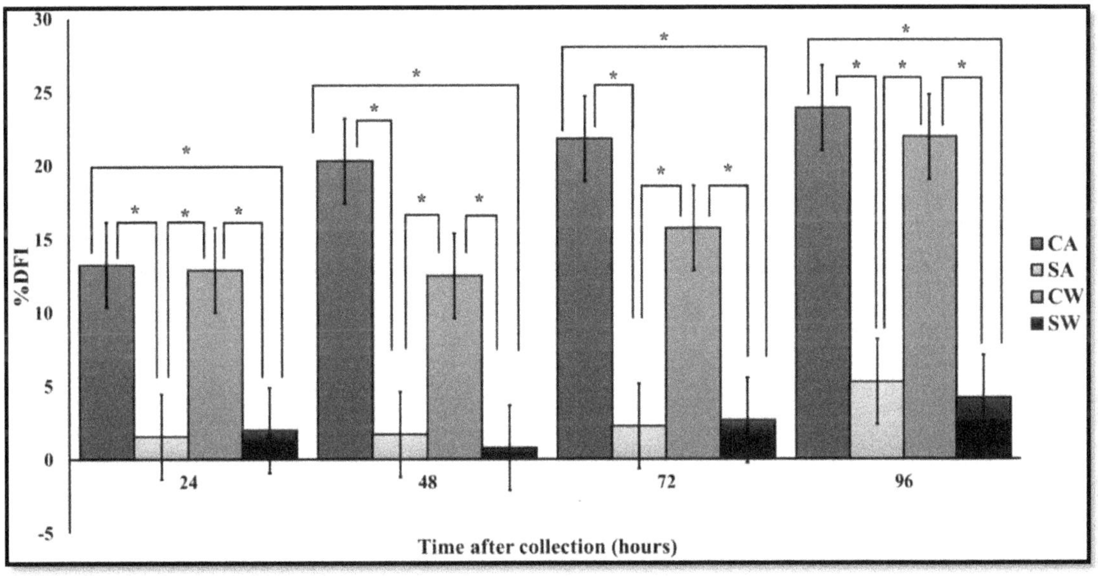

Figure 4. DNA fragmentation index for control and MSLC samples, with and without antibiotics (Least squares means ± SE; $n = 18$). Note: * $P < 0.05$; it was not possible to analyze samples at 0 h. Abbreviations: CA, control with antibiotics; SA, modified single layer centrifugation with antibiotics; CW, control without antibiotics; SW, modified single layer centrifugation without antibiotics.

3.5. Bacteriology

Figure 5 shows the proportion of total bacterial colony counts in all samples relative to CA (=1 arbitrary unit). There was a higher number of culturable bacteria in CW than in CA, but a lower number in SA and SW. The number of colonies depended on the type of plate and corresponding culture conditions (aerobic, microaerobic or anaerobic; 33 °C or 37 °C).

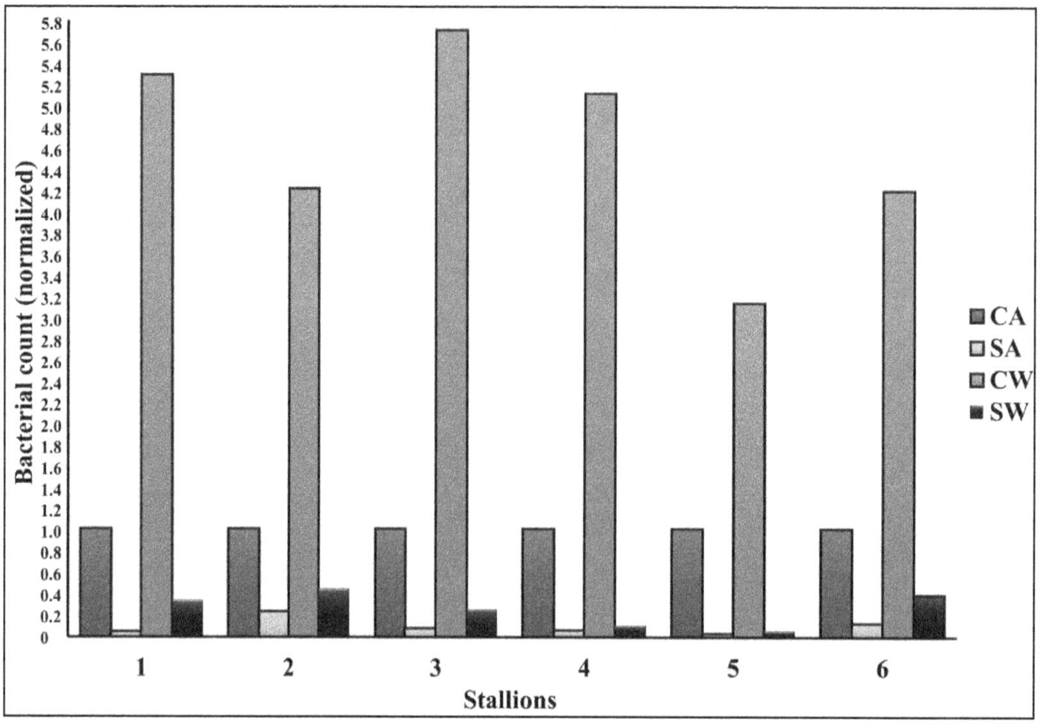

Figure 5. Total bacterial colony counts per treatment group relative to control with antibiotics (at 0 h); control with antibiotics has been normalized to 1 arbitrary unit. Abbreviations: CA, control with antibiotics; SA, modified single layer centrifugation with antibiotics; CW, control without antibiotics; SW, modified single layer centrifugation without antibiotics.

There was a significant negative correlation ($P < 0.05$) between total bacterial colony counts in the sample and PM (Figure 6). There were no other significant correlations between total bacterial load and sperm quality.

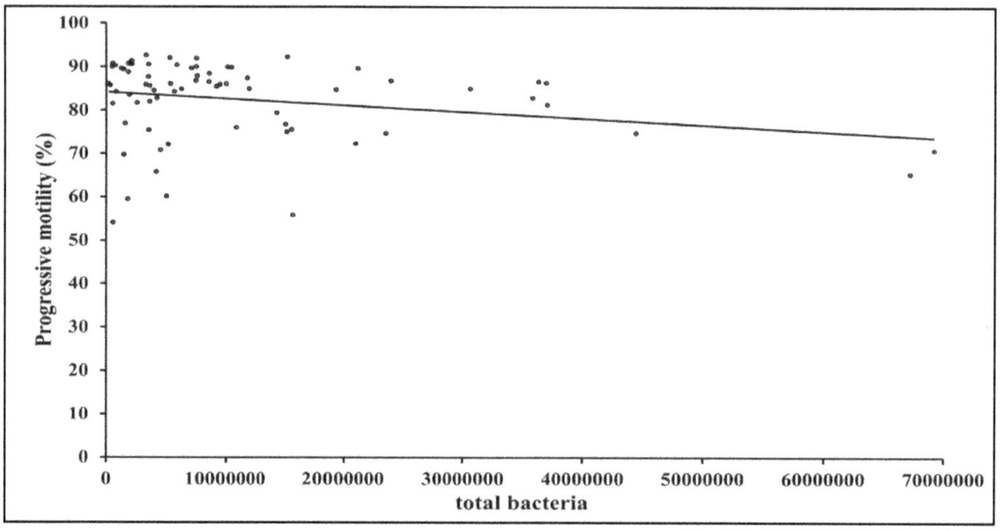

Figure 6. Correlation between total bacterial colony counts per sample and progressive motility at 0 h ($r = -0.24$; $P < 0.05$).

4. Discussion

The study was designed to test the effect of the presence or absence of antibiotics in the semen extender on sperm quality, and also the effect of removal of bacteria by MSLC. The presence or absence of antibiotics did not affect sperm characteristics in this study. However, MSLC did have an effect on sperm characteristics, since most parameters evaluated were higher in MSLC than in controls: e.g., TM and PM were higher in MSLC samples than in control samples, even after storage. Sperm viability was higher in MSLC samples than controls, and remained so during storage. Similarly, MMP was higher in MSLC than controls.

Our present results are in agreement with those of [18], who showed that 11 out of 30 samples of frozen commercial bull semen still contained viable bacteria despite the presence of antibiotics. Another study on stallion semen in a commercial extender demonstrated that a large number of bacteria were detectable in extended stallion semen 24–48 h after preparation [19], indicating that the presence of antibiotics does not guarantee absence of viable bacteria. In contrast, in a study on ram semen, all bacteria in the semen were sensitive to gentamicin and to ceftiofur [20]. These authors also showed that there was a significant reduction in sperm motility, velocity and viability during storage in semen containing *Escherichia coli.* Similar results were observed by [6], who noted that stallion sperm quality deteriorated during cooled storage if certain bacteria were present; this reduction in sperm quality was not altered by the presence of gentamicin.

Other studies have reported that the presence of antibiotics affects both bacteria and spermatozoa [21]. A high dose of amikacin in semen extender resulted in a decrease in PM in stallion semen [22]. A study on cooled stallion semen also showed a decrease in PM when gentamicin sulfate was included [5]. No improvement in motility parameters was reported when gentamicin was added to stored stallion semen spiked with different bacteria [6]. In buffalo (*Bubalus bubalis*) semen *Klebsiella pneumoniae, Staphylococcus aureus* and *Pseudomonas aeruginosa* were isolated, which were resistant to benzylpenicillin and streptomycin [23].

Several studies with colloid centrifugation have shown a reduction in bacterial contamination. Density gradient centrifugation improved sperm viability and reduced the bacterial contamination in human semen [24]. A substantial reduction in bacterial contamination was reported in boar semen samples processed by SLC [12]. In a similar study, approximately 90% of the bacterial load in stallion semen could be removed with SLC [11]. However, only 50% of the bacterial load could be removed with a higher g force [25].

The current results are in agreement with many other studies in which SLC-selected sperm samples show improved sperm characteristics in comparison to controls [26,27]. Improvements in motility and %DFI in SLC samples in stallion sperm samples compared to controls at all time points were reported by [14,27,28]. In a study with donkey semen, the use of SLC improved TM, PM, viability and normal sperm morphology after 24 h of cooled storage [29].

There was an improvement in sperm motility, sperm viability and sperm chromatin integrity in samples prepared by SLC at 0 h, 24 h and 48 h [28]. In addition, there was improved survival of stallion spermatozoa for 96 h after SLC when stored at 4 °C [30]. The present study showed similar improvements in sperm quality. Fertility was also maintained even after cooled storage for up to 96 h [31]. It is interesting to note that MSLC selected samples showed lower velocities than the controls at all time points, despite having a higher mitochondrial membrane potential, indicating higher mitochondrial activity. Similar results have been seen in other species, although the velocity measurement recorded does depend on the CASA instrument and settings used. With the SpermVision instrument, SLC-selected spermatozoa show a straighter but slower pattern of motility than controls, with less pronounced head movements than unselected spermatozoa. This motility pattern does not appear to be related to mitochondrial membrane potential, which is higher in selected spermatozoa than in controls. However, since the fertility of selected spermatozoa is higher than unselected spermatozoa [32], the lower velocity of the selected spermatozoa does not seem to reflect a problem with their ability to traverse the female reproductive tract.

According to the results of this present experiment, there was no difference in sperm quality between samples with or without antibiotics, but samples prepared with MSLC had better quality, and also lower content of bacteria than controls, even those with added antibiotics. These results indicate that MSLC can be used to improve the quality of stallion semen, and that this quality is maintained during storage regardless of whether antibiotics are included in the extender or not. These results are potentially very interesting with regard to decreasing usage of antibiotics in semen extenders although further studies are needed to determine the circumstances under which antibiotics could be excluded. Although sperm quality is thought to be improved by some other methods of sperm selection, none of these other methods has been shown to reduce bacterial contamination [32].

5. Conclusions

Use of MSLC with pony stallion semen improved sperm quality compared to controls, and this improvement was maintained during prolonged storage at 6 °C. The presence of antibiotics neither improved nor adversely affected sperm quality. Therefore, MSLC may be useful for controlling bacterial contamination in stallion semen but in vivo studies are needed to assess the effects on the mare.

Acknowledgments: We would like to thank the ministry of Higher Education and Scientific Research, Iraq (Z.A.-K.), and the Foundation for Equine Research, Stockholm (grant number H 14-47-008; J.M.M. and A.J.) for financial support for this work. In addition, special thanks to the people working in the Center for Artificial Insemination and Embryo Transfer, Vetmeduni Vienna, Austria, for their help with this study.

Author Contributions: J.M.M., Z.A.-K., A.J. and C.A. conceived and designed the experiments; all authors contributed to the performance of the experiments; Z.A.-K., J.S., A.J. and J.M.M. analyzed the data; all authors contributed reagents/materials/analysis tools; Z.A.-K. drafted the paper and all authors contributed to the final version.

References

1. Baumber, J. Evaluation of Semen. In *Equine Reproduction*, 2nd ed.; John Wiley & Sons: Hoboken, NJ, USA, 2011; pp. 1278–1291.
2. Lindeberg, H.; Karjalainen, H.; Koskinen, E.; Katila, T. Quality of stallion semen obtained by a new semen collection phantom (Equidame) versus a Missouri artificial vagaina. *Theriogenology* **1999**, *51*, 1157–1173. [CrossRef]
3. Bennett, D.G. Therapy of Endometritis in Mares. *J. Am. Vet. Med. Assoc.* **1986**, *188*, 1390–1392. [PubMed]
4. Johansson, A.; Greko, C.; Engstrom, B.E.; Karlsson, M. Antimicrobial susceptibility of Swedish, Norwegian and Danish isolates of Clostridium perfringens from poultry, and distribution of tetracycline resistance genes. *Vet. Microbiol.* **2004**, *99*, 251–257. [CrossRef] [PubMed]
5. Jasko, D.J.; Bedford, S.J.; Cook, N.L.; Mumford, E.L.; Squires, E.L.; Pickett, B.W. Effect of antibiotics on motion characteristics of cooled stallion spermatozoa. *Theriogenology* **1993**, *40*, 885–893. [CrossRef]
6. Aurich, C.; Spergser, J. Influence of bacteria and gentamicin on cooled-stored stallion spermatozoa. *Theriogenology* **2007**, *67*, 912–918. [CrossRef] [PubMed]
7. Barratt, C.L. Semen analysis is the cornerstone of investigation for male infertility. *Practitioner* **2007**, *251*, 8–17. [PubMed]
8. Rodriguez-Martinez, H. Semen evaluation techniques and their relationship with fertility. *Anim. Reprod. Sci.* **2013**, *10*, 148–159.
9. Quintero-Moreno, A.; Miro, J.; Rigau, A.T.; Rodriguez-Gil, J.E. Identification of sperm subpopulations with specific motility characteristics in stallion ejaculates. *Theriogenology* **2003**, *59*, 1973–1990. [CrossRef]
10. Hossain, M.S.; Johannisson, A.; Wallgren, M.; Nagy, S.; Siqueira, A.P.; Rodriguez-Martinez, H. Flow cytometry for the assessment of animal sperm integrity and functionally: State of the art. *Asian J. Androl.* **2011**, *13*, 406–419. [CrossRef] [PubMed]
11. Morrell, J.; Klein, C.; Lundeheim, N.; Erol, E.; Troedsson, M. Removal of bacteria from stallion semen by colloid centrifugation. *Anim. Reprod. Sci.* **2014**, *145*, 47–53. [CrossRef] [PubMed]
12. Morrell, J.M.; Wallgren, M. Removal of bacteria from boar ejaculates by Single Layer Centrifugation can reduce the use of antibiotics in semen extenders. *Anim. Reprod. Sci.* **2011**, *123*, 64–69. [CrossRef] [PubMed]
13. Morrell, J.M.; Wallgren, M. Alternatives to antibiotics in semen extenders: A review. *Pathogens* **2014**, *3*, 934–946. [CrossRef] [PubMed]

14. Johannisson, A.; Morrell, J.M.; Thoren, J.; Jönsson, M.; Dalin, A.M.; Rodriguez-Martinez, H. Colloidal centrifugation with Androcoll-ETM prolongs stallion sperm motility, viability and chromatin integrity. *Anim. Reprod. Sci.* **2009**, *116*, 119–128. [CrossRef] [PubMed]
15. Morrell, J.M.; Lagerqvist, A.; Humblot, P.; Johannisson, A. Effect of Single Layer Centrifugation on reactive oxygen species and sperm mitochondrial membrane potential in cooled stallion semen. *Reprod. Fertil. Dev.* **2017**, *29*, 1039–1045. [CrossRef] [PubMed]
16. Johannisson, A.; Lundgren, A.; Humblot, P.; Morrell, J.M. Natural and stimulated levels of reactive oxygen species in cooled stallion semen destined for artificial insemination. *Animal* **2014**, *8*, 1706–1714. [CrossRef] [PubMed]
17. Wang, Z.; Goonewardene, L.A. The use of MIXED models in the analysis of animal experiments with repeated measures data. *Can. J. Anim. Sci.* **2004**, *84*, 1–11. [CrossRef]
18. Zampieri, D.; Santos, V.G.; Braga, P.A.; Ferreira, C.R.; Ballottin, D.; Tasic, L.; Basso, A.C.; Sanches, B.V.; Pontes, J.H.F.; Da Silva, B.P.; et al. Microorganisms in cryopreserved semen and culture media used in the in vitro production (IVP) of bovine embryos identified by matrix-assisted laser desorption ionization mass spectrometry (MALDI-MS). *Theriogenology* **2013**, *80*, 337–345. [CrossRef] [PubMed]
19. Althouse, G.C.; Skaife, J.; Loomis, P. Prevalence and types of contamination in extended, chilled equine semen. *Anim. Reprod. Sci.* **2010**, *121S*, 224–225.
20. Yaniz, J.L.; Marco-Aguado, M.A.; Mateos, J.A.; Santolaria, P. Bacterial contamination of ram semen, antibiotic sensitivities, and effects on sperm quality during storage at 15 °C. *Anim. Reprod. Sci.* **2010**, *122*, 142–149. [CrossRef] [PubMed]
21. Bussalleu, E.; Yeste, M.; Sepulveda, L.; Torner, E.; Pinart, E.; Bonet, S. Effects of different concentrations of enterotoxigenic and verotoxi-genic *E. coli* on boar sperm quality. *Anim. Reprod. Sci.* **2011**, *127*, 176–182. [CrossRef] [PubMed]
22. Arriola, J.; Foote, R.H. Effects of amikacin sulfate on the motility of stallion and bull spermatozoa at different temperatures and intervals of storage. *J. Anim. Sci.* **1982**, *54*, 1105–1110. [CrossRef] [PubMed]
23. Akhter, S.; Ansari, M.S.; Andrabi, S.M.; Ullah, N.; Oayyum, M. Effect of antibiotics in extender on bacterial and spermatozoal quality of cooled buffalo (bubalus bubalis) bull semen. *Reprod. Domest. Anim.* **2008**, *43*, 272–278. [CrossRef] [PubMed]
24. Nicholson, C.M.; Abramsson, L.; Holm, S.E.; Bjurulf, E. Bacterial contamination and sperm recovery after semen preparation by density gradient centrifugation using silane-coated silica particles at different g forces. *Hum. Reprod.* **2000**, *15*, 662–666. [CrossRef] [PubMed]
25. Guimaraes, T.; Lopes, G.; Pinto, M.; Silva, E.; Miranda, C.; Correia, M.J.; Damasio, L.; Thompson, G.; Rocha, A. Colloid centrifugation of fresh stallion semen before cryopreservation decreased microorganism load of frozen- thawed semen without affecting seminal kinetics. *Theriogenology* **2015**, *83*, 186–191. [CrossRef] [PubMed]
26. Morrell, J.M.; Dalin, A.M.; Rodriguez-Martinez, H. Prolongation of stallion sperm survival by centrifugation through coated silica colloids: A preliminary study. *Anim. Reprod.* **2008**, *5*, 121–126.
27. Morrell, J.M.; Rodriguez-Martinez, H.; Johannisson, A. Single layer centrifugation of stallion spermatozoa consistently selects the most robust spermatozoa from the rest of the ejaculate in a large sample size. *Equine Vet. J.* **2010**, *42*, 579–585. [CrossRef] [PubMed]
28. Morrell, J.M.; Johannisson, A.; Dalin, A.M.; Rodriguez-Martinez, H. Single Layer Centrifugation with Androcoll^{TM}—E can be scaled-up to allow large volumes of stallion ejaculate to be processed easily. *Theriogenology* **2009**, *72*, 879–884. [CrossRef] [PubMed]
29. Ortiz, I.; Dorado, J.; Ramirez, L.; Morrell, J.M.; Acha, D.; Urbano, M.; Galvez, M.J.; Carrasco, J.J.; Gomez-Arrones, V.; Calero-Carretero, R.; et al. Effect of single layer centrifugation using Androcoll-E-Large on the sperm quality parameters of cooled-stored donkey semen doses. *Animal* **2014**, *8*, 308–315. [CrossRef] [PubMed]
30. Morrell, J.M.; Alsina, M.S.; Abraham, M.C.; Sjunnesson, Y. Practical applications of sperm selection techniques for improving reproduction efficiency. *Anim. Reprod.* **2016**, *13*, 340–345. [CrossRef]

31. Lindahl, J.; Dalin, A.M.; Stuhtmann, G.; Morrell, J.M. Stallion spermatozoa selected by single layer centrifugation are capable of fertilization after storage for up to 96 h at 6 °C prior to artificial insemination. *Acta Vet. Scand.* **2012**, *54*. [CrossRef] [PubMed]
32. Morrell, J.M.; Rodriguez-Martinez, H. Colloid Centrifugation of Semen: Applications in Assisted Reproduction. *J. Anal. Chem.* **2016**, *7*, 597–610. [CrossRef]

14

Probiotics for the Prevention of Antibiotic-Associated Diarrhea in Outpatients

Sara Blaabjerg *, Daniel Maribo Artzi * and Rune Aabenhus *

The Research Unit for General Practice and Section of General Practice, University of Copenhagen, 1014 Copenhagen K, Denmark

* Correspondence: wck913@alumni.ku.dk (S.B.); fsm593@alumni.ku.dk (D.M.A.); runeaa@sund.ku.dk (R.A.)

Academic Editor: Christopher C. Butler

Abstract: A common adverse effect of antibiotic use is diarrhea. Probiotics are living microorganisms, which, upon oral ingestion, may prevent antibiotic-associated diarrhea (AAD) by the normalization of an unbalanced gastrointestinal flora. The objective of this systematic review was to assess the benefits and harms of probiotics used for the prevention of AAD in an outpatient setting. A search of the PubMed database was conducted and yielded a total of 17 RCTs with 3631 participants to be included in the review. A meta-analysis was conducted for the primary outcome: the incidence of AAD. The pooled results found that AAD was present in 8.0% of the probiotic group compared to 17.7% in the control group (RR 0.49, 95% CI 0.36 to 0.66; $I^2 = 58\%$), and the species-specific results were similar regarding the probiotic strains *L. rhamnosus* GG and *S. boulardii*. However, the overall quality of the included studies was moderate. A meta-analysis of the ten trials reporting adverse events demonstrated no statistically significant differences in the incidence of adverse events between the intervention and control group (RD 0.00, 95% CI −0.02 to 0.02, 2.363 participants). The results suggests that probiotic use may be beneficial in the prevention of AAD among outpatients. Furthermore, the use of probiotics appears safe.

Keywords: primary care; antibiotic-associated diarrhea; probiotics; *Lactobacillus*; *Bifidobacterium*; *Saccharomyces*

---

1. Introduction

Diarrhea is a common adverse effect of systemic antibiotic treatment. Antibiotic-associated diarrhea (AAD) occurs in 5% to 39% of patients, from the beginning and up to two months after the end of treatment [1]. Any type of antibiotics can cause AAD. In particular, aminopenicillins, cephalosporins, and clindamycin that act on anaerobes are associated with a high risk of AAD [2]. The symptoms range from mild and self-limiting diarrhea to severe diarrhea, the latter particularly in *Clostridium difficile* infections.

The primary care sector is responsible for the bulk of antibiotic consumption in humans [3]. Reports suggest that a major part of this antibiotic use may, in fact, be inappropriate, and efforts to reduce and target antibiotics are rightly promoted. However, when antibiotic therapy is deemed necessary, it is useful to have an easily available, cost effective, and safe method to prevent side effects associated with the issued antibiotic.

Probiotics are defined as "live microorganisms which when administered in adequate amounts confer a health benefit on the host" [4]. The rationale behind the administration of probiotics in gastrointestinal disorders is based on the hypothesis that they may assist a normalization of an unbalanced gastrointestinal flora. There are many proposed mechanisms by which probiotics enhance intestinal health, including the stimulation of immunity, competition for nutrients, the inhibition of the epithelial and mucosal adherence of pathogens, the inhibition of epithelial invasion, and the production of antimicrobial substances [5].

Numerous probiotic species have been tested, most commonly the *Lactobacillus* genus, *Bifidobacterium* genus, and *Saccharomyces* genus. Previous reviews suggest that probiotics are useful in the prevention of AAD, especially in a pediatric population (RR 0.46; 95% CI 0.35 to 0.61) with a NNT of 10 [6]. However, these reviews have mainly focused on the prevention of AAD in inpatients from secondary care settings, which was likely influenced by the intensity of antibiotic treatment (intravenous vs. oral), the type of infection, and the microbial pathogens, in turn making the translation of the results into the primary care sector less straightforward.

The objective of this systematic review and meta-analysis was thus to assess the benefits and harms of probiotics used for the prevention of antibiotic-associated diarrhea in outpatients of all ages.

2. Results

2.1. Description of Studies

2.1.1. Results of the Search

A total of 637 studies were identified through MEDLINE/PubMed. An independent review of these titles and abstracts identified 53 potentially relevant studies for full-text reviews. Of these studies, 17 met the inclusion criteria. The details of the study flow, including reasons for exclusion, are documented in the study flow diagram in Supplementary Materials File S1.

2.1.2. Design

All included studies were prospective, randomized, controlled trials with placebo, active, or no treatment control arms. Additional information about each study can be found in the Characteristics of Included Studies table in Supplementary Materials File S2.

2.1.3. Patient Population

The 17 studies included a total of 3631 patients. The patient population was restricted to outpatients taking oral antibiotics, as trials randomizing hospitalized patients were excluded. The recruitment and evaluation of patients took place in private practices, pharmacies, or hospitals (ambulatory settings, outpatient clinics, etc.).

All studies included both males and females.

2.1.4. Interventions

Probiotics:

The trials tested the prevention of AAD with *Lactobacilli* spp., *Lactococcus* spp., *Bacillus* spp., *Bifidobacterium* spp., *Saccharomyces* spp., *Leuconostoc cremoris*, *Clostridium* spp., or *Streptococcus* spp. Eight studies (N = 1638; Tankanow 1990, Park 2007, Conway 2007, Kim 2008, Merenstein 2009, De Vrese 2011, Chatterjee 2013, Fox 2014) used a combination of two or more probiotic strains as intervention. Additional information about the type of probiotic(s) that were used, including the dosages and treatment durations, can be found in Table 1.

Table 1. Probiotic(s) used, dosages, and treatment durations.

RCT	Probiotic(s) Used (Genus and Strain)	Dosage	Duration of Treatment
Tankanow et al., 1990 [7]	*Lactobacillus acidophilus* *Lactobacillus bulgaricus*	5.1×10^8 CFU, four times daily	10 days
Vanderhoof et al., 1999 [8]	*Lactobacillus rhamnosus GG*	Children < 12 kg: 1×10^{10} CFU, once daily Children > 12 kg: 2×10^{10}, once daily	10 days
Arvola et al., 1999 [9]	*Lactobacillus rhamnosus GG*	2×10^{10} CFU, twice daily	Seven to 10 days
Erdeve et al., 2004 [10]	*Saccharomyces boulardii*	Not mentioned	Not mentioned
Duman et al., 2005 [11]	*Saccharomyces boulardii*	500 mg, twice daily	14 days
Park et al., 2007 [12]	*Bacillus subtilis* *Streptococcus faecium*	two capsules three times a day: 2.5×10^9 CFU (*Bacillus subtilis*) 22.5×10^9 CFU (*Streptococcus faecium*)	Eight weeks
Cindoruk et al., 2007 [13]	*Saccharomyces boulardii*	500 mg, twice daily	14 days
Conway et al., 2007 [14]	*Lactobacillus acidophilus* *Streptococcus thermophilus* *Bifidobacterium animalis lactis*	10^9 CFU, once daily	12 days
Imase et al., 2008 [15]	*Clostridium butyricum*	1×10^7 CFU per tablet Group B: two tablets, three times daily Group C: 4 tablets, three times daily	Seven days
Kim et al., 2008 [16]	*Lactobacillus acidophilus* *Lactobacillus casei* *Bifidobacterium longum* *Streptococcus thermophilus*	One bottle (150 mL) per day: $>1 \times 10^5$ CFU/mL (*L. acidophilus*) $>1 \times 10^5$ CFU/mL (*L. casei*) $>1 \times 10^6$ CFU/mL (*B. longum*) $>1 \times 10^8$ CFU/mL (*S. themophilus*)	At least three weeks

Table 1. *Cont.*

RCT	Probiotic(s) Used (Genus and Strain)	Dosage	Duration of Treatment
Merenstein et al., 2009 [17]	*Lactococcus lactis* *Lactococcus plantarum* *Lactococcus rhamnosus* *Lactococcus casei* *Lactococcus lactis subspecies diacetylactis* *Leuconostoc cremoris* *Bifidobacterium longum* *Bifidobacterium breve* *Lactobacillus acidophilus* *Saccharomyces florentinus*	One bottle (150 mL) per day, amount of CFU not mentioned	10 days
De Vrese et al., 2011 [18]	*Lactobacillus acidophilus LA-5* *Bifidobacterium lactis BB-12*	>1 × 10^6 CFU/g, 125 g, twice daily	Five weeks
Ojetti et al., 2013 [19]	*Lactobacillus reuteri*	1 × 10^8 CFU, three times daily	14 days
Chatterjee et al., 2013 [20]	*Lactobacillus acidophilus La-5,* *Bifidobacterium Bb-12*	4 × 10^9 CFU	14 days
Zojaji et al., 2013 [21]	*Saccharomyces boulardii*	250 mg twice daily, amount of CFU not mentioned	14 days
Fox et al., 2014 [22]	*Lactobacillus rhamnosus, G.G.;* *Lactobacillus acidophilus LA-5,* *Bifidobacterium Bb-12*	5.2 × 10^9 CFU (*L. rhamnosus*) 5.9 × 10^9 CFU (*B. Bb-12*) 8.3 × 10^9 CFU (*L. acidophilus LA-5*)	Number of days not mentioned ("From the start to the end of their antibiotic treatment")
Olek et al., 2017 [23]	*Lactobacillus plantarum* DSM9843 (LP299V)	1 × 10^{10} CFU/capsule	Five to 10 days during antibiotic treatment and one week after (±two days)

Antibiotics:

The patients were treated with oral antibiotics for various clinical indications, but the most common reason was *H. pylori* eradication with a combination of clarithromycin and amoxicillin (seven studies: $N = 1450$; Duman 2005, Park 2007, Cindoruk 2007, Imase 2008, Kim 2008, De Vrese 2011, Zojaji 2013). One study (Ojetti 2012) used a combination of levofloxacin and amoxicillin for *H. pylori* eradication therapy. Two studies (Tankanow 1990, Erdeve 2004) reported the use of single beta-lactam antibiotics, while others included several antibiotics or were otherwise unspecified.

Aside from *H. pylori* infection, the most common indications for treatment with antibiotics were upper and lower respiratory tract infections, otitis media, and throat infections.

2.1.5. Comparison

Most RCTs randomized a moderate number of participants (median, 174.0; mean [SD], 205.3 [130.2]) to either probiotics vs. placebo (nine studies: $N = 1557$; Tankanow 1990, Arvola 1999, Vanderhoof 1999, Cindoruk 2007, Merenstein 2009, De Vrese 2011, Chatterjee 2013, Fox 2014, Olek 2017) or probiotics vs. no treatment (eight studies: $N = 2074$; Erdeve 2004, Duman 2005, Park 2007, Conway 2007, Kim 2008, Imase 2008, Ojetti 2012, Zojaji 2013).

2.1.6. Outcomes

All of the included studies provided data on the main outcome: the incidence of AAD. The outcomes were patient-reported. The definitions of diarrhea varied in each study in regard to the number of bowel movements per day and the consistency of stools ("semi-solid", "watery", "liquid", "abnormally loose", etc.). Seven studies ($N = 1724$; Arvola 1999, Duman 2005, Conway 2007, De Vrese 2011, Chatterjee 2013, Fox 2014, Olek 2017) applied the WHO definition of diarrhea ("the passage of three or more loose or liquid stools per day") [24]. Three studies ($N = 561$; Cindoruk 2007, Kim 2008, Ojetti 2012) categorized diarrhea into groups ("none", "mild", "moderate", and "severe"), but did not include the frequency or consistency of bowel movements. Four studies ($N = 656$; Park 2007, Imase 2008, Merenstein 2009, Zojaji 2013) did not provide any definition of diarrhea. The individual studies' definitions of diarrhea can be seen in Table 2.

Table 2. The individual studies' definitions of diarrhea.

RCT	Definition of Diarrhea
Tankanow et al., 1990	One or more abnormally loose bowel movements/day throughout the study period of one to 10 days (parental reports)
Vanderhoof et al., 1999	The presence of at least two liquid stools/day during at least two observation periods during the course of the study
Arvola et al., 1999	At least three watery or loose stools/day for a minimum of two consecutive days
Erdeve et al., 2004	Three or more watery stools/day during antibiotic treatment
Duman et al., 2005	A change in bowel habits with at least three semi-solid or watery bowel movements/day for at least two consecutive days
Park et al., 2007	Not specified (self-report)
Cindoruk et al., 2007	Not specified (modified *De Boer* questionnaire categorizing diarrhea into "none", "mild", "moderate" and "severe")
Conway et al., 2007	Three or more loose stools/day over at least two consecutive days during the 12-day follow-up period
Imase et al., 2008	"Loose or mostly loose stools", not specified further
Kim et al., 2008	Not specified other than categorized in groups ("none", "mild", "moderate", "severe")
Merenstein et al., 2009	Not specified (parental reports)
De Vrese et al., 2011	Three or more watery stools for at least one day (where at least one episode lay within the eradication week)
Ojetti et al., 2013	Not specified other than categorized in groups ("none", "mild", "moderate", "severe")
Chatterjee et al., 2013	Passage of at least three or more watery or loose stools/day for at least two consecutive days
Zojaji et al., 2013	Not specified (self-report)
Fox et al., 2014	Categories:
	"A" (stool consistency ≥ 5, ≥ 2 stools/day for ≥ 2 days)
	"B" (stool consistency ≥ 5, ≥ 3 stools/day for ≥ 2 days)
	"C" (stool consistency ≥ 6, ≥ 2 stools/day for ≥ 2 days)
	"D" (stool consistency ≥ 6, ≥ 3 stools/day for ≥ 2 days)
Olek et al., 2017	≥ 3 loose/watery stools/24 h starting after the initiation of antibiotic treatment

Ten studies (N = 2363; Tankanow 1990, Arvola 1999, Vanderhoof 1999, Duman 2005, Conway 2007, Kim 2008, Merenstein 2009, Chatterjee 2013, Fox 2014, Olek 2017) reported the incidence of adverse events (i.e., the number of participants with at least one adverse event of any type). The definitions of adverse events varied widely. Four studies (N = 762; Vanderhoof 1999, Arvola 1999, De Vrese 2011, Chatterjee 2013) reported the mean duration of diarrhea, but the data was not sufficient to make a quantitative analysis of this outcome. Instead these are summarized qualitatively and/or by descriptive statistics.

2.2. Risk of Bias in Included Studies

The risk of bias is categorized into three categories: high risk of bias, low risk of bias, and unclear. The individual studies' results of the risk of bias assessment are shown in Figure 1.

The quality of reporting was low; 11 trials lacked adequate information to assess one or more of the parameters, thus making the risk of bias "unclear". This was the case particularly regarding allocation concealment and blinding methods. For the blinding of participants, nearly half of the studies were evaluated as having a "high risk of bias" because the participants in the control group did not receive any kind of placebo matching the probiotic(s) given to the intervention group.

	Random sequence generation (selection bias)	Allocation concealment (selection bias)	Blinding of participants and personnel (performance bias)	Blinding of outcome assessment (detection bias)	Incomplete outcome data (attrition bias)	Selective reporting (reporting bias)	Other bias
Arvola et al., 1999	+	?	+	?	−	+	+
Chatterjee et al., 2013	+	+	+	?	+	+	+
Cindoruk et al., 2007	+	?	+	+	+	+	+
Conway et al., 2007	+	+	−	+	+	+	+
De Vrese et al., 2011	?	?	+	?	+	+	+
Duman et al., 2005	?	−	−	−	?	+	+
Erdeve et al., 2004	?	?	?	?	−	+	+
Fox et al., 2014	+	+	+	?	+	+	+
Imase et al., 2008	?	?	−	?	+	+	+
Kim et al., 2008	−	−	−	−	+	+	+
Merenstein et al., 2009	+	+	+	+	+	+	+
Ojetti et al., 2012	+	?	−	?	+	+	+
Olek et al., 2017	+	+	+	+	+	+	+
Park et al., 2007	?	+	−	?	+	+	+
Tankanow et al., 1990	?	?	−	?	−	+	−
Vanderhoof et al., 1999	+	+	−	+	+	+	−
Zojaji et al., 2013	?	?	−	?	+	+	+

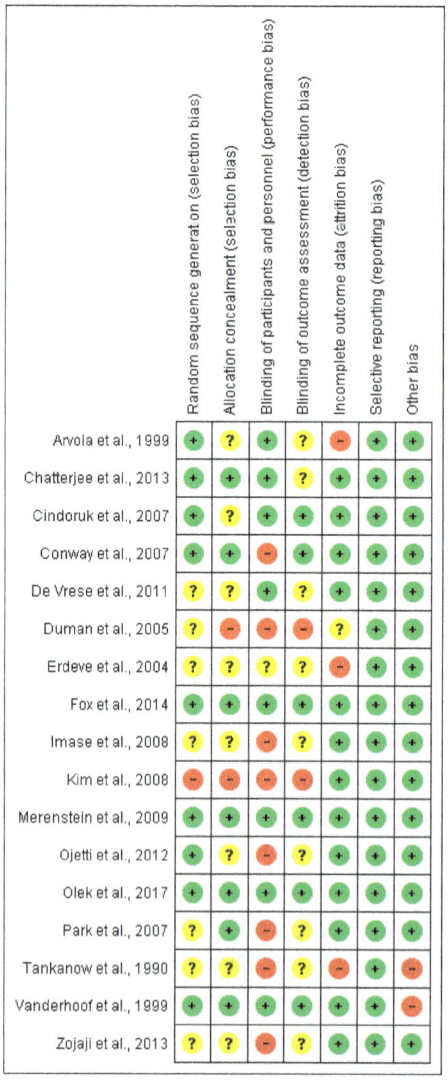

Figure 1. Risk of bias summary.

Loss to follow-up was substantial (i.e., >20%) in three trials (Tankanow 1990, Arvola 1999, Erdeve 2004). 11 studies (Tankanow 1990, Arvola 1999, Vanderhoof 1999, Erdeve 2004, Duman 2005, Cindoruk 2007, Imase 2008, De Vrese 2011, Zojaji 2013, Fox 2014) did not perform an intention-to-treat analysis.

Loss to follow-up was substantial (i.e., >20%) in three trials (Tankanow 1990, Arvola 1999, Erdeve 2004). 11 studies (Tankanow 1990, Arvola 1999, Vanderhoof 1999, Erdeve 2004, Duman 2005, Cindoruk 2007, Imase 2008, De Vrese 2011, Zojaji 2013, Fox 2014) did not perform an intention-to-treat analysis.

Visual inspection of the funnel plot (Figure 2) for the primary outcome identified minor asymmetries for the smaller studies, but the relationship between the risk ratio and standard error did not appear substantially skewed, in turn suggesting that a possible publication bias is not likely to markedly affect the results.

Visual inspection of the funnel plot (Figure 2) for the primary outcome identified minor asymmetries for the smaller studies, but the relationship between the risk ratio and standard error did not appear substantially skewed, in turn suggesting that a possible publication bias is not likely to markedly affect the results.

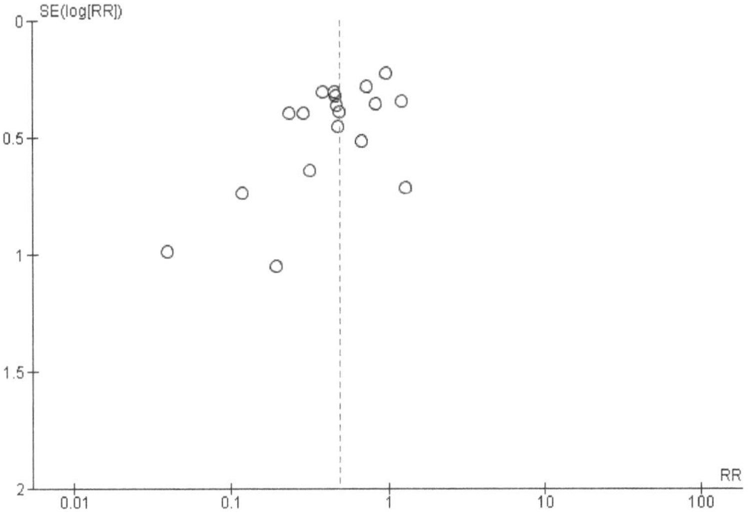

Figure 2. Funnel plot.

Figure 2. Funnel plot.

2.3. Effects of Interventions

2.3.1. Main Outcome: Incidence of Antibiotic-Associated Diarrhea

2.3. Effects of Interventions

2.3.1. Main Outcome: Incidence of Antibiotic-Associated Diarrhea

All of the 17 included studies reported the incidence of diarrhea and the number of patients randomized to each group. The incidence of AAD in the probiotic group was 8.0%, compared to 17.7% in the control group. The overall pooled results showed that the use of probiotics produced a statistically significant reduction in the incidence of AAD (RR 0.49, 95% CI 0.36 to 0.66). The forest plot can be seen in **Supplementary Materials File S3**. Statistically significant heterogeneity was detected (p = 0.001) and this was moderate (I^2 = 58%). A GRADE analysis (Supplementary Materials File S4) indicated that the overall quality of evidence for this outcome was moderate due to moderate heterogeneity and high risk of bias of trials.

In addition to the pooled analysis of any probiotic, a strain-specific meta-analysis (Figure 3) was conducted on eight of the included studies with three subgroups of the following probiotic strain(s): two studies using *L. rhamnosus GG* (*N* = 307; Arvola 1999, Vanderhoof 1999), four studies using *S. boulardii* (*N* = 1139; Erdeve 2004, Duman 2005, Cindoruk 2007, Zojaji 2013), and two studies using a combination of *L. acidophilus La-5* and *B. lactis Bb-12* (*N* = 455; De Vrese 2011, Chatterjee 2013).

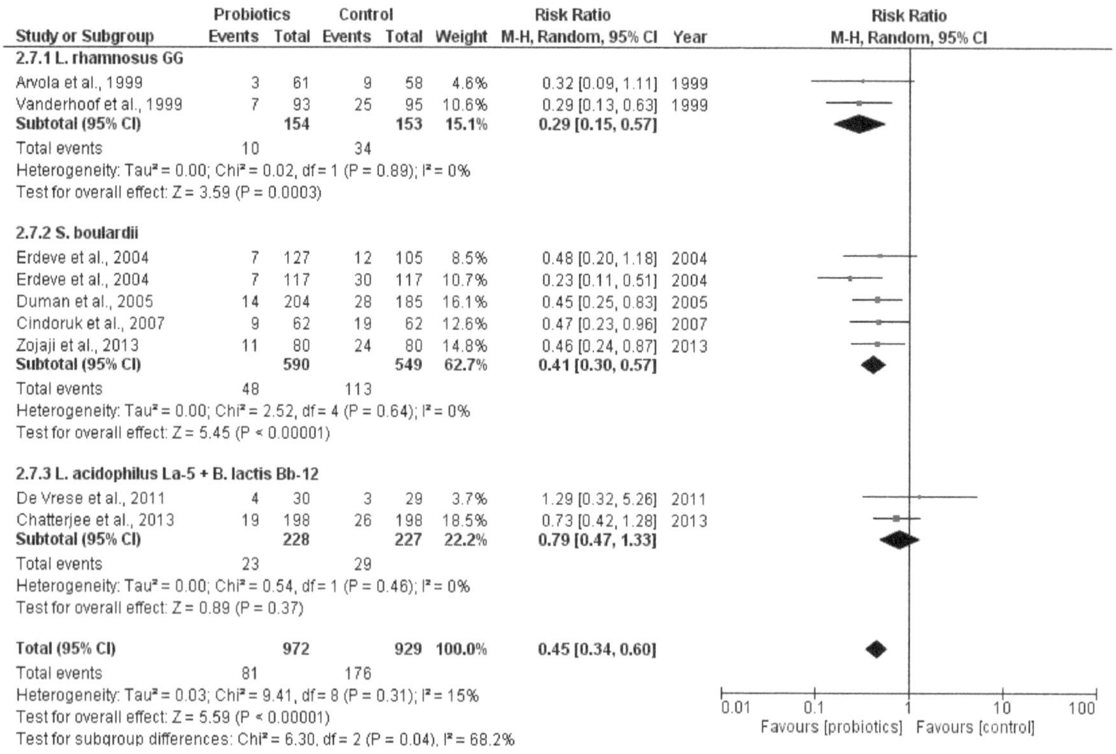
Probiotics
Control
Risk Ratio
Risk Ratio
Study or Subgroup Events Total Events Total Weight M-H, Random, 95% CI Year
M-H, Random, 95% CI
2.7.1 L. rhamnosus GG
Arvola et al., 1999 3 61 9 58 4.6% 0.32 [0.09, 1.11] 1999
Vanderhoof et al., 1999 7 93 25 95 10.6% 0.29 [0.13, 0.63] 1999
Subtotal (95% CI) 154 153 15.1% 0.29 [0.15, 0.57]
Total events 10 34
Heterogeneity: Tau² = 0.00; Chi² = 0.02, df = 1 (P = 0.89); I² = 0%
Test for overall effect: Z = 3.59 (P = 0.0003)
2.7.2 S. boulardii
Erdeve et al., 2004 7 127 12 105 8.5% 0.48 [0.20, 1.18] 2004
Erdeve et al., 2004 7 117 30 117 10.7% 0.23 [0.11, 0.51] 2004
Duman et al., 2005 14 204 28 185 16.1% 0.45 [0.25, 0.83] 2005
Cindoruk et al., 2007 9 62 19 62 12.6% 0.47 [0.23, 0.96] 2007
Zojaji et al., 2013 11 80 24 80 14.8% 0.46 [0.24, 0.87] 2013
Subtotal (95% CI) 590 549 62.7% 0.41 [0.30, 0.57]
Total events 48 113
Heterogeneity: Tau² = 0.00; Chi² = 2.52, df = 4 (P = 0.64); I² = 0%
Test for overall effect: Z = 5.45 (P < 0.00001)
2.7.3 L. acidophilus La-5 + B. lactis Bb-12
De Vrese et al., 2011 4 30 3 29 3.7% 1.29 [0.32, 5.26] 2011
Chatterjee et al., 2013 19 198 26 198 18.5% 0.73 [0.42, 1.28] 2013
Subtotal (95% CI) 228 227 22.2% 0.79 [0.47, 1.33]
Total events 23 29
Heterogeneity: Tau² = 0.00; Chi² = 0.54, df = 1 (P = 0.46); I² = 0%
Test for overall effect: Z = 0.89 (P = 0.37)
Total (95% CI) 972 929 100.0% 0.45 [0.34, 0.60]
Total events 81 176
Heterogeneity: Tau² = 0.03; Chi² = 9.41, df = 8 (P = 0.31); I² = 15%
Test for overall effect: Z = 5.59 (P < 0.00001)
Test for subgroup differences: Chi² = 6.30, df = 2 (P = 0.04), I² = 68.2%
0.01
0.1
1
10
100
Favours [probiotics] Favours [control]

Figure 3. Efficacy results of probiotic use: eight RCTs by three probiotic subgroups (outcome: incidence of antibiotic-associated diarrhea (AAD)).

The results were similar to the overall pooled analysis and showed a beneficial effect of probiotics in the prevention of AAD. This effect was statistically significant in two of the three subgroups.

The subgroup analyses on *L. rhamnosus GG* and *S. boulardii* showed a statistically significant lower risk of AAD, while this was not the case regarding the combination probiotic supplement of *L. acidophilus La-5* and *B. lactis Bb-12* (RR 0.79; 95% CI 0.47 to 1.33). The high level of heterogeneity in the overall pooled results could no longer be detected in these three subgroups ($I^2 = 0\%$). A GRADE analysis (Supplementary Materials File S4) indicated that the overall quality of evidence for this outcome was high.

2.3.2. Secondary Outcome: Incidence of Antibiotic-Associated Diarrhea Using the Criteria Defined by WHO

Seven studies ($N = 1724$; Arvola 1999, Duman 2005, Conway 2007, De Vrese 2011, Chatterjee 2013, Fox 2014, Olek 2017) applied the WHO definition of diarrhea, and the pooled results showed that the use of probiotics produced a statistically significant reduction in the incidence of AAD: RR 0.54; 95% CI 0.36 to 0.82 (Figure 4).

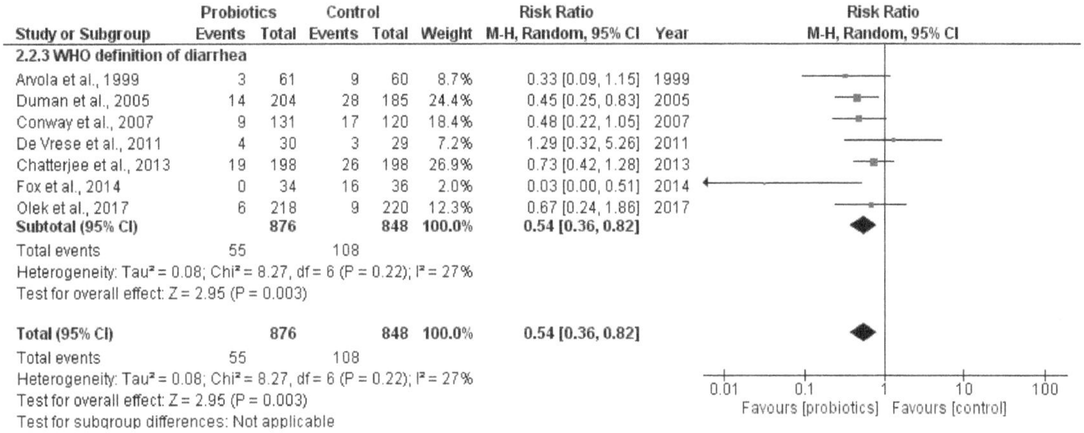

Figure 4. Efficacy results of probiotic use by study (secondary outcome: incidence of AAD using the criteria defined by WHO).

No statistically significant heterogeneity was detected ($p = 0.22$; $I^2 = 27\%$). A GRADE analysis (Supplementary Materials File S4) indicated that the overall quality of evidence for this outcome was high.

2.3.3. Secondary Outcome: Mean Duration of Diarrhea

Four studies ($N = 762$; Vanderhoof 1999, Arvola 1999, De Vrese 2011, Chatterjee 2013) reported the mean duration of diarrhea (MDD). The results can be seen in Table 3. The standard deviations (SD) for these trials were not reported so a quantitative analysis for this outcome was not possible. One study (Arvola 1999) showed a similar duration of diarrhea in both groups, while the other three all showed a positive effect on the MDD in the intervention group. Combining these four studies, the average MDD in the intervention group was 2.93 days, while the average was 4.65 days in the control group.

Table 3. Mean duration of diarrhea (MDD).

	MDD (Days)	Range	Probiotic Group (N)	MDD (Days)	Range	Control Group (N)
Vanderhoof et al., 1999	4.70	N/A	93	5.88	N/A	95
Arvola et al., 1999	4.00	2–8	61	4.00	2–8	58
De Vrese et al., 2011	1.00	N/A	30	4.70	N/A	29
Chatterjee et al., 2013	2.00	1–3	198	4.00	3–5.5	198

2.3.4. Secondary Outcome: Incidence of Adverse Events

None of the 17 included studies specifically defined adverse events prior to enrolment of participants. Ten trials ($N = 2363$; Tankanow 1990, Arvola 1999, Vanderhoof 1999, Duman 2005, Conway 2007, Kim 2008, Merenstein 2009, Chatterjee 2013, Fox 2014, Olek 2017) reported the number of participants with adverse events in each group. Adverse events consisted of a variety of different symptoms such as metallic taste, nausea, loss of appetite, epigastric discomfort, headache, flu-like symptoms, rash, etc. There were no serious adverse effects leading to major disabilities, hospitalization, or death. Three trials (Kim 2008, Fox 2004, Olek 2017) found a statistically significant difference in adverse events between groups; one favors placebo and two favor probiotics. Kim et al. found a difference in the presence of metallic taste between the intervention group (16.7%) and the control group (7.3%). Fox et al., as well as *Olek* et al., reported more adverse events in their placebo-controlled patient group, and these were abdominal pain, loss of appetite, nausea, pyrexia, headache, and rash.

A meta-analysis of the ten trials reporting on any adverse events (Figure 5) demonstrated no statistically significant differences in the incidence of adverse events between the intervention and control groups (RD 0.00, 95% CI −0.02 to 0.02, 2363 participants).

Study or Subgroup	Probiotics Events	Probiotics Total	Control Events	Control Total	Weight	Risk Difference M-H, Random, 95% CI	Year
Tankanow et al., 1990	3	15	0	23	0.8%	0.20 [-0.01, 0.41]	1990
Vanderhoof et al., 1999	0	93	0	95	16.7%	0.00 [-0.02, 0.02]	1999
Arvola et al., 1999	0	61	0	60	13.3%	0.00 [-0.03, 0.03]	1999
Duman et al., 2005	3	204	3	185	15.5%	-0.00 [-0.03, 0.02]	2005
Conway et al., 2007	0	131	0	120	18.2%	0.00 [-0.02, 0.02]	2007
Kim et al., 2008	69	168	47	179	3.3%	0.15 [0.05, 0.25]	2008
Merenstein et al., 2009	1	61	1	64	10.0%	0.00 [-0.04, 0.04]	2009
Chatterjee et al., 2013	4	198	0	198	16.3%	0.02 [-0.00, 0.04]	2013
Fox et al., 2014	3	34	11	36	1.1%	-0.22 [-0.40, -0.04]	2014
Olek et al., 2017	39	218	60	220	4.8%	-0.09 [-0.17, -0.02]	2017
Total (95% CI)		**1183**		**1180**	**100.0%**	**0.00 [-0.02, 0.02]**	
Total events	122		122				

Heterogeneity: Tau² = 0.00; Chi² = 26.39, df = 9 (P = 0.002); I² = 66%
Test for overall effect: Z = 0.27 (P = 0.78)

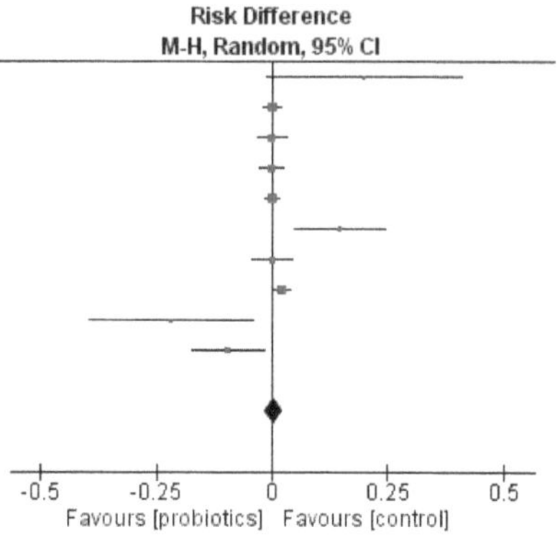

Figure 5. Adverse events.

A GRADE analysis indicated that the overall quality of evidence for this outcome was low due to heterogeneity and indirectness (Supplementary Materials File S4).

2.3.5. Dose-Response Analysis

The analysis regarding dose-response relationships included ten studies of different probiotic species. The pooled effect size for doses larger than 5×10^9 CFU/day was RR 0.18 (95% CI 0.08 to 0.42; $I^2 = 41\%$), and, for doses less than 5×10^9 CFU/day, it was RR 0.61 (95% CI 0.42 to 0.90; $I^2 = 40\%$). The difference in response rates between high-dose and low-dose probiotics were statistically significant ($p < 0.002$) by Fisher's exact test). The forest plot is provided in Supplementary Materials File S5.

2.4. *Subgroup Analyses*

Prespecified subgroup analyses for the main outcome were conducted on (1) age groups; (2) trials with *H. pylori* eradication; (3) low risk of bias; and (4) intention-to-treat analyses. Forest plots from each subgroup analysis can be seen in (Supplementary Materials Files S6–S9).

2.4.1. Age Groups

Two subgroups were based on the age of the participants, including children (<15 years of age) and adults (>15 years of age). Seven trials ($N = 1446$; Tankanow 1990, Arvola 1999, Vanderhoof 1999, Erdeve 2004, Merenstein 2009, Fox 2014, Olek 2017) targeted children specifically, and their results showed a statistically significant lower risk of AAD but with considerable heterogeneity (RR 0.42; 95% CI 0.23 to 0.77; $I^2 = 76\%$).

Nine trials ($N = 1936$; Duman 2005, Park 2007, Cindoruk 2007, Imase 2008, De Vrese 2011, Ojetti 2012, Zojaji 2013, Chatterjee 2013) targeting adults also showed a statistically significant reduction in the risk of AAD and moderate heterogeneity (RR 0.53; 95% CI 0.37 to 0.76; $I^2 = 47\%$).

One trial (Conway 2007) included both children and adults and therefore was not included in this subgroup analysis.

2.4.2. Trials with *H. pylori* Eradication Therapy

In the seven trials using a combination of clarithromycin and amoxicillin for *H. pylori* eradication therapy ($N = 1450$; Duman 2005, Park 2007, Cindoruk 2007, Kim 2008, Imase 2008, De Vrese 2011, Zojaji 2013), adjunct probiotic use was also associated with a lower risk of AAD (RR 0.52; 95% CI 0.32 to 0.85; $I^2 = 53\%$).

2.4.3. Low Risk of Bias

The trial quality was generally low, and only three studies (N = 633; Merenstein 2009, Fox 2014, Olek 2017) were evaluated as having a low risk of bias. Combining these three low risk studies in a meta-analysis showed a non-significant lower risk of AAD and considerable heterogeneity (RR 0.36; 95% CI 0.08 to 1.64; I^2 = 82%).

2.4.4. Intention-To-Treat Analyses

A meta-analysis combining the six studies using intention-to-treat analyses (N = 1561; Park 2007, Conway 2007, Kim 2008, Merenstein 2009, Ojetti 2012, Chatterjee 2013) showed similar results to the overall pooled analysis, with a significantly lower risk of AAD and moderate heterogeneity (RR 0.58; 95% CI 0.36 to 0.94; I^2 = 60%).

3. Discussion

The results of this review point towards a protective effect of the use of probiotics as adjunct therapy to prevent antibiotic-associated diarrhea in outpatients of all ages. Data from 17 studies with a total of 3631 patients found that the use of a probiotic may reduce the risk of AAD by 51% (RR 0.49; 95% CI 0.36 to 0.66; I^2 = 58%), with no apparent increase in the risk of side effects (RD 0.00, 95% CI −0.02 to 0.02, 2.363 participants). The number needed to treat (NNT) to prevent one case of diarrhea was 11 (95% CI 6 to 13). The quality of evidence for the main outcome was categorized as moderate due to a moderate degree of heterogeneity and a high risk of bias in some trials.

A strain-specific subgroup analysis combining data from eight of the included trials showed a similar protective effect of probiotics in the prevention of AAD when compared to the overall pooled analysis. The most effective probiotic strain was *L. rhamnosus GG* (RR 0.29; 95% CI 0.15 to 0.57; 307 participants), followed by *S. boulardii* (RR 0.41; 95% CI 0.30 to 0.57; 1.139 participants). Furthermore, with this subgroup analysis, the heterogeneity from the pooled analysis (I^2 = 58%) disappeared in each of the three subgroups (I^2 = 0%).

Data from the seven studies applying the definition of diarrhea defined by WHO showed a similar protective effect of probiotic use to prevent AAD (RR 0.54; 95% CI 0.36 to 0.82) but with no statistically significant heterogeneity (I^2 = 27%; p = 0.22). This explains some of the statistical heterogeneity, and it also demonstrates the importance of having clear and consistent definitions of outcomes in clinical trials. The quality of evidence for this outcome was categorized as high.

We also provide preliminary evidence of a possible dose-response relationship, as results indicate that higher doses were associated with fewer ADD events (higher than 5×10^9 CFU 3.6% vs. less than 5×10^9 CFU 8.9%; $p < 0.002$). However, this result should be interpreted with caution as the analysis was on any probiotic species and not on specific strains. A review investigating different treatment regimens of probiotics in human studies concluded that a dose-response relationship exists within the commonly studied range of 10^8 to 10^{11} CFU, meaning that, within this range, a higher dose will lead to a better response [25]. However, the previously-mentioned Cochrane review on the prevention of pediatric AAD did not find any statistically significant difference in the use of high versus low dose probiotics (over or under 5×10^9 CFU/day) [6].

We did not find evidence to suggest an increase in effect when more than one probiotic strain was used to prevent AAD.

Our result was fairly consistent across a number of subgroup analyses in which RRs ranged from 0.36 to 0.58. All but two subgroup analyses yielded a statistically significant result. Of note, the analysis of studies with a low risk of bias did not produce a statistically significant result. This is concerning, and although in part may be ascribed to a low number of trials (three), this finding calls for caution in its interpretation. Nevertheless, our results are in line with a previous Cochrane review [6] on the prevention of pediatric AAD (RR 0.46, 95% CI 0.35 to 0.61, I^2 = 55%, 3898 participants), as well as a review, including hospitalized patients [26], on the prevention and treatment of AAD regardless of age (RR 0.58, 95% CI 0.50 to 0.68, $I^2 = 54\%$, 11,811 participants).

Subgroup analyses did not further explain the substantial amount of heterogeneity across studies as heterogeneity remained evident throughout all these analyses. Combining data into a meta-analysis by probiotic species and strain level from all included studies would have been preferred, but this was not possible due to varying species, strains, and combinations of strains used in the included studies.

In most of the included studies, the types of infections/diagnoses of the subjects in the included studies were not specified. This was due to inadequate reporting of the trials. Likewise, the antibiotics used were rarely specified, but, by excluding inpatients from the analysis, some similarity regarding the diagnoses of subjects can be expected. The five most important causes of antibacterial prescribing in primary care are upper respiratory tract infection, lower respiratory tract infection, sore throat, urinary tract infection, and otitis media [27]. Outpatients being prescribed antibiotics are likely to experience less severe and relatively common types of infections than inpatients because the latter requires hospitalization. Also, outpatients were not exposed to intravenous antibiotics. The decision to include only outpatients was made in order to lower the degree of heterogeneity and to have a patient group that more closely represents primary care patients.

Probiotics can be found in the form of yoghurt, tablets, and capsules, e.g., in dietary supplements and as non-prescription drugs from pharmacies. This makes the use of probiotics an easily available and relatively simple method of AAD prophylaxis. Furthermore, the ingestion of probiotics seems safe, and our meta-analysis found no increased risk of adverse events, including serious adverse events. This result is in line with a previous review on the safety of probiotics [28]. The majority of adverse events that occurred such as abdominal pain, loss of appetite, nausea, headache and flu-like symptoms were most likely due to antibiotic side effects or were symptoms from the underlying infection.

4. Materials and Methods

4.1. Criteria for Selecting Studies for This Review

4.1.1. Types of Studies

All randomized controlled trials in which probiotics were given to prevent antibiotic-associated diarrhea and in which the use of probiotics was compared to either a placebo or an active alternative prophylaxis or in which no treatment were considered for inclusion. Trials were also included if probiotics were given together with antibiotics in *H. pylori* eradication, if the incidence of AAD was reported. Trials testing probiotics for the treatment of diarrhea were not included.

4.1.2. Types of Participants

Studies with outpatients of all ages being administered antibiotic therapy for any indication were considered for inclusion. An outpatient can be defined as "a person who goes to a health-care facility for a consultation, and who leaves the facility within three hours of the start of consultation. An outpatient is not formally admitted to the facility" [29]. Trials with *H. pylori* eradication therapy for otherwise healthy adults were also included, and the subjects were assumed to be outpatients (if not directly stated as inpatients) due to the nature of the trials because this kind of treatment is normally done in an ambulatory setting.

Trials with inpatients were not included in this review because this patient group a priori was different with regard to the severity of their illness, the presence of comorbidity, and equally more comprehensive treatment (e.g., administration of broad-spectrum antibiotics given intravenously to an inpatient vs. narrow-spectrum antibiotics taken orally by an outpatient).

4.1.3. Types of Interventions

Intervention:

The administration of an identified probiotic agent of any specified strain or dose, regardless of the administration form (e.g., yoghurt, capsules, tablets, etc.).

Control:

Administration of placebo or an active comparator or no treatment.

4.1.4. Types of Outcome Measures

Primary outcome:

- Incidence of antibiotic-associated diarrhea (AAD)

This analysis used the original study's definition of diarrhea.
An overall pooled meta-analysis, as well as a strain-specific subgroup analysis, was conducted.

Secondary outcomes:

- Incidence of AAD using the criteria defined by WHO:

This analysis used the definition of diarrhea authored by WHO. Diarrhea is defined as "the passage of three or more loose or liquid stools per day (or more frequent passage than is normal for the individual)" [24]. Antibiotic-associated diarrhea was considered in cases of a subject having diarrhea in relation to their treatment with antibiotics. A specific time factor in this regard was not considered.

- Mean duration of diarrhea (MDD) in days
- Number and types of adverse events

4.2. Search Methods for Identification of Studies

On the 20th of July 2017 a search was conducted of the MEDLINE/PubMed database to identify relevant RCTs. Combinations of the keywords "probiotics", "prevention", "antibiotics", and "diarrhea" were used.

The exact search terms for PubMed can be seen in Supplementary Materials File S10.

4.3. Data Collection and Analysis

4.3.1. Study Selection

Two independent investigators screened all the titles and abstracts from the search results and retrieved the relevant articles. The articles were then assessed for inclusion according to the selection criteria defined previously.

4.3.2. Data Extraction and Management

Data extraction and management was conducted by two independent investigators. The following data were extracted from each study: author, year of publication, patient characteristics (age group and mean age), country, study setting, diagnosis, antibiotic(s) administered, probiotic(s) used, comparator, outcome measures (incidence of diarrhea, mean duration of diarrhea, number and type of adverse events), the study's definition of diarrhea, the number of patients allocated to each group, the presence/absence of intention-to-treat analysis, and the number of participants lost to follow-up or withdrawn from the study (including the reasons for this).

4.3.3. Quality Assessments

Methodological quality assessment using the Cochrane Collaboration's tool for assessing risk of bias [30] was also done by two independent investigators. Each of the included studies were evaluated for sequence generation, allocation concealment, blinding of participants and personnel, blinding of outcome assessment, incomplete outcome data, selective outcome reporting, and other sources of bias. The risk of bias was visualized in a risk of bias summary and a risk of bias graph.

The overall quality of the evidence supporting the main outcome (incidence of AAD) and the secondary outcomes (incidence of AAD using the criteria defined by WHO; adverse events) was evaluated using "the Grading of Recommendations, Assessment, Development and Evaluations" (GRADE) criteria [31]. RCTs are by default regarded as high quality evidence but may be downgraded on the basis of five categories of limitations: (1) risk of bias; (2) inconsistency; (3) indirectness; (4) imprecision; and (5) publication bias. The quality of evidence can be categorized as either high (we are very confident that the true effect lies close to the estimated effect); moderate (we are moderately confident in the effect estimate; the true effect is likely to be close to the estimated effect, but there is a possibility that new evidence will affect the estimated effect size); low (our confidence in the effect estimate is limited; new evidence may be substantially different from the estimated effect); very low (we have very little confidence in the effect estimate; the true effect is likely to be substantially different from the estimated effect). The data were entered into GRADEpro GDT [32] for analysis of the quality of evidence.

4.3.4. Statistical Analysis

Dichotomous data (antibiotic-associated diarrhea vs. no diarrhea and adverse events vs. no adverse events) were combined in a random effects meta-analysis using a pooled risk ratio (RR) or risk difference (RD) along with the corresponding 95% confidence interval (95% CI). All models were weighted based on study size. The number needed to treat (NNT) was calculated for the main outcome. The data were entered into Review Manager 5.3 [33] for statistical analysis.

A high degree of heterogeneity was expected because of the broad inclusion criteria (e.g., differences in types of participants, interventions, and definitions of AAD), and this was investigated using the I^2 statistic, wherein a value of >50% may represent substantial heterogeneity [34]. To explore possible explanations for heterogeneity, prespecified subgroup analyses were conducted on (1) the WHO definition of diarrhea; (2) age groups; (3) studies with *H. pylori* eradication; (4) probiotic genus; (5) low risk of bias; and (6) intention-to-treat analyses.

To evaluate the potential for publication bias, a funnel plot was applied for the efficacy outcome (incidence of AAD).

5. Conclusions

Using probiotics for the prevention of antibiotic-associated diarrhea reduces the risk of AAD by 51% (RR 0.49; 95% CI 0.36 to 0.67) with a moderate quality of evidence according to GRADE. This result was confirmed in analyses of specific strains, namely *Lactobacillus rhamnosus GG* and *Saccharomyces boulardii*. Furthermore, we found preliminary evidence to suggest a dose-response relationship.

The use of probiotics appears safe. However, our study still suggests that caution be applied prior to widespread introduction of probiotic treatment for AAD as only 18% of the included studies had a low risk of bias, and these studies did not find a statistical significant reduction in the prevention of AAD.

Limitations to the findings include the paucity of data on probiotic strain level, and future studies on probiotics to prevent AAD should focus on identifying the most effective agent(s) preferable in head-to-head comparisons and follow a stringent approach to definitions of outcomes, as well as clinical scenarios, prior to the widespread recommendation of probiotics as adjunct therapy to antibiotics. Also, more data are needed to determine the safety of probiotics, and trials should define potential adverse events in advance.

Acknowledgments: The authors received no funding.

Author Contributions: S.B. and R.A. conceived and designed the study. S.B. and D.M.A. performed the search and data extraction. All authors analyzed the data. S.B. wrote the first draft of the paper.

References

1. McFarland, L.V. Epidemiology, risk factors and treatments for antibiotic-associated diarrhea. *Dig. Dis. (Basel Switz.)* **1998**, *16*, 292–307. [CrossRef]
2. Wistrom, J.; Norrby, S.R.; Myhre, E.B.; Eriksson, S.; Granstrom, G.; Lagergren, L.; Englund, G.; Nord, C.E.; Svenungsson, B. Frequency of antibiotic-associated diarrhoea in 2462 antibiotic-treated hospitalized patients: A prospective study. *J. Antimicrob. Chemother.* **2001**, *47*, 43–50. [CrossRef] [PubMed]
3. Goossens, H.; Ferech, M.; Vander Stichele, R.; Elseviers, M. Outpatient antibiotic use in Europe and association with resistance: A cross-national database study. *Lancet (Lond. Engl.)* **2005**, *365*, 579–587. [CrossRef]
4. Food and Agriculture Organization of the United Nation/World Health Organization. *Report of a Joint FAO/WHO Working Group on Drafting Guidelines for the Evaluation of Probiotics in Food*; FAO/WHO: London, ON, Canada, 2002.
5. Rolfe, R.D. The role of probiotic cultures in the control of gastrointestinal health. *J. Nutr.* **2000**, *130*, 396s–402s. [PubMed]
6. Goldenberg, J.Z.; Lytvyn, L.; Steurich, J.; Parkin, P.; Mahant, S.; Johnston, B.C. Probiotics for the prevention of pediatric antibiotic-associated diarrhea. *Cochrane Database Syst. Rev.* **2015**, Cd004827. [CrossRef]
7. Tankanow, R.M.; Ross, M.B.; Ertel, I.J.; Dickinson, D.G.; McCormick, L.S.; Garfinkel, J.F. A double-blind, placebo-controlled study of the efficacy of Lactinex in the prophylaxis of amoxicillin-induced diarrhea. *DICP* **1990**, *24*, 382–384. [CrossRef] [PubMed]
8. Vanderhoof, J.A.; Whitney, D.B.; Antonson, D.L.; Hanner, T.L.; Lupo, J.V.; Young, R.J. Lactobacillus GG in the prevention of antibiotic-associated diarrhea in children. *J. Pediatr.* **1999**, *135*, 564–568. [CrossRef]
9. Arvola, T.; Laiho, K.; Torkkeli, S.; Mykkanen, H.; Salminen, S.; Maunula, L.; Isolauri, E. Prophylactic Lactobacillus GG reduces antibiotic-associated diarrhea in children with respiratory infections: A randomized study. *Pediatrics* **1999**, *104*, e64. [CrossRef] [PubMed]
10. Erdeve, O.; Tiras, U.; Dallar, Y. The probiotic effect of Saccharomyces boulardii in a pediatric age group. *J. Trop. Pediatr.* **2004**, *50*, 234–236. [CrossRef] [PubMed]
11. Duman, D.G.; Bor, S.; Ozutemiz, O.; Sahin, T.; Oguz, D.; Istan, F.; Vural, T.; Sandkci, M.; Işksal, F.; Simşek, I.; et al. Efficacy and safety of Saccharomyces boulardii in prevention of antibiotic-associated diarrhoea due to Helicobacterpylori eradication. *Eur. J. Gastroenterol. Hepatol.* **2005**, *17*, 1357–1361. [CrossRef] [PubMed]
12. Park, S.K.; Park, D.I.; Choi, J.S.; Kang, M.S.; Park, J.H.; Kim, H.J.; Cho, Y.K.; Sohn, C.I.; Jeon, W.K.; Kim, B.I. The effect of probiotics on Helicobacter pylori eradication. *Hepatogastroenterology* **2007**, *54*, 2032–2036. [PubMed]
13. Cindoruk, M.; Erkan, G.; Karakan, T.; Dursun, A.; Unal, S. Efficacy and safety of Saccharomyces boulardii in the 14-day triple anti-Helicobacter pylori therapy: A prospective randomized placebo-controlled double-blind study. *Helicobacter* **2007**, *12*, 309–316. [CrossRef] [PubMed]
14. Conway, S.; Hart, A.; Clark, A.; Harvey, I. Does eating yogurt prevent antibiotic-associated diarrhoea? A placebo-controlled randomised controlled trial in general practice. *Br. J. Gen. Pract.* **2007**, *57*, 953–959. [CrossRef] [PubMed]

15. Imase, K.; Takahashi, M.; Tanaka, A.; Tokunaga, K.; Sugano, H.; Tanaka, M.; Ishida, H.; Kamiya, S.; Takahashi, S. Efficacy of Clostridium butyricum preparation concomitantly with Helicobacter pylori eradication therapy in relation to changes in the intestinal microbiota. *Microbiol. Immunol.* **2008**, *52*, 156–161. [CrossRef] [PubMed]
16. Kim, M.N.; Kim, N.; Lee, S.H.; Park, Y.S.; Hwang, J.H.; Kim, J.W.; Jeong, S.H.; Lee, D.H.; Kim, J.S.; Jung, H.C.; et al. The effects of probiotics on PPI-triple therapy for Helicobacter pylori eradication. *Helicobacter* **2008**, *13*, 261–268. [CrossRef] [PubMed]
17. Merenstein, D.J.; Foster, J.; D'Amico, F. A randomized clinical trial measuring the influence of kefir on antibiotic-associated diarrhea: The measuring the influence of Kefir (MILK) Study. *Arch. Pediatr. Adolesc. Med.* **2009**, *163*, 750–754. [CrossRef] [PubMed]
18. De Vrese, M.; Kristen, H.; Rautenberg, P.; Laue, C.; Schrezenmeir, J. Probiotic lactobacilli and bifidobacteria in a fermented milk product with added fruit preparation reduce antibiotic associated diarrhea and Helicobacter pylori activity. *J. Dairy Res.* **2011**, *78*, 396–403. [CrossRef] [PubMed]
19. Ojetti, V.; Bruno, G.; Ainora, M.E.; Gigante, G.; Rizzo, G.; Roccarina, D.; Gasbarrini, A. Impact of Lactobacillus reuteri Supplementation on Anti-Helicobacter pylori Levofloxacin-Based Second-Line Therapy. *Gastroenterol. Res. Pract.* **2012**, *2012*, 740381. [CrossRef] [PubMed]
20. Chatterjee, S.; Kar, P.; Das, T.; Ray, S.; Gangulyt, S.; Rajendiran, C.; Mitra, M. Randomised placebo-controlled double blind multicentric trial on efficacy and safety of Lactobacillus acidophilus LA-5 and Bifidobacterium BB-12 for prevention of antibiotic-associated diarrhoea. *J. Assoc. Phys. India* **2013**, *61*, 708–712.
21. Zojaji, H.; Ghobakhlou, M.; Rajabalinia, H.; Ataei, E.; Jahani Sherafat, S.; Moghimi-Dehkordi, B.; Bahreiny, R. The efficacy and safety of adding the probiotic *Saccharomyces boulardiito* standard triple therapy for eradication of *H.pylori*: A randomized controlled trial. *Gastroenterol. Hepatol. Bed. Bench* **2013**, *6*, S99–S104. [PubMed]
22. Fox, M.J.; Ahuja, K.D.; Robertson, I.K.; Ball, M.J.; Eri, R.D. Can probiotic yogurt prevent diarrhoea in children on antibiotics? A double-blind, randomised, placebo-controlled study. *BMJ Open* **2015**, *5*, e006474. [CrossRef] [PubMed]
23. Olek, A.; Woynarowski, M.; Ahren, I.L.; Kierkus, J.; Socha, P.; Larsson, N.; Önning, G. Efficacy and Safety of Lactobacillus plantarum DSM 9843 (LP299V) in the Prevention of Antibiotic-Associated Gastrointestinal Symptoms in Children-Randomized, Double-Blind, Placebo-Controlled Study. *J. Pediatr.* **2017**, *186*, 82–86. [CrossRef] [PubMed]
24. WHO. Diarrhoeal Disease. Available online: http://www.who.int/mediacentre/factsheets/fs330/en/ (accessed on 1 June 2017).
25. Ouwehand, A.C. A review of dose-responses of probiotics in human studies. *Benef. Microbes* **2016**, *8*, 143–151. [CrossRef] [PubMed]
26. Hempel, S.; Newberry, S.J.; Maher, A.R.; Wang, Z.; Miles, J.N.; Shanman, R.; Johnsen, B.; Shekelle, P.G. Probiotics for the prevention and treatment of antibiotic-associated diarrhea: A systematic review and meta-analysis. *JAMA* **2012**, *307*, 1959–1969. [PubMed]
27. Petersen, I.; Hayward, A.C. Antibacterial prescribing in primary care. *J. Antimicrob. Chemother.* **2007**, *60*, i43–i47. [CrossRef] [PubMed]
28. Hempel, S.; Newberry, S.; Ruelaz, A.; Wang, Z.; Miles, J.N.; Suttorp, M.J.; Johnsen, B.; Shanman, R.; Slusser, W.; Fu, N.; et al. *Safety of Probiotics Used to Reduce Risk and Prevent or Treat Disease*; Evidence Report/Technology Assessment No. 200; Agency for Healthcare Research and Quality: Rockville, MD, USA, 2011.
29. WHO. Appendix 1, Definitions of health-care settings and other related terms. In *Guidelines on Hand Hygiene in Health Care: First Global Patient Safety Challenge Clean Care Is Safer Care*; World Health Organization: Geneva, Switzerland, 2009. Available online: https://www.ncbi.nlm.nih.gov/books/NBK144006/ (accessed on 1 June 2017).
30. Higgins, J.P.T. *Cochrane Handbook for Systematic Reviews of Interventions, Chapter 8: Assessing Risk of Bias in Included Studies*; Higgins, J.P.T., Green, S., Eds.; John Wiley & Sons: Chichester, UK, 2008.
31. The GRADE Working Group. *GRADE Handbook for Grading Quality of Evidence and Strength of Recommendations*; Schünemann, H., Brożek, J., Guyatt, G., Oxman, A., Eds.; Updated October 2013. The GRADE Working Group, 2013. Available online: https://gdt.gradepro.org/app/handbook/handbook.html (accessed on 1 June 2017).
32. GRADEpro GDT: GRADEpro Guideline Development Tool [Software]. McMaster University, 2015. (Developed by Evidence Prime, Inc.). Available online: https://gradepro.org./ (accessed on 5 October 2017).

33. *Review Manager (RevMan) [Computer program]. Version 5.3*; The Nordic Cochrane Centre: The Cochrane Collaboration: Copenhagen, Denmark, 2014.
34. *Cochrane Handbook for Systematic Reviews of Interventions Version 5.1.0 [Updated March 2011]*; Higgins, J.P.T.; Green, S., Eds.; The Cochrane Collaboration: Copenhagen, Denmark, 2011; Available online: www.handbook.cochrane.org (accessed on 1 June 2017).

15

Parallel Colorimetric Quantification of Choline and Phosphocholine as a Method for Studying Choline Kinase Activity in Complex Mixtures

Tahl Zimmerman * and Salam A. Ibrahim

Food Microbiology and Biotechnology Laboratory, Food and Nutritional Sciences Program, North Carolina A & T State University, 1601 East Market Street, Greensboro, NC 27411, USA; ibrah001@ncat.edu

* Correspondence: tzimmerman@ncat.edu

Abstract: Choline kinase (Chok) is an enzyme found in eukaryotes and Gram-positive bacteria. Chok catalyzes the production of phosphocholine from choline and ATP. This enzyme has been validated as a drug target in *Streptococcus pneumonia,* but the role Chok enzymatic activity plays in bacterial cell growth and division is not well understood. Phosphocholine production by Chok and its attenuation by inhibitors in the context of complex samples such as cell extracts can currently be quantified by several methods. These include choline depletion measurements, radioactive methods, mass-spectrometry, and nuclear magnetic resonance. The first does not measure phosphocholine directly, the second requires elaborate safety procedures, and the third and fourth require significant capital investments and technical expertise. For these reasons, a less expensive, higher throughput, more easily accessible assay is needed to facilitate further study in Gram-positive Choks. Here, we present the development of a triiodide/activated charcoal/molybdenum blue system for detecting and quantifying choline and phosphocholine in parallel. We demonstrate that this system can reliably quantify changes in choline and phosphocholine concentrations over time in Chok enzymatic assays using cell extracts as the source of the enzyme. This is an easily accessible, convenient, robust, and economical method for studying Chok activity in complex samples. The triiodide/activated charcoal/molybdenum blue system opens new doors into the study choline kinase in Gram-positive pathogens.

Keywords: choline kinase; *S. pneumonia*; choline; phosphocholine; colorimetric methods; enzymes; gram-positive bacteria

---

1. Introduction

Choline kinase (Chok) is an enzyme that catalyzes the production of phosphocholine (PCho) from choline (Cho) and ATP [1]. Chok enzymes play a key role in cell growth and division in eukaryotic cells [2] and are also oncogenic drug targets for cancer cells [3] as well as for parasites such as *Plasmodium falciparum* [4]. However, the role Chok plays in bacterial cell division and growth is less clear, although it is known to be involved in the pathway leading to the production of lipoteichoic acid (LTA) and cell wall teichoic acid (CTA) [5,6]. *Streptococcus pneumoniae* is a pathogen known to express Chok [7]. Experimentally unconfirmed sequence predictions suggest that other Gram-positive pathogens, such as *Stapholooccus aureus*, *Bacillus subtilis*, *Clostridium perfringens*, and *Clostridium botulinum* also produce Chok isoforms. Importantly, the choline kinase of *Streptococcus pneumoniae* (sChok) has recently been established as a drug target [8], and inhibiting sChok was found to effectively slow cell growth and division in this species. However, Chok activity is confirmed in *S. pneumoniae* alone and has not yet been well characterized in this species of bacteria. Consequently, further studies on the enzymatic activity of sChok as well as other bacterial Choks are warranted, as is the development of tools designed to facilitate these studies.

When adding a cell extract containing Chok to a solution of ATP and Cho, the resulting activity generates a complex mixture containing choline, ATP, PCho and Cho. The rate of the PCho production can be inferred indirectly from the rate of Cho consumption through colorimetric methods involving triiodide precipitation [1,9] or Cho conversion to betaine aldehyde by choline oxidase [10]. Phosphocholine can be directly detected by utilizing ^{14}C Cho substrate in an enzymatic reaction, followed by a thin layer chromatography step to separate the reactants from products, followed by detection using a phosphoimager [4]. Organic chemistry fractionation techniques can also be used to separate the reactants from the products [11]. Radioactive methods require added safety procedures because, if ingested, ^{14}C Cho can accumulate in organs, exposing cells directly to emissions, causing DNA damage. For example, a separate space in the laboratory is necessary for dispensing radioactive reagents, as well as shielding. Double gloves need to be used when handling isotopes, and workspaces must be monitored regularly with Geiger counters. In addition, accessibility is limited because a specialized infrastructure is required to monitor individuals for contamination using dosage monitors and urine testing [12,13]. While highly sensitive, radioactive methods for measuring PCho lead to only relative, rather than absolute quantities. Much safer and quantitative methods for measuring PCho include mass spectrometry [8], and nuclear magnetic resonance [14]. However, these techniques are not accessible or economical because they require specialized training and significant capital investments. Moreover, all the non-colorimetric methods for measuring PCho or choline are time consuming because the number of samples that can be tested in parallel is limited. To study choline kinase function in greater detail, a method that is accessible and economical is needed to quantify the production of PCho. In addition, a convenient, more quantitative benchtop alternative to radioisotope methods is needed that requires fewer safety procedures. We present here the development of an easy-to-implement colorimetric method to detect and quantify both Cho and PCho using absorbance at wavelengths in the visible range.

2. Results

Development of the Detection Method

In our initial search of viable methods for the colorimetric detection of PCho, we encountered a past study which demonstrated that PCho could be precipitated as a complex with a molybdenum blue dye (MBD) with 90% efficiency [15], resuspended in an acetone/HCl solution, and then quantified by absorbance at 725 nm. The lower limit of sensitivity of the MBD was 100 μM. However, this dye was also found to precipitate Cho (data not shown), ATP (Figure 1B), and ADP (Figure 1B). Due to its promiscuity, use of MBD alone was not deemed sufficient to reliably quantify PCho. To employ the MBD dye to detect PCho, the contaminants Cho, ATP, and ADP had to first be filtered out of the solution.

To accomplish the ADP/ATP filtration step, activated carbon prepared in 0.1 N HCl was used as a highly efficient nucleotide filter [16]. Using this method ATP and ADP were filtered out to levels undetected by the MBD (see Figure 1B).

Meanwhile, Cho was filtered out using a method adapted from Appleton et al. [9]. This method employed a triiodide solution to convert Cho to choline iodide, which was then precipitated by centrifugation, leaving only PCho in solution. Significantly, the triiodide method could be used to quantify Cho, because, as reported, the amount of precipitate was proportional to the concentration of Cho in solution. After resuspension of the choline iodide in ethylene dichloride, absorbance was measured at 365 nm [9]. A standard curve correlating known amounts of Cho with the measure of absorbance was constructed for use in elucidating unknown quantities of Cho (see Figure 2A). This method was sensitive to a lower limit of 50 μM.

Therefore, the complete PCho/Cho detection method for ChoK enzymatic reactions had three principle steps: (1) filtration of ATP/ADP by activated charcoal; (2) Cho quantification (and removal) using a triiodide solution; and (3) PCho quantification using an MBD solution.

However, three important questions had to be answered to determine if this method was robust: (1) Did triiodide cross-react with any other component of the reaction (PCho, ADP, ATP)? (2) Did the initial activated charcoal and triiodide steps filter out the confounding agents (Cho/ADP/ATP) to levels undetectable by the MBD dye so that only PCho was detected? (3) Was there a detectable loss of Cho or PCho during the filtration steps which could confound the measurements?

As a first step, we determined that the triiodide precipitated Cho but did not precipitate ATP, ADP, or PCho (Figure 1A). As seen in Figure 1B, the combined activated charcoal and triiodide steps removed the sChok inhibitor Hemicholinium-3 (HC-3) and Cho to levels that were undetectable by the MBD agent. Meanwhile, ATP and ADP were efficiently filtered by the activated charcoal step alone ((Figure 1B, ATP (F) and ADP (F)). As a result, all confounding agents were removed in the filtration steps leaving PCho alone to be detected by the MBD. In addition, the filtration steps did not lead to meaningful losses of Cho or PCho (Figure 1C).

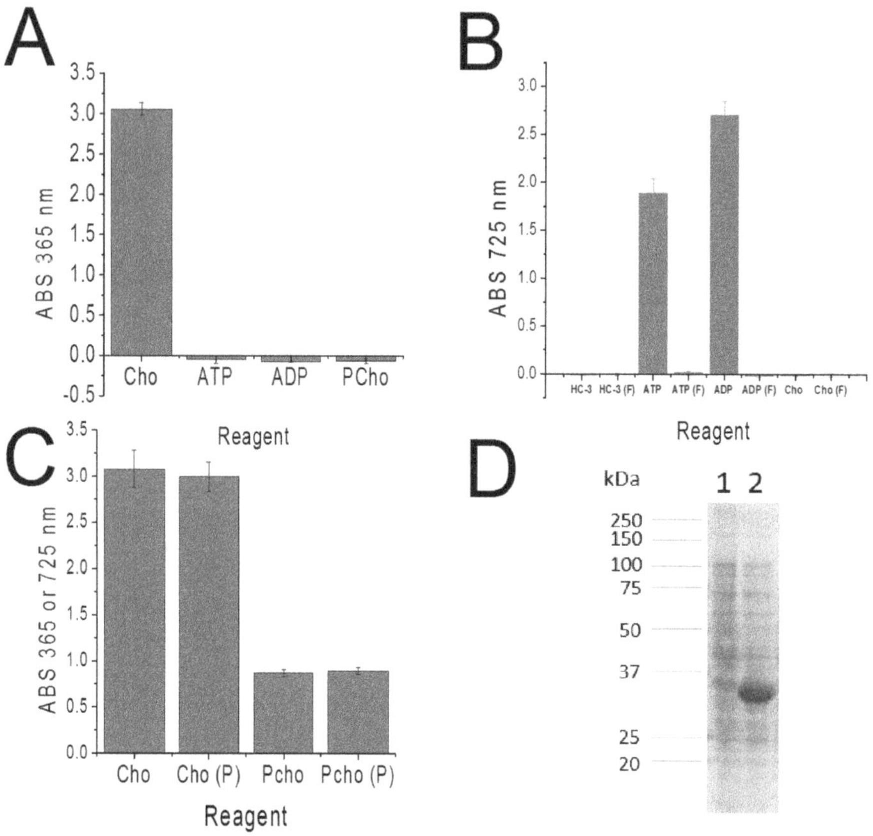

Figure 1. Validation of the colorimetric method. A 1 mM concentration of each reagent was assayed, except for 2.7 mM of HC-3. (**A**) Triiodide reactions with each component of the Chok reaction: choline (Cho), ATP, and phopshocholine (PCho). (**B**) Analysis of MBD absorbance measurements after processing of each compound with triiodide step alone and the combined steps of triiodide and charcoal (marked with an (F)). (**C**) Absorbance values of PCho and Cho samples detected with and without processing (P). (**D**) SDS-PAGE of extracts of uninduced (1) and induced (2) BL21 (DE3) cells transformed with *S. pneumoniae LicA*, the gene coding for sChok.

The primary objective of this study was to develop a colorimetric method for detecting the amount of PCho generated from Cho and ATP using a complex protein mixture as the Chok source. As a model, we selected the sChok expressed in *E. coli* [7]. The *S. pneumoniae LicA* gene overexpressed well in BL21(DE3) cells (Figure 1D). The SDS-Page analysis clearly showed a strong band at around the expected size (35.5 kDa) in the induced sample, indicating that Cho kinase was overproduced against a background of endogenous proteins.

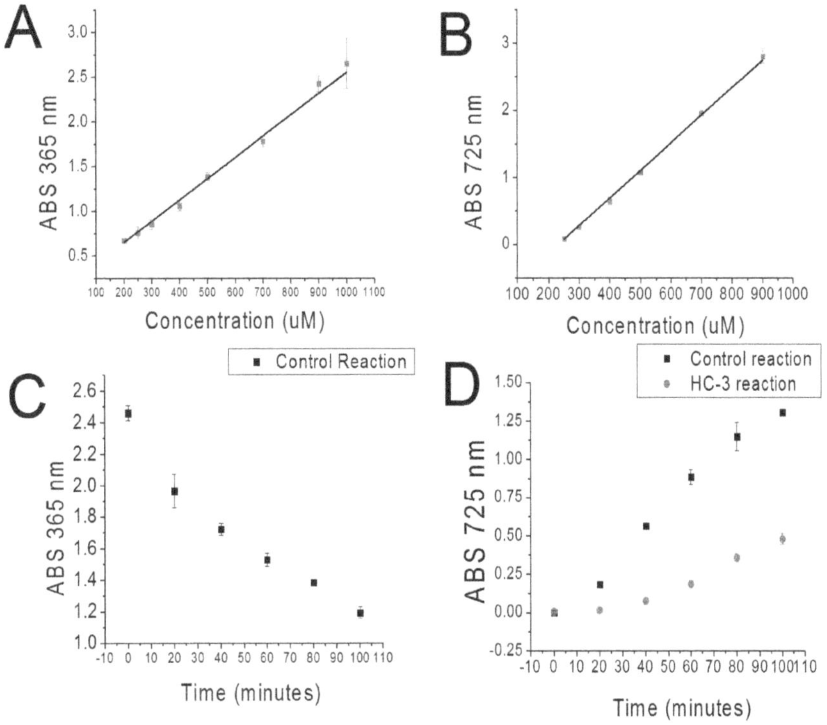

Figure 2. Standard concentration vs absorbance curves of Cho and PCho and colorimetric absorbance at different time points in an sChok enzymatic assay. (**A**) Standard curve of [Cho] vs absorbance derived from known quantities of Cho. (**B**) Standard curve of [PCho] vs. absorbance derived from known quantities of PCho. (**C**) Absorbance changes over time derived triiodide analysis of an sChok enzymatic assay (Control Reaction). (**D**) Absorbance changes over time derived from MBD analysis of an sChok enzymatic assay with (HC-3 reaction) and without (Control Reaction) sChok inhibitor HC-3.

A time course of enzymatic activity was performed over a period of 100 min using cell extracts of sChok overexpressed in BL21 (DE3). Samples were taken every 20 min. In addition, a second time course was performed using HC-3, a known inhibitor of sChok [8], for comparison purposes. A second objective of this study was to demonstrate that this system was a viable method for drug screening against bacterial Chok enzymes. A linear reduction of Cho was observed over time in parallel with an observed increase in PCho (see Figure 2C,D). Quantification of Cho and PCho demonstrated that the two separate measurements corresponded with minor deviations when the concentration of Pcho was inferred from the concentration of Cho (see Table 1, [PCho] vs inverse [Cho]). Cho quantification was confounded in the case of the reaction containing HC-3 because this compound precipitated alongside Cho in the triiodide step. Nevertheless, HC-3 was no longer present in quantities that interfered with the MBD step (See Figure 1B). This meant that PCho could be reliably measured even when HC-3 was included in an enzymatic reaction. However, Cho could not be measured in the case HC-3 was added to the reaction. As a final validation step, the concentration of Cho and PCho found at 60, 80, and 100 min time points was measured by mass spectrometry (MS). MS values were found to be comparable to the colorimetric values. The results of the MS assays also confirmed that the catalysis of choline was inhibited in the presence of HC-3 (Table 1). Consequently, overall, this colorimetric method could be considered to be validated.

Table 1. Comparisons between PCho and Cho colorimetric measurements, as well as the PCho measurement as inferred from the Cho measurement (inverse [Cho]), from both the control and the HC-3 reactions. Asterisks are shown in places where a calculation could not be made due to limitations in the sensitivity of the MBD method. Bars are shown where measurements were not made.

	Control Reaction (μM)					HC-3 Reaction (μM)		
Minutes	[PCho]	Inverse [Cho]	[Cho]	[Cho] MS	[PCho] MS	[Pcholine]	[Cho] MS	[Pcho] MS
0	*	72.6	927.4	-	-	*	-	-
20	284.3	270.4	729.6	-	-	*	-	-
40	374.8	367.7	632.3	-	-	258.5	-	-
60	451.7	445.2	554.8	521.1	422.2	284.9	741.1	295.2
80	514.4	502.5	497.5	478.7	540.9	325.5	693.1	326.2
100	551.7	579.2	420.8	462.6	549.5	354.3	668.9	375.3

3. Discussion

We have presented here a combined MBD/activated charcoal/triiodide method for the simultaneous quantification of Cho and PCho for use in measuring changes in Cho and PCho concentration during choline kinase enzymatic assays.

The Cho and PCho quantification overlapped in the control enzymatic reaction. This meant that the method was self-verifying. In addition, this dual quantification method is flexible enough to overcome sensitivity limitations. Since the initial amount of Cho in an enzymatic reaction is fixed, the amount of Cho measured at any time point is inversely related to the amount of PCho. Therefore, even when the MBD cannot quantify PCho directly because the concentration of PCho does not meet the sensitivity threshold for this dye, an indirect reading is still possible using the triiodide, and vice versa. Most importantly, this system is redundant and, as such, measurements can be made in a way that prevents the confounding effects of inhibitors. If a tested inhibitor interferes with one set of measurements, as in the case of HC-3 and Cho, by definition this inhibitor cannot interfere with the second set of measurements because the inhibitor will have precipitated in only one of the steps. That is, the interfering molecule is precipitated either with the MBD or the triiodide, but not both. In addition, the activated charcoal itself removed a large part of the HC-3 (data not shown). It is likely that many other aromatic molecules could be filtered out to some degree. In our case, the amount of HC-3 was simply too elevated (2.7 mM) for the activated charcoal to handle alone, and the rest was precipitated by the triiodide. However, the activated charcoal alone may be sufficient to remove aromatic inhibitors that are effective in the μM range. Therefore, this colorimetric system could feasibly be used for medium throughput screening of choline kinase inhibitors.

This is the first known colorimetric method for quantifying phosphocholine. We have demonstrated here a robust, highly accessible, and economical method for the quantification of both Cho and PCho. In addition, we have shown that this method can be used to monitor the consumption of Cho in parallel with the production of PCho in enzymatic reactions using cell extracts as the source of the ChoK enzyme. Using this method, ChoK enzyme inhibition can be monitored and characterized and can be studied as part of a complex mixture without prior enrichment. This colorimetric technique requires only a few simple reagents and three pieces of equipment that are available in most biochemistry laboratories: a scale for measuring reagents, a centrifuge to remove precipitants, and a spectrophotometer to carry out measurements. This method is optimized for use in quantifying the generation of PCho enzymatic reactions using cell extracts as the enzyme source. The development of this method also supports exploration into the role of Choks in Gram-positive strains as well as bacterial pathogens already known to express Chok and provides a simple method for medium-throughput screening for potential inhibitors of bacterial ChoKs. This result is accomplished without resorting to the use of methods that require a high capital investment or specialized training. Radioactive methods are highly sensitive, reaching the picomole range [11]. Our method can be used to detect choline and phosphocholine at 50 μM and 200 μM, respectively, and is therefore far less sensitive. Nevertheless, this colorimetric method is more quantitative and can be used without the need for the elaborate safety procedures required for the use of radioisotopes. Use of this technique will thus facilitate clarification of the role Chok plays in Gram-positive bacteria.

4. Materials and Methods

All chemical reagents were purchased from Sigma-Aldrich, unless otherwise noted.

4.1. Preparation of Enzyme Extracts

The *S. pneumoniae* LicA gene expressing sChok had been previously cloned into the pET28a plasmid [7]. This construct was generously provided to us by the group of Dr. Yuxing Chen. The plasmid was transformed into BL21(DE3) cells (New England Biolabs). These cells were then used to inoculate 10 mL of Luria Broth (LB) which was incubated overnight at 37 °C. The next morning, a 10 mL of fresh LB was inoculated to 2% with the overnight culture and then incubated at 37 °C until an $O.D._{600}$ of 0.6 was reached. The culture was cooled on ice, and IPTG was added to a final concentration of 1 mM to induce production of sChok. The culture was then incubated overnight at room temperature after which it was centrifuged for 10 min at 3500 *g*, resuspended in 1 mL 100 mM Tris pH 8 and transferred to an Eppendorf tube. Three mg of Glasperlen beads (Sartorius Stedim) were added to the resuspension and lysis was performed using a Bead-Beater 16 (Biospec products). The lysate was centrifuged at 20,000 *g* for 30 min at 4 °C. The supernatant was removed, aliquoted into Eppendorf tubes, and stored at −20 °C. An aliquot was defrosted on ice when needed for use in an enzymatic reaction.

4.2. sChok Enzymatic Reaction

Four microliters of Chok enzyme extract were added per 15 mL reaction buffer (RB: 100 mM Tris, 10 mM $MgCl_2$, 1 mM Cho, 1 mM ATP) with or without 2.7 mM HC-3, and the reactions were incubated in a water bath at 37 °C for 100 min. One-milliliter samples were removed in duplicate every 20 min and placed in Eppendorf tubes on ice. The samples were immediately heated to 95 °C in a heat block for 3 min to stop the reaction. Samples were then placed on ice again for a minimum of 10 min.

4.3. Activated Charcoal Filtration of ATP

Activated charcoal was suspended in 0.1 N HCl for a total of 2.5 g/50 mL and then mixed by inversion and centrifuged at 4000 *g* for 20 min at 4 °C. The supernatant was removed and the charcoal pellet was resuspended in fresh 0.1 N HCl. This sequence was repeated 3 times, and the charcoal was resuspended in 50 mL 0.1 N HCl/2.5 g. The suspension was stored at 4 °C until needed.

Three-hundred microliters of this suspension were added to the enzymatic reaction sample and mixed by inversion at 1 min intervals for 10 min and then centrifuged in tubes at 20,000 *g* 4 °C for 1 h to remove the charcoal and denatured protein. One milliliter of supernatant was transferred to a clean 1.5 milliliter Eppendorf tube. The Cho in these samples was then quantified.

4.4. Triiodide Quantification/Removal of Cho

A solution of potassium triiodide was prepared using the following reagents (per 100 mL deionized water): 15.7 g of reagent grade iodine and 20 g of reagent grade potassium iodide. The solution was stored at 4 °C until immediately before use.

Four-hundred microliters of triiodide solution were added to each charcoal supernatant sample after which the mixture was immediately placed on ice for 1 h. The samples were then centrifuged at room temperature for 15 min at 20,000 *g*. One milliliter of each sample in triiodide solution was then set aside in fresh Eppendorf tubes for the subsequent PCho quantification. The remainder of the supernatant was discarded without disturbing the pellet which exhibited a dark red color. Because chlorine iodide decays quickly [9], 1 mL 1,2-Dichloroethane, was added immediately.

The pellets were then dissolved by vortexing. Some charcoal fines were occasionally left over from the previous step. However, these did not dissolve and were left for 1 min to settle to the bottom of the tube before continuing with the procedure. As previously reported, the residual triiodide solution did not interfere with subsequent measurements. Forty microliters of each sample were aliquoted into wells of Greiner Bio-one CellStar® U-bottom 96 well-plates. One hundred sixty microliters 1,2-Dichloroethane were then added to each sample-containing well. Two hundred microliters 1,2-Dichloroethane were added to an empty well in the plate and used as the blank. Absorbance was measured at 365 nm in a BioTek Synergy HT microplate reader.

4.5. MBD Quantification of PCho

Molybdenum blue dye (MBD) was prepared fresh daily two hours before use. One and two-tenths of a gram of Phosphomolybdic acid hydrate (Sigma-Aldrich, St. Louis, MO, USA) and 0.2 g Stannous chloride (Fisher Scientific, Hampton, NH, USA) were dissolved in 2.5 N HCl by vortexing for 1 min. Ten milliliters of deionized water were added, and the mixture was vortexed for 1 more min. The resulting solution was then filtered using a 0.2 M GPF/CA membrane non-sterile syringe filter (Phenomenex, Torrance, CA, USA).

Four hundred microliters of MBD were added to 1 mL enzymatic assay samples in triiodide. The samples were placed on ice for two hours and then centrifuged at 20,000 *g* for 3 min at room temperature. The pellets had a dark blue color. The supernatants were discarded and 1 mL of a 1:1 solution of 2.5 N HCl:acetone was added to the pellet resulting in a blue solution whose intensity increased with concentration. Two hundred microliters of each resuspension were aliquoted onto a well in a Greiner Bio-one CellStar® U-bottom 96-well plate. Absorbance readings were immediately made at 725 nm using a BioTek Synergy HT microplate reader.

4.6. Mass Spectrometry

Enzymatic assay samples were spiked with stable labeled internal standards of all the analytes and extracted using a modified method from [17]. Samples were extracted with 4 volumes of methanol/chloroform (2:1, *v*/*v*) containing internal standards. The mixture was vortexed and stored at 4 °C for 2–24 h. Samples were centrifuged, supernatants were transferred to microcentrifuge tubes, and the pellets were re-extracted with methanol/chloroform/water (2:1:0.8, *v*/*v*/*v*). After vortexing and centrifugation, the supernatants were collected and combined with the first supernatant. Water and chloroform were added to induce phase separation. After centrifugation, 50 µL of the aqueous phase (containing choline and phosphocholine) were transferred to HPLC vials containing 100 µL acetonitrile for instrumental analysis. A series of standards of known concentration containing the corresponding internal standards were prepared and treated identically to the samples.

Quantification of the analytes was performed using liquid chromatography-stable isotope dilution-multiple reaction monitoring mass spectrometry (LC-SID-MRM/MS). Chromatographic separations were performed on an Acquity HILIC 1.6 µm 2.1 × 50 mm column (Waters Corp, Milford, MA, USA) using a Waters ACQUITY UPLC system. The column was warmed to 40 °C, and the flow rate maintained at 0.37 mL/min. The mobile phases were: A-100% water with 0.1% formic acid, and B-90% acetonitrile/10% water with 10 mM ammonium formate and 0.125% formic acid.

The gradient was 0% A/100% B, to 40% A/60% B to 2.5 min, to 70% A/30% B to 4.5 min, and 0% A/100% B to 5 min (total run = 5 min). The analytes and their corresponding isotopes were monitored on a Waters TQ detector using characteristic precursor-product ion transitions indicated in Table 2. Concentrations of each analyte in the samples were determined using the peak area ratio of the analyte to its isotope (response), and read off a standard curve of response values versus standard concentration for each analyte.

Table 2. Precursor-product ion transitions.

Name	Precursor *m*/*z*	Product *m*/*z*
Choline	104	45
Phosphocholine	184	86

Acknowledgments: This research was funded in part, by the NIFA through the Agricultural Research Program at North Carolina Agricultural and Technical State University (Evans-Allen Program, project number NC.X-291-5-15-170-1). We would also like to express our gratitude to the group of Yuxing Chen of the Hefei National Laboratory for Physical Sciences at the Microscale and School of Life Sciences, at the University of Science and Technology of China for their generous donation of the *LicA* construct.

Author Contributions: T.Z. and S.I. were involved in the research design; T.Z. designed and performed the experiments and analyzed the results; T.Z. wrote the paper; and S.I. contributed reagents and supplies andrevised the manuscript.

References

1. Wittenberg, J.; Kornberg, A. Choline phosphokinase. *J. Biol. Chem.* **1953**, *202*, 431–444. [PubMed]
2. Lacal Sanjuan, J.C. Choline kinase as a precision medicine target for therapy in cancer, autoimmune diseases and malaria. *Precis. Med.* **2015**, *1*, 2.
3. Lacal, J.C. Choline kinase is a novel prognostic marker and a therapeutic target in human cancer. *EJC Suppl.* **2008**, *6*, 121. [CrossRef]
4. Zimmerman, T.; Moneriz, C.; Diez, A.; Bautista, J.M.; Gomez Del Pulgar, T.; Cebrian, A.; Lacal, J.C. Antiplasmodial activity and mechanism of action of RSM-932A, a promising synergistic inhibitor of Plasmodium falciparum choline kinase. *Antimicrob. Agents Chemother.* **2013**, *57*, 5878–5888. [CrossRef] [PubMed]
5. Whiting, G.C.; Gillespie, S.H. Incorporation of choline into Streptococcus pneumoniae cell wall antigens: Evidence for choline kinase activity. *FEMS Microbiol. Lett.* **1996**, *138*, 141–145. [CrossRef] [PubMed]
6. Grundling, A.; Schneewind, O. Synthesis of glycerol phosphate lipoteichoic acid in Staphylococcus aureus. *Proc. Natl. Acad. Sci. USA* **2007**, *104*, 8478–8483. [CrossRef] [PubMed]
7. Wang, L.; Jiang, Y.L.; Zhang, J.R.; Zhou, C.Z.; Chen, Y.X. Structural and Enzymatic Characterization of the Choline Kinase LicA from Streptococcus pneumoniae. *PLoS ONE* **2015**, *10*, e0120467. [CrossRef] [PubMed]
8. Zimmerman, T.; Ibrahim, S. Choline Kinase, A Novel Drug Target for the Inhibition of Streptococcus pneumoniae. *Antibiotics* **2017**, *6*, 20. [CrossRef] [PubMed]
9. Appleton, H.D.; La Du, B.N., Jr.; Levy, B.; Steele, J.M.; Brodie, B.B. A chemical method for the determination of free choline in plasma. *J. Biol. Chem.* **1953**, *205*, 803–813. [PubMed]
10. Wu, W.L.; Adams, C.E.; Stevens, K.E.; Chow, K.H.; Freedman, R.; Patterson, P.H. The interaction between maternal immune activation and alpha 7 nicotinic acetylcholine receptor in regulating behaviors in the offspring. *Brain Behav. Immun.* **2015**, *46*, 192–202. [CrossRef] [PubMed]
11. Murray, J.J.; Dinh, T.T.; Truett, A.P.; Kennerly, D.A. Isolation and Enzymatic Assay of Choline and Phosphocholine Present in Cell-Extracts with Picomole Sensitivity. *Biochem. J.* **1990**, *270*, 63–68. [CrossRef] [PubMed]
12. Elmer, P. Guide to the Safe Handling of Radioactive Materials in Research. 2007. Available online: https://ehsucsfedu/sites/ehsucsfedu/files/documents/2011Guide%20Safe%20HandlingRAD2pdf (accessed on 13 March 2018).
13. Services UDS. Safe Handling of Radioisotopes. 2015. Available online: http://safetyservicesucdavisedu/article/safe-handling-radioisotopes (accessed on 15 March 2108).
14. Shah, T.; Wildes, F.; Penet, M.F.; Winnard, P.T., Jr.; Glunde, K.; Artemov, D.; Ackerstaff, E.; Gimi, B.; Kakkad, S.; Raman, V.; et al. Choline kinase overexpression increases invasiveness and drug resistance of human breast cancer cells. *NMR Biomed.* **2010**, *23*, 633–642. [CrossRef] [PubMed]
15. Makoto Hayashi, T.U.; Komei, Miyaki. Colorimetric Method for the Determination of Phosphorylcholine. *Yakugaku Zasshi* **1961**, *81*, 1039. [CrossRef]
16. Mo, J.; Duncan, J.A. Assessing ATP binding and hydrolysis by NLR proteins. *Methods Mol. Biol.* **2013**, *1040*, 153–168. [PubMed]

16

Ubiquitous Nature of Fluoroquinolones: The Oscillation between Antibacterial and Anticancer Activities

Temilolu Idowu [1,*] and Frank Schweizer [1,2]

[1] Department of Chemistry, University of Manitoba, Winnipeg, MB R3T 2N2, Canada; frank.schweizer@umanitoba.ca
[2] Department of Medical Microbiology and Infectious Diseases, University of Manitoba, Winnipeg, MB R3T 1R9, Canada
* Correspondence: Temilolu.Idowu@umanitoba.ca

Abstract: Fluoroquinolones are synthetic antibacterial agents that stabilize the ternary complex of prokaryotic topoisomerase II enzymes (gyrase and Topo IV), leading to extensive DNA fragmentation and bacteria death. Despite the similar structural folds within the critical regions of prokaryotic and eukaryotic topoisomerases, clinically relevant fluoroquinolones display a remarkable selectivity for prokaryotic topoisomerase II, with excellent safety records in humans. Typical agents that target human topoisomerases (such as etoposide, doxorubicin and mitoxantrone) are associated with significant toxicities and secondary malignancies, whereas clinically relevant fluoroquinolones are not known to exhibit such propensities. Although many fluoroquinolones have been shown to display topoisomerase-independent antiproliferative effects against various human cancer cells, those that are significantly active against eukaryotic topoisomerase show the same DNA damaging properties as other topoisomerase poisons. Empirical models also show that fluoroquinolones mediate some unique immunomodulatory activities of suppressing pro-inflammatory cytokines and super-inducing interleukin-2. This article reviews the extended roles of fluoroquinolones and their prospects as lead for the unmet needs of "small and safe" multimodal-targeting drug scaffolds.

Keywords: antibacterial; antiproliferative; antitumor; fluoroquinolone; gyrase; immunomodulation; topoisomerase

---

1. Introduction

Antibiotics are not made, they are simply discovered, and the discovery process is a mixed bag of profound scientific exploration and/or fortunate coincidences. Our current arsenal is mainly made up of compounds that were derived from natural sources, the very source of their woes, and their semi-synthetic derivatives. Microorganisms often secrete trace amount of antibiotics primarily as warfare agents to kill other bacteria or fungi in the evolutionary struggle to gain an advantage over other species that are competing for the same ecological niche [1]. Nature's laboratory is therefore a good reservoir of antibiotic scaffolds that have been evolutionarily optimized to suit the physicochemical requirements for activity in microorganisms, especially against Gram-negative bacteria. However, given the need for the organism producing an antibiotic to protect itself against the harmful effects of such an antibiotic and the defensive mechanism evolved by other bacteria to the agent, antibiotic-resistance mechanisms to natural products are presumed to be already present in the bacterial community [2]. This phenomenon significantly shortens the time between when an isolated antibiotic is introduced into the clinic and when full-fledged resistance is observed. It is therefore imperative to develop new molecules that have not been previously encountered by microorganisms.

Quinolones (Figure 1) are the first class of fully synthetic antibacterial agents to be "discovered", representing the first set of anti-infective agents that were not modeled knowingly after any natural antibiotics. The scaffold was later optimized to fluoroquinolones (FQs) and has remained an integral part of treating Gram-positive and Gram-negative bacteria infections to date. Only a handful of current antimicrobial agents have broad spectrum of activity across both Gram-positive and Gram-negative bacteria. FQs are a class of privileged antibiotics that enjoy a wide acceptability due to their broad spectrum of bactericidal activity at clinically achievable doses, a wide therapeutic index, comparatively tolerable resistance levels, and their synthetic tractability [3,4]. They act by binding to an intracellular target in the cytosol of bacterial cells where they inhibit the activities of topoisomerase II enzymes (Top II, i.e., gyrase and Top IV), with a high selectivity for prokaryotic enzymes [5]. The inherent physicochemical properties of FQs and their ability to traverse the orthogonal lipid bilayers of Gram-negative bacteria, a feat that some naturally-occurring antibiotics are unable to achieve, is noteworthy. These intrinsic capabilities i.e., intracellular target and suitable physicochemical properties, contributed immensely to the success story of fluoroquinolones and made them desirous as reference scaffold for the development of ideal antibacterial agents.

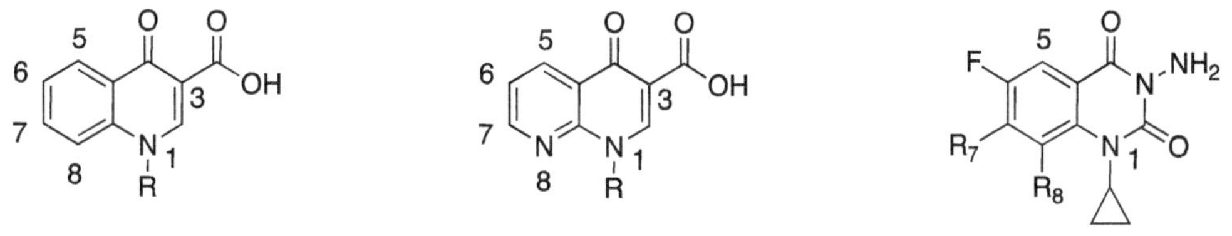

quinolone core **1,8-naphthyridone core** **Quinazolinedione core**

Figure 1. Core structures of the quinolone class of drugs.

On the other hand, cancer is a more devastating chronic disease that claims millions of lives every year worldwide [6]. It is a class of disease in which a group of aberrant cells exhibit uncontrollable growth, invade neighboring tissues or organs, and sometimes metastasize [7]. There are several classes of drugs currently in use for managing this disease, but of interest are those that target and act on mammalian topoisomerases. Etoposide (Figure 2) is an antitumor agent that displays a mechanism of action (in eukaryotic cells) that is similar to that of FQs (in prokaryotic cells). They both act on topoisomerases [8–11]. However, clinically relevant FQs are able to distinguish between bacterial and mammalian topoisomerases, and avoid cross-reactivity with human type II enzyme even at concentrations well beyond their therapeutic doses [5]. Interestingly, some clinically relevant FQs have been shown to be potent antiproliferative agents at much lower concentrations than is needed for their antibacterial activity [12]. It should be noted that FQs that are significantly active against eukaryotic enzymes exhibit the same DNA damaging properties as other topoisomerase poisons [13,14]. Since clinically relevant FQs are known to be safe in humans, how then do they discriminate cancer cells from healthy cells? What can we learn from their physicochemical properties? Moreover, the endowment of quinolones with other "non-classical" biological activities such as anti-HIV-1 integrase [15], cannabinoid receptor-2 agonist/antagonist [16,17], anxiolytic agents [18,19], anti-ischemic activities [20], antiviral effects [21], etc. is continually injecting new enthusiasm towards this scaffold of drug. This article aims to articulate the biological properties of FQs, how they perform their extended roles *viz-a-viz* their structural basis, and their prospects as a promising drug scaffold.

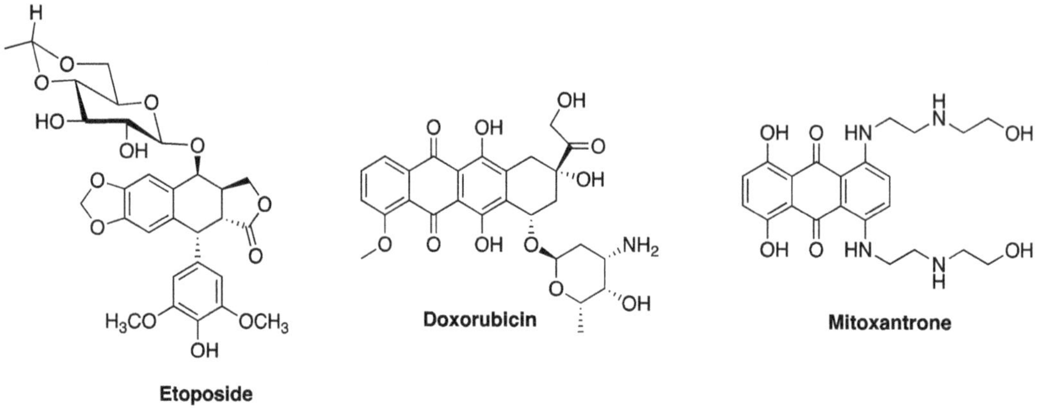

Figure 2. Examples of eukaryotic topoisomerase II poisons.

2. Discovery and Development of Fluoroquinolones

Before the discovery of quinolones in the 1960s, antibiotics were majorly sourced from natural products. They were either obtained from plants and animals in the form of host defence peptides that were produced as a part of their innate immunity (e.g., cecropins, defensins, magainins, cathelicidins) [22–25], or isolated directly from microorganism cultures themselves (e.g., penicillin, aminoglycosides, polymyxins, etc.) [1,26,27]. The accidental discovery of 7-chloroquinolone as an impurity in a distillate during the chemical synthesis of the antimalarial drug, chloroquine, made them the first class of synthetic antibiotics [28]. Although the exact account of how 7-chloroquinolone evolved to 1,8-naphthyridone core (Figure 1) (as in nalidixic acid), and back to quinolone core (as in ciprofloxacin), has been laced with gaps and counter-arguments, George Lesher (the acknowledged discoverer) and his coworkers at Sterling Drugs (now part of Sanofi) are credited as being the first to report the antibacterial activities of this class of drugs in the 1960s [28]. A recent article attempts to shed some lights on the mystery surrounding the discovery process of quinolones, and concluded based on original documents and Lab notes, that Sterling Drugs and Imperial Chemical Industries (now part of AstraZeneca) might have independently discovered this scaffold around the same time [29].

Nonetheless, Lesher and coworkers established the anti-Gram-negative bacteria potency of 7-chloroquinolone during biological screening [28], but the compound had limited usefulness due to its high protein binding (approximately 90%) and short half-life (about 90 min) [30]. The lead compound was therefore optimized to nalidixic acid (Figure 3) in 1962, and was used extensively for over 30 years to treat urinary tract infections (UTIs) that are caused by Gram-negative bacteria, mainly *Escherichia coli*. This optimization marked the beginning of an active campaign of chemical synthesis to refine the structure-activity relationship of FQs, such that biological activity and pharmacokinetics could be improved and toxicity and drug interactions diminished [30]. A further introduction of fluorine atom at position-6 of the bicyclic ring system was found to significantly increase tissue penetration, giving rise to the first FQ, flumequine (Figure 3). Quinolone is a generic term that loosely refers to a class of drugs that include quinines, naphthyridines, fluoroquinolones, quinazolines, isothiazoloquinolones, and related agents. FQs (except for enoxacin and gemifloxacin) differ from nalidixic acid in that they have the same quinolone core as the 7-chloroquine impurity, with the addition of a fluorine atom at the sixth position, while nalidixic acid, gemifloxacin, and enoxacin have 1,8-naphthyridone core (Figure 1). The rationale for the back and forth switch in core scaffold is unknown, perhaps due to intellectual property concerns [29], but the addition of fluorine conferred more potent antibiotic action and broader spectrum of activity on this class of drugs [4].

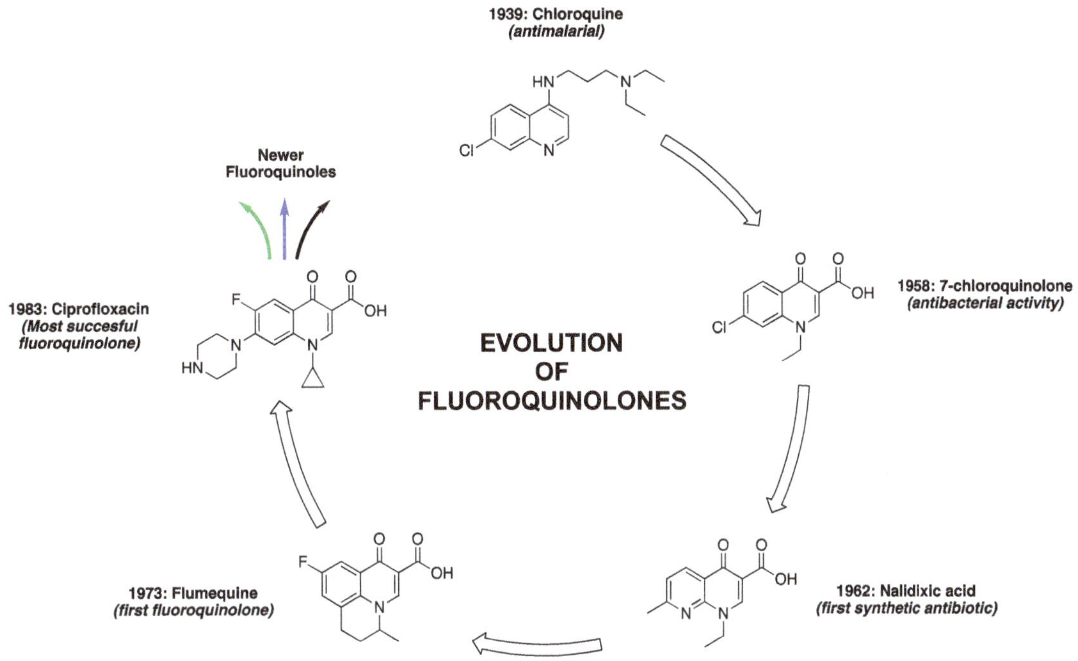

Figure 3. Landmark developmental trends of fluoroquinolones.

In a bid to further improve the spectrum of activity against Gram-positive species, lower potency, higher frequency of spontaneous bacterial resistance, shorter half-lives, and lower serum concentrations of early FQs [31], several modifications, such as side-chain nuclear manipulations and mono- or bicyclic ring substitutions, were done. The newer FQs were found to exhibit longer elimination half-lives, high oral bioavailability, high potency, extensive tissue penetration, and lower incidences of resistance when compared to the earlier ones [32]. Being a fully synthetic class of drug, the development of FQs has been gradual and systematic (Figure 3). Each generation seems to impart new potencies in a trend that has seen them acquire excellent efficacy towards Gram-positive bacteria in addition to their now optimized potency against Gram-negative bacteria. Remarkably, the newer FQs also display activity against anaerobes [33]. Anaerobes are organisms that do not require oxygen for survival, thereby making drugs that require an oxygen transport into ribosomes (e.g., aminoglycosides) ineffective and never taken up by these organisms [34,35].

Based on their systematic structure optimization process and developmental trends, FQs can be distinctly classified into four generations (Table 1).

Table 1. Comparison of fluoroquinolone generations (Adapted from refs [4,36,37]).

Generations	Microbiologic Activity	Administration and Characteristics	Indications
First generation Nalidixic acid, Cinoxacin (*Discontinued*), Flumequine	Enterobacteriaceae	Oral administration. Low serum and tissue drug concentrations. Narrow gram-negative coverage	Uncomplicated urinary tract infections Not for use in systemic infections
Second generation *Class I* Lomefloxacin (*Discontinued*), Norfloxacin, Enoxacin *Class II* Ofloxacin Ciprofloxacin	Enterobacteriaceae. Enterobacteriaceae, atypical pathogens; *Pseudomonas aeruginosa* (ciprofloxacin only), Pneumoccoci	Oral administration. Low serum and tissue drug concentrations. Improved gram-negative coverage, limited gram-positive coverage. Oral and intravenous administration. Higher serum, tissue, and intracellular drug concentrations, coverage of atypical pathogens	Uncomplicated urinary tract infections. Not for use in systemic infections. Complicated urinary tract and catheter-related infections. Gastroenteritis with severe diarrhea, prostatitis, nosocomial infections, sexually transmitted diseases

Table 1. *Cont.*

Generations	Microbiologic Activity	Administration and Characteristics	Indications
Third generation Levofloxacin, Sparfloxacin (Discontinued) Gatifloxacin (Discontinued)	Enterobacteriaceae, atypical pathogens, streptococci. Pneumoccoci MIC: 0.25–0.5 μg/mL	Oral and intravenous administration, similar to class II second-generation but with modest streptococcal coverage. Increased hepatic metabolism (sparfloxacin)	Similar indications as for second-generation. Community-acquired pneumonia in hospitalized patients or if atypical pathogens are strongly suspected
Fourth generation Trovafloxacin (Discontinued) Moxifloxacin Gemifloxacin	Enterobacteriaceae, *P. aeruginosa*, atypical pathogens, MSSA, streptococci, anaerobes, Pneumoccoci	Oral and intravenous administration. Similar to third-generation, but with improved gram-positive and anaerobic coverages	Consider for treatment of intra-abdominal infections

3. Classical Antimicrobial Activity of Fluoroquinolones

The antimicrobial activity of FQs against a wide range of organisms and their clinical use in the treatment of urinary tract infections (UTIs), prostatitis, bacterial enteric infections, biliary tract infections, sexually transmitted diseases, prophylaxis in immune-compromised neutropenic patients, and a host of other clinical conditions confirm their broad-spectrum of activity [38,39]. While efficacy and spectrum of activity have improved across the generations, tolerability and pharmacokinetic parameters, such as tissue penetration, bioavailability, and serum half-life have also been optimized [40]. The antimicrobial spectrum of the first-generation was largely limited to aerobic Gram-negative bacillary infections, particularly in the urinary tract, while the second generation FQs have enhanced activity (1000-fold) against aerobic Gram-negative and Gram-positive bacteria [41,42]. Ciprofloxacin, a second generation FQ, is the most successful of all FQs to date, both economically and clinically [3]. Newer FQs, such as gatifloxacin, levofloxacin, gemifloxacin, moxifloxacin, etc. (Figure 4) offer enhanced activity against aerobic Gram-negative bacilli and improved Gram-positive activity over ciprofloxacin (e.g., against *Streptococcus pneumoniae* and *Staphylococcus aureus*) [43], but ciprofloxacin and moxifloxacin maintain the best in vitro activity against *Pseudomonas aeruginosa* [43,44]. It is interesting to note that *P. aeruginosa* produces 2-heptyl-3-hydroxy-4(1*H*)-quinolone (PQS), a quorum-sensing signal molecule that shares some core structural features with fluoroquinolones, to regulate numerous virulence genes, including those involved in iron scavenging [45]. In terms of potency, moxifloxacin is more effective against Gram-positive and anaerobes than ciprofloxacin and levofloxacin. Moxifloxacin is often considered as a "respiratory quinolone" because of its significant potency against the respiratory pathogen *S. pneumoniae* [46]. It is currently being investigated as a BPaMZ (bedaquiline + pretomanid + moxifloxacin + pyrazinamide) regimen for the treatment of multidrug resistant tuberculosis, an effort that could shorten the duration of tuberculosis treatment from six to four months if successful [47,48]. When compared to other FQs, moxifloxacin appears to be less affected by the bacterial efflux system because of its bulky C-7 substituents [49–52] and their optimized 8-methoxy substituent (Figure 4) [53,54].

The newer generations FQs display potent activity against penicillin-resistant and multidrug-resistant (MDR) pneumococcus and anaerobes, while still retaining their activity against aerobes [55,56]. Several quinolones, most of which are FQs, are also currently at different stages of clinical development. For example, nemonoxacin (Figure 5) is a non-fluorinated broad spectrum quinolone (isothiazoloquinolone) that displays comparable in vitro Gram-negative activity as ciprofloxacin, levofloxacin, and moxifloxacin, but an enhanced potency against Gram-positive bacteria (including MRSA and MDR *S. pneumoniae*) [57]. It is currently under development for oral and intravenous treatment of community acquired pneumonia (approved in Taiwan), as well as the oral treatment of diabetic foot ulcer infections and skin and soft tissue infections [57]. Also, in 2014, finafloxacin (Figure 5) was approved by FDA as a topical otic suspension for the treatment of acute otitis eterna (swimmer's ear), which is caused by susceptible strains of *P. aeruginosa* and *S. aureus* [58]. Delafloxacin (Figure 5) was approved in 2017 for the systemic treatment of acute bacterial skin and skin structure infections caused by a range of susceptible Gram-positive and Gram-negative bacteria (including ESKAPE pathogens) in adults [59]. The "ESKAPE" pathogens—encompassing *Enterococcus faecium*, *S. aureus*, *Klebsiella pneumonia*, *Acinetobacter baumanii*, *P. aeruginosa*, and *Enterobacter* spp—are responsible for many serious infections in hospitals [60]. Interestingly, unlike ciprofloxacin, moxifloxacin, and levofloxacin, which exhibit reduced activity at slightly acidic pH (5.0–6.5), finafloxacin and delafloxacin exhibit enhanced potency at this pH level, making them suitable for the eradication of *S. aureus* found in acidic environment.

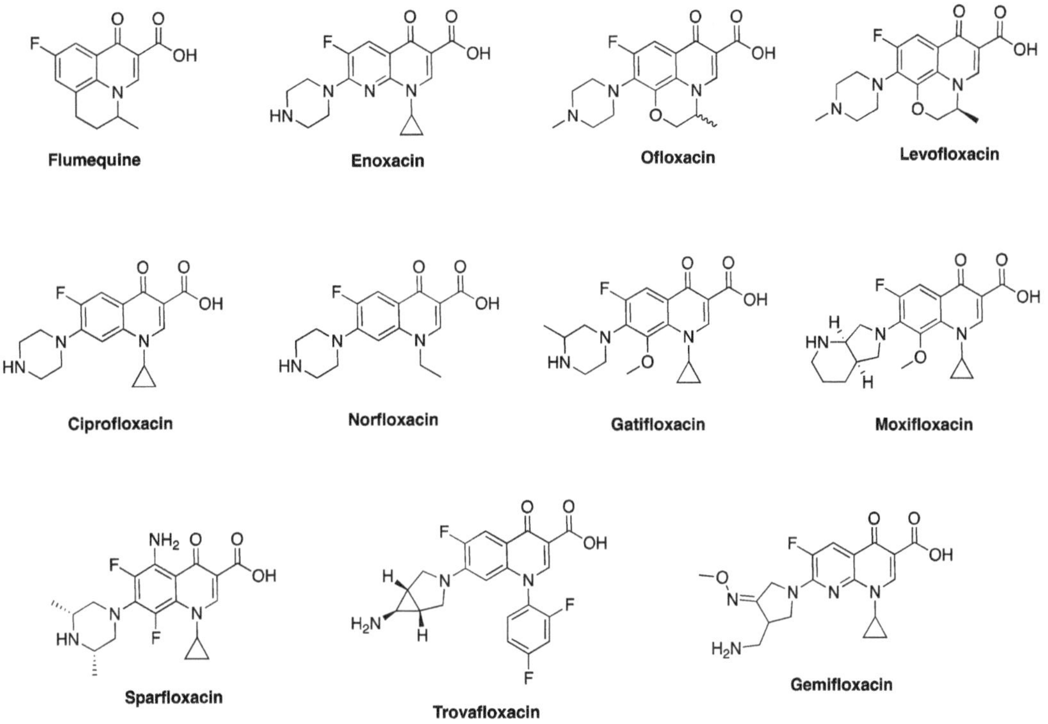

Figure 4. Structures of select fluoroquinolones.

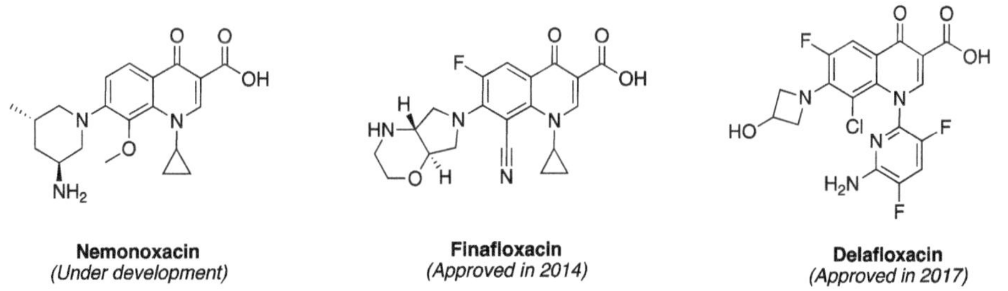

Figure 5. Structures of two recently approved quinolones and one in clinical development.

The comprehensive knowledge of the SAR of FQs (Figure 6) is central to the optimization of this class of drugs [43,61–63]. The pharmacophoric group of quinolones has been identified as a central bicyclic ring with hydrogen at position-2, a carboxyl group at position-3 and a keto group at position-4. This is known as the quinolone core (Figure 1) and it cannot be altered in any way without losing potency [43,64]. However, quinazolinediones (Figure 1) that share similar structural homology but lack the C3/C4 keto acid have now been demonstrated to be capable of overcoming quinolone resistance [65–67]. Mechanistic studies revealed that quinazolinediones overcome resistance via additional drug-enzyme contacts mediated by their "unusual" C7 substituent [5,65–67], and that substituents at position-7 greatly influence potency, spectrum, and safety of FQs [43]. These substituents are considered as the portion that bind to the subunit B of the DNA-enzyme complex, and changes at C-7 and C-8 of quinolones appear to play a significant role in the target preferences of this class of drugs [68].

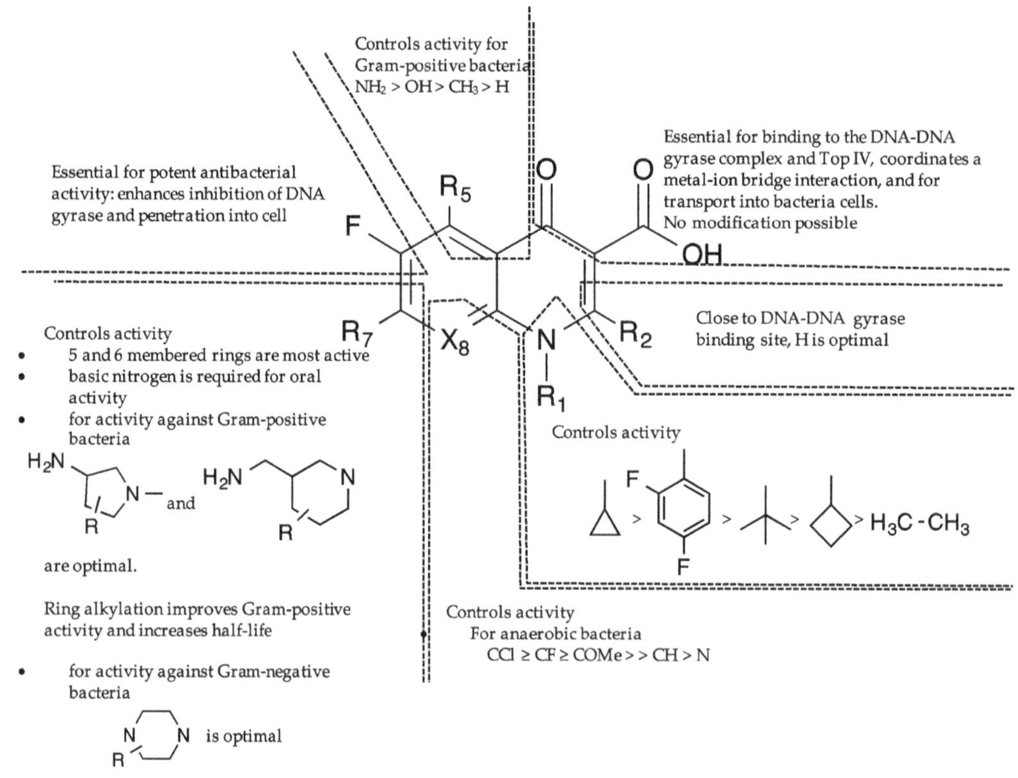

Figure 6. Structure-activity relationships of fluoroquinolones (adapted from reference [43]).

4. Non-Classical Antiproliferative Activity of Fluoroquinolones

FQs were optimized and developed as antimicrobial agents, but several reports have shown that their potentials might be more than just antimicrobial actions [69]. Some FQs have been reported to display in vitro antiproliferative properties by inducing apoptosis, disrupting biochemical transformation of potentially cancerous cells, enhancing the uptake of other chemotherapeutic agents, and/or mediating immunomodulatory responses [70–72].

4.1. *Ciprofloxacin*

The antitumor efficacy of ciprofloxacin has been attributed to both intrinsic apoptosis and cell cycle arrest that could be reversed upon removal of the quinolone [12]. It was shown that ciprofloxacin induced a time- and dose-dependent growth inhibition, and apoptosis of various carcinoma, osteosarcoma, and leukemia cell lines [72]. The inhibition of mammalian cell growth by ciprofloxacin via the induction of tumor growth factor (TGF) β-1 by colonic epithelial cells was reported at concentration as low as 10 $\mu g \cdot mL^{-1}$ [12]. This is a clinically achievable concentration in human tissues using standard dosing regimen [12]. Moreover, of all of the different FQs that were tested in a cell free system, ciprofloxacin was the most potent inhibitor of mammalian DNA topoisomerase and polymerase [73]. Similarly, ciprofloxacin has been found to induce cell cycle arrest at the S and G2/M phases of androgen-independent carcinoma PC3, while sparing non-tumorigenic prostate epithelial cells [74]. This is particularly interesting because most chemotherapeutic agents that were used for treating advanced hormone resistant prostate cancer often result in 100% mortality, with a mean survival time of 7–8 months, as well as several associated toxicities [74].

4.2. *Enoxacin*

Enoxacin, a second-generation FQ, is one of the few FQs that retain the original 1,8-naphthyridone core of nalidixic acid. It has been used to treat bacterial infections ranging from gonorrhea to urinary tract infections [75] but has now been discontinued in the United States due to its severe side effects of insomnia and ability to trigger seizures or lower seizure threshold [76,77]. The human breast cancer cell line, MCF-7, was shown to be highly responsive to treatment with enoxacin, and growth inhibition was dose- and time-dependent, and irreversible in nature [78]. This is in contrast to ciprofloxacin, where its effect could be reversed upon the removal of the drug [12]. A separate study also showed that enoxacin was able to enhance the production of micro ribonucleic acids (miRNAs) that suppresses the tumor by binding to the miRNA biosynthesis protein, trans-activation response RNA-binding protein-2 (TRBP) [79]. MicroRNAs are small RNA molecules that regulate gene expression at the post-transcriptional level and are critical for many cellular pathways, with their disruption often being associated with the development of human tumors [80–82]. Unexpectedly, of the ten FQs that were analyzed, enoxacin was the only one that was capable of selectively stimulating miRNA expression with a median effective concentration of ~30 μM [83]. Importantly, enoxacin was found to be relatively non-toxic even at a high concentration of 150 μM [83], which is lower than its clinical dose [84]. The effect of enoxacin was also observed in vivo using a transgenic mouse line, and its miRNA-enhancing activity was TRBP-dependent [83]. Modifications and substitutions at the *N*-1, *C*-6, and *C*-7 positions of enoxacin significantly interfered with its miRNA-enhancing activity, suggesting that the compound forms a specific complex that is distinct from known targets of quinolones [83]. It also hints that the miRNA biogenesis-enhancing activity of enoxacin might probably not depend on the general FQ activities, but rather on the unique chemical structure of enoxacin. The cancer-selective properties of this molecule and its proposed cell cycle arrest of enhancing miRNA machinery could therefore represent a unique step towards the potential application of miRNA-based therapy in the treatment of human cancer [79].

4.3. Moxifloxacin

Moxifloxacin is a fourth-generation FQ antibiotic that differs mainly from ciprofloxacin, in that the piperazine moiety in ciprofloxacin has been replaced by a (1*S*,2*S*)-2,8-diazabicyclo[4.3.0]nonyl moiety. Moxifloxacin is also available in ophthalmic formulations that is widely used as prophylaxis for managing endophthalmitis after cataract surgery [85,86]. However, intraocular penetration of moxifloxacin was found to be inefficient for postoperative bacterial endopthalmitis, hence its use via an intracameral route of administration [87,88]. Based on this different route of drug delivery, the effect and safety of moxifloxacin on retinal ganglion cells (RGC5) of rats were examined. Moxifloxacin was found to exhibit both cytotoxic and anti-proliferative activity in vitro at a concentration >50 μg/mL [89]. Although a little higher than the expected prophylactic concentration of ≤50 μg/mL, an apparent lack of toxicity to other normal cellular activities [87,90] revealed the prospects of moxifloxacin to treat glaucoma patients with an increased risk of ganglion cell damage, where they may be used at such concentration advisedly.

4.4. Other Quinolones

Several novel tetracyclic FQs have been found to display anticancer properties against various human cells, such as breast cancer (MCF-7) and non-small cell lung cancer (A549), and were non-toxic to normal human-derm fibroblasts (HuDe) [68]. For example, 6,8-difluoroquinolones have been shown to be potent effectors of eukaryotic topoisomerase, as evident in the increased level of cleavage intermediates without impairing the DNA religation reaction of the enzyme [91]. One of the difluoro compounds examined, CP-115,953, (Figure 7) was twice as potent as etoposide at enhancing Top 2-mediated DNA cleavage in eukaryotic cells, while retaining potency against DNA gyrase [92]. Tasquinimod (Figure 7), a novel small-molecule inhibitor and second-generation oral quinolone-3-carboxamide, has also been reported to have anti-angiogenic properties and tumor growth-inhibiting activities against human prostate cancer. It is believed to mediate its activities via angiogenesis and immunomodulation, with a potency of about 30- to 60-times of its structural analog, linomide [93,94].

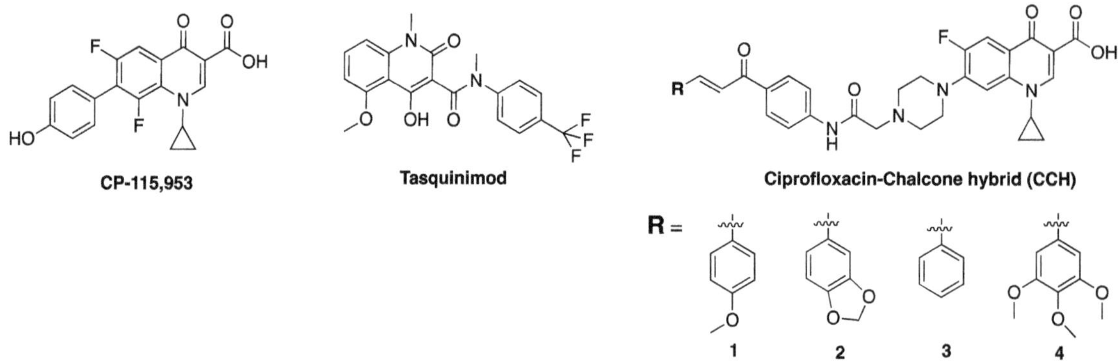

Figure 7. Structures of some fluoroquinolone-derivatives with enhanced antiproliferative activity.

In summary, most FQs tend to induce nearly similar types of morphological alterations where cells become rounded, detached, and show cell membrane blebbing, a typical morphological change that signals the initiation of apoptotic processes [95].

5. Topoisomerases as Targets for Fluoroquinolone Actions: Prokaryotes versus Eukaryotes

Topoisomerases are large proteins found in humans and bacteria, with functional sizes of their enzyme-complex assembly ranging from 70 to 400 kDa [96]. Since the circumference of an average mammalian cell nucleus is almost one million times smaller than the length of the genome that needs to be packed into it, DNA compaction is necessary to squeeze these base pairs into the nucleus. Specifically, the entire genome of a single human cell (3×10^9 base pairs, corresponding to approximately 1.8 m) needs to be squeezed into a nucleus with an average diameter of 6 μm [96]. Even the smaller circular *E. coli* genome (4.7×10^6 base pairs) needs to be compacted within the nucleoid space of bacteria whose average circumference is 3000 times smaller [96]. The primary function of topoisomerases is therefore to introduce positive and/or negative supercoil during DNA transcription and replication to avoid super-helical tension and knots. Both human and bacteria topoisomerases are divided into type I and II, each with further subdivisions (Figure 8). Surprisingly, despite little or no sequence homology, both type IA and type IIA from prokaryotes and the type 2A enzymes from eukaryotes share structural folds that appear to reflect functional motifs within the critical regions of the enzymes [97]. Several excellent reviews have been published on DNA topoisomerases and their inhibitors [98–102]. FQs are safe in humans because they can discriminate between prokaryotic and eukaryotic topoisomerase targets. Whereas, gyrase and Top IV appear to be the preferential targets of FQs in Gram-negative and Gram-positive bacteria, respectively [69,103], other studies indicate that the primary targets of FQs are more drug-dependent than Gram-classification-dependent [104–106]. However, both prokaryotic enzymes can be targeted simultaneously due to the high degree of homology between them. Inhibition of eukaryotic Top 2 correlates with cytotoxicity in those cells, and clinically-relevant FQs are known to be safe and tolerated at concentrations that far exceed their cytotoxic threshold without bearing cytotoxic, genotoxic or carcinogenic potential. Since FQs also mediate antitumor activities in humans at clinically achievable concentrations, how they perform these extended roles is unclear.

5.1. Prokaryotic Topoisomerase Type IIA

In contrast to most anti-infective drugs, quinolones do not kill bacteria by interfering with a critical cellular process, rather, they corrupt the activities of two essential enzymes: DNA gyrase and Top IV, and subsequently induce them to kill cells by generating high levels of double-stranded DNA breaks [5,96,107–111]. Ordinarily, the relaxed bacterial DNA is too long to fit inside a bacterial cell, and must therefore be folded and compacted. Supercoiling (overwind or unwind) is an essential process during chromosome compaction, but also during transcription, replication, and DNA repair [111]. Due to the strain that is generated during unwinding, DNA gyrase transiently nicks each chromosomal domain, introduces a negative supercoil, and rapidly seals the nicked DNA before Top IV separates the linked daughter DNA molecules after replication. Both DNA gyrase and Top IV are classified as prokaryotic Top II (Figure 8), and they play two essential roles: (i) supercoiling (involved in chromosome replication) and (ii) decatenation (involved in chromosome partitioning such as topological resolution and topographical segregation) [96]. Crystal structures show that quinolones bind to the ternary complexes formed between Top II and the supercoiled DNA, hence, stabilizing a process that should have otherwise been very transient [108–110,112]. This stabilization effectively impedes the normal breaking-passing-resealing processes of the bacterial DNA by converting topoisomerases into physiological toxins. The extensive DNA fragmentation therefore becomes overwhelming for the bacterial repair mechanisms, thus leading to bacteria cell death [110,111].

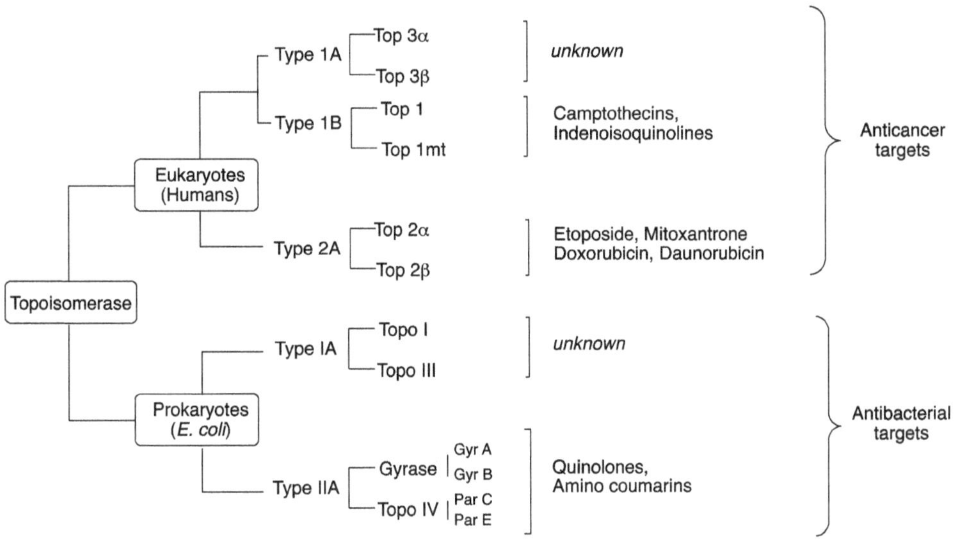

Figure 8. Classification of topoisomerases and their poisons.

Several theories have been propounded as the molecular basis by which quinolones interact with DNA-enzyme complex. One model proposes that quinolones interfere with DNA gyrase activity by selectively and directly interacting with the substrate DNA, rather than to gyrase [113–115]. This implies that the enzyme only plays a passive role in the inhibition mechanism [113]. However, the revised and widely accepted model is that quinolones do not bind directly to DNA, but to an enzyme-DNA complex [5,96,108–111]. The gyrase itself is believed to bind directly to the DNA, thereby creating a suitable pocket for quinolones to bind and stabilize the complex [116,117]. Stabilization of this ternary complex prolongs the normal transient nicking of the chromosome, thus leading to an extensive fragmentation of the DNA. The C3/C4 keto acid of quinolones (Figure 6) have long been known to chelate a divalent metal ion, but it was not until recently that this was captured in a crystal structure of a ternary *A. baumannii* Top IV-cleaved DNA-moxifloxacin complex [112]. The chelated Mg^{2+} ion appeared to be coordinated to four water molecules; two of which were situated close enough to Ser84 and Glu88 (equivalent of GyrA Ser83 and Glu87 in *E. coli*) to form hydrogen bonds [112]. The serine (Ser83 in *E. coli*) and acidic amino acid (Glu87 in *E. coli*) residues act as the anchor points that coordinate the bridge to the enzyme. Mutations at these highly conserved residues in the A subunit of Gyrase or Top IV are therefore the dominant mechanism of the resistance to FQs [5,64]. This supports the observation that water-metal ion interaction that bridges FQ to the enzyme plays a significant role in mediating quinolone activity [64]. The moxifloxacin binding model gives a structural explanation for key quinolone structure-activity relationships (Figure 6) [3] and the bulky substituent at position 7 of moxifloxacin was found to occupy a large and open pocket between the DNA and the ParE subunit [112]. This is consistent with the C7 position being the most versatile position for substitution in quinolones [44], suggesting that the basic substituent at this position possibly interacts with ParE/GyrB, thus explaining the effect of a ParE/GyrB mutation on quinolone sensitivity [118]. On the contrary, a recent crystal structure of gyrase-FQ cleaved complexes from *Mycobacterium tuberculosis* showed that moieties appended to the C7 position of FQs have no specific interactions with any Gyr B residue, but that the quinolone resistance-determining region (QRDR) of Gyr B provides a complementary van der Waals surface that can favorably accommodate fairly large moieties [119]. The exact orientation and interactions between FQs, DNA, and enzyme within the cleavage complex has however remained controversial [62,110,112,115,120,121].

5.2. Eukaryotic Topoisomerase Type IIA

Similar to prokaryotic topoisomerases, eukaryotic DNA topoisomerases control DNA topology and play an important role in the regulation of the physiological function of the genome and DNA processes such as replication, transcription, recombination repair, chromosome decondensation, and sister chromatid [122]. The human genome encodes six isoforms of topoisomerases, as opposed to four in *E. coli* (Figure 8). Type 1 enzymes cleave one DNA strand at a time, while type 2 cleave both strands to perform their catalytic functions [96]. Clinically used anticancer agents, such as camptothecins, target eukaryotic type 1B topoisomerases, whereas human type 2A topoisomerases are the targets of etoposide, anthracyclines (doxorubicin, daunorubicin), and mitoxantrone [96].

Since the major pharmacological breakthrough of identifying type 2A topoisomerase as the crucial target point of activity of etoposide and doxorubicin, targeting DNA Top 2 in cancer chemotherapy has been extensively researched towards the discovery of newer anticancer molecules [123–125]. In contrast to lower eukaryotes such as yeast and *Drosophila,* which encode a single type 2 enzyme [126,127], vertebrates have two isoforms of this enzyme, α and β. These two isoforms, which display similar enzymatic activities and share almost 70% amino acid sequence identity, are encoded by separate genes and differ in their physiological regulation and cellular functions. Top 2β is required for proper neurological development in mouse embryos and vertebrate cells can survive in their absence, while Top 2α is an essential enzyme primarily responsible for cell growth during DNA replication and mitosis [128–130].

Remarkably, clinically relevant quinolones, such as ciprofloxacin and moxifloxacin, display very little activity against human type 2 topoisomerases even at concentrations beyond their therapeutic doses [5]. The selectivity of FQs for bacterial topoisomerases was found to be 1000-fold more than human topoisomerases [131,132], although the basis for this has remained largely unexplained. However, unlike gyrase and Top IV, human Top 2α and 2β lack the serine and acidic amino acid residues present in prokaryotic Top II. Both of these residues are methionine in eukaryotic Top 2α isoform [5]. Since the primary interaction of FQs with bacterial type II enzymes is mediated through a water-metal bridge ion anchored by serine and acidic amino acid residues, the loss of the bridge anchors in Top 2α and 2β has been proposed as a possible underlying basis for discriminating between bacterial and human type II enzymes [5]. In effect, the human enzyme is the equivalent of a quinolone-resistant topoisomerase IV.

Anticancer drugs that target Top 2 (such as etoposide, doxorubicin, mitoxantrone, and ellipticine) generate DNA damage that interferes with crucial cellular processes by stabilizing the breaking-passing-resealing complex [10,11]. This lead to severe damage that overwhelms the repair pathways of the human cells, and that they are thus referred to as topoisomerase poisons [11,96]. The ability to specifically and selectively disrupt these pathways in cancer cells, but not in normal cells, leading to improved clinical responses, remains a challenge. DNA Top 2-targeting anticancer drugs are usually associated with secondary malignancies and non-specific tissue cytotoxicity [11]. How then do FQs mediate their activities in human cancer cells but not in normal cells?

5.3. Interfacial Inhibition of Topoisomerases by Fluoroquinolones

Whereas, Top 2β is expressed in both dividing and non-dividing cells, Top 2α is tightly linked to cell proliferation and is orders of magnitude higher in rapidly proliferating cells than quiescent cells [96]. Top 2α relaxes positively supercoiled DNA more efficiently than negatively supercoiled DNA, while Top 2β acts on both equally [133]. Drugs that target Top 2 are classified as either Top 2 poisons or Top 2 catalytic inhibitors. Top 2 poisons effectively block transcription and replication [11]. They interfere with Top 2 cleavage complexes (Top 2cc) by either inhibiting DNA religation (e.g., etoposide, doxorubicin) or enhancing the formation of Top 2cc (e.g., quinolone CP-115,953, ellipticines, azatoxins). However, drug-induced Top 2cc alone is not sufficient to rationalize the anticancer activity of Top 2 poisons as both normal and cancer cells express Top 2. For example, the cytotoxicity of etoposide was found to be decreased by RNA synthesis inhibitor [134], suggesting that it interferences between trapped Top 2cc and transcription might play a prominent role in cytotoxicity. On the other hand, Top 2 catalytic inhibitors do not interfere with crucial cellular processes and do not generate an increase in the levels of Top 2cc, rather, they are thought to kill cells through the elimination of essential enzymatic activities of Top 2 by inhibiting the ATP-driven energy transduction component, e.g., bisdioxopiperazines [11,135].

The mechanism of action of FQs in eukaryotic cancer cells is unknown, but studies have shown that the yeast Top 2 could be made sensitive to FQs, and that point mutations in eukaryotic Top 2 occurs in the region that is homologous to the QRDR of prokaryotic Gyr A [136]. Similarly, *E. coli* could be rendered sensitive to eukaryotic topoisomerase poisons by point mutations at Ser83 of Gyr A [137]. Typical eukaryotic Top 2 poisons (such as etoposide) exhibit significant toxicities against proliferating cells, but they also generate enzyme-mediated DNA damage [11]. Although the ability of FQs to target eukaryotic topoisomerases have been shown [13,14], it is unclear whether clinically used FQs (e.g., ciprofloxacin) indeed mediate their antiproliferative actions against cancer cells via topoisomerase interaction since they are relatively safe in human. Other reported mechanisms of action of FQs against rapidly proliferating cells (that spare non-tumorigenic cells), such as apoptosis and regulation of tumor growth factors [72,74], microRNA production [79,83], etc. suggest that intrinsic defects in DNA and checkpoints, which are landmarks of cancer cells [138], are likely the Achilles' heels of cancer cells exposed to FQs. Physiologic and genetic changes in protein compositions/assembly in cancer cells, such as hyperactive DNA-enzyme machinery and their aggressively-proliferating nature, perhaps contribute to the more pronounced effect of clinically used FQs (such as ciprofloxacin) against cancer cells as opposed to normal cells. The mechanism of action of FQs on prokaryotic topoisomerases appears to be consistent with the mechanism of action of Top 2 poisons on eukaryotic topoisomerase. Indeed, some experimental FQ-derivatives (such as CP-115,953) have been shown to be as potent as etoposide at enhancing Top 2-mediated DNA cleavage in eukaryotic cells [92]. Note that these FQ analogs with significant activity against eukaryotic enzymes display similar toxicities that are associated with eukaryotic Top 2 poisons [13,14]. It is therefore unlikely that FQs with potent eukaryotic Top 2 activities will be useful as antibacterial agents going forward. The future of eukaryotic Top 2 as a drug target, as aptly discussed in an excellent review [11], will depend on whether isotype-specific agents can be developed. The ability of FQs to interact with eukaryotic Top 2β [13,14], impacting negatively on neurological development [129], is perhaps another reason why FQs should only be used in neonates and growing infants with great caution [139].

Based on this premise, many attempts have been made to modify antibacterial fluoroquinolones to produce novel antitumor agents [68,92,140–143]. A virtual screen of around 70,000 compounds revealed some quinolones to be potent inhibitors of human protein casein kinase (CK) 2 [144]. CK2 participates in the development of some type of cancers, and it is also implicated in viral infections and inflammatory failures [145], justifying some of the non-classical biological activities associated with FQs.

6. Immunomodulatory Properties of Fluoroquinolones

There is growing evidence that some antibiotics exert their beneficial effects not only by killing or inhibiting the growth of bacteria, but also indirectly by immunomodulation [146–148]. The first findings on the potential immunomodulatory properties of FQs were published in the late 1980s [149,150]. Whereas, the mechanism of antibacterial activity and effects of FQs on topoisomerase type II in prokaryotic and eukaryotic cells have been extensively investigated in vitro and in vivo, the mechanism underlying their immunomodulatory activities is still vague. However, possible cascade of intracellular processes leading to stimulatory or inhibitory effects on cytokines, chemokines, and other components of the immune system have been proposed [151,152].

The immune system can be thought of as a surveillance system that scans and ensures that tissues of the body are free of invading organisms and pathogens. When bacteria adhere to and colonize epithelial surfaces in their host macroorganism, they stimulate inflammatory responses and trigger the complex cytokine network. This is due to the released exoenzymes, exotoxins, polysaccharide, lipoteichoic and teichoic acid, peptidoglycan, and even DNA fragments, which are all proinflammatory [153,154]. One of the ways by which the immune system attack and get rid of foreign tissues/cells in such a complex environment is by induction of inflammation at the site of perturbation, which is by itself not a disease but a physiological response to a diseased state leading to the production of chemokines.

Chemokines (a large multifunctional family of cytokines; CHEMOtactic cytoKINES) are signaling proteins produced at the sites of infection or injury and act as chemoattractants to guide the migration of immune cells (such as lymphocytes) to their site of production [155]. Chemokines that are formed or produced under pathological conditions (such as infections and physical injury) are known as 'inflammatory chemokines', while those that are constitutively produced in certain tissues and that are responsible for leucocytes migration are known as "homeostatic chemokines". The release of inflammatory chemokines is often stimulated by pro-inflammatory stimuli, such as interleukin-1 (IL-1), tumor necrosis factor (TNF)-α, lipopolysaccharides (LPS), or viruses, while homeostatic chemokines are produced and secreted without any need to stimulate their source cells [156,157].

FQs have been observed to interact with bacterial adherence to and colonization of epithelial surfaces, as well as alter the release of proinflammatory bacterial products [151,152]. Ciprofloxacin, moxifloxacin, levofloxacin, trovafloxacin, and grepafloxacin have all been shown to dose-dependently inhibit the synthesis of IL-1 and TNF-α at therapeutic concentrations in LPS-stimulated monocytes, while at the same time super-induce interleukin-2 (IL-2) in vitro [152]. Ciprofloxacin was seen to directly exhibit a concentration-dependent inhibition of LPS activity [158]. In vivo assessment of the effects of ciprofloxacin, rufloxacin, difloxacin, tremafloxacin, and trovafloxacin in a preclinical *Bacteroides fragilis* intra-abdominal infection model showed the elimination of this pathogen in 66% of treated animals at subtherapeutic doses [159–164]. FQs are inactive against *B. fragilis* in vitro, suggesting that their protective effect was not due to their antibacterial efficacy but probably due to the modulation of TNF production in vivo.

Moreover, the T-cell growth factor IL-2 belongs to the set of "early expressed" genes that are produced within few hours upon activation, and two to three days before initiation of cell division. Since this governs cell proliferation, it has been hypothesized that the IL-2 super-inducing activities of quinolones [150,165] enhance drug uptake during this crucial stage of cell division and ultimately modulate the rate of proliferation, as observed in the pulsing of phytohemagglutinin-stimulated peripheral blood lymphocytes (PBL) with ciprofloxacin [166].

The benefits and implications of these immunomodulatory properties are obvious and far-reaching. Inhibiting monokine synthesis, specifically IL-1 and TNF-α, could be advantageous in combating septicemia and septic shock where overstimulation of inflammation by LPS is a major virulence factor of hard-to-treat Gram-negative organisms. Moreover, the super-induction of IL-2 synthesis could be relevant in immunocompromised cancer patients that might need some form of external assistance for regulation of cell proliferation [151].

However, there appears to be a need for co-stimulants, trigger, or stress, to be applied to cells or experimental animals for FQs to mediate immunomodulatory actions. Administration of quinolones to intact animals or healthy volunteers, and/or in vitro exposure of various cells to quinolones alone did not exert, in general, any measurable immunomodulatory effect [151,152]. Thus, the potential therapeutic relevance of FQs should be interpreted with great caution, as it may be of relatively low importance compared to their intrinsic antibacterial activities.

7. Selectivity and Amplification of Desirable Properties in Fluoroquinolones

The SAR of FQs (Figure 6) is well known and all of the clinically relevant analogs have been optimized to suit antibacterial activities [3,43]. However, structural requirements and/or optimization for non-classical activities are also beginning to emerge. For instance, reports show that increasing the lipophilicity of FQs results in a commensurate improvement in antiproliferative efficacy [167]. This is consistent with published evidences that support the correlation between lipophilicity of compounds and antitumor efficacy [168–174]. Several derivatives of ciprofloxacin have been shown to display more potent in vitro antitumor activity than the parent compound, culminating into analogs whose inhibitory concentration (IC_{50}) values are as low as $\leq$10 μM in various cancer cell lines [175]. Interestingly, novel *N*-4-piperazinyl-ciprofloxacin-chalcone hybrids (CCH) 1 and 2 (Figure 7) showed remarkable eukaryotic Top 2 activity that is comparable to etoposide, while CCH 3 and 4 displayed broad spectrum antitumor activity and high selectivity towards leukemia subpanel, respectively [167]. These show that lipophilicity plays a major role in the antiproliferative potentials of FQs.

Furthermore, fluoroquinolones with cyclopropyl moiety at position *N*1 (such as ciprofloxacin, sparfloxacin, and clinafloxacin) have been observed to exert increased production of interleukin 3 and granulocyte-macrophage colony-stimulating factor (GM-CSF) at clinically relevant dosing regimens, in contrast to those lacking the moiety [176]. GM-CSF stimulates stem cells to produce granulocytes (neutrophils, eosinophils, and basophils) and monocytes as part of the immune/inflammatory cascade crucial for fighting infections, and is clinically used to treat neutropenia in cancer patients undergoing chemotherapy, in AIDS patient during therapy, and in patients after bone marrow transplantation [177].

8. Limitations to the Development and Use of Fluoroquinolones

Early generation FQs, especially ciprofloxacin, have been very successful, but modifications that have led to optimization of pharmacokinetic properties and enhanced spectrum of activity have not been without their own costs. For example, specific idiosyncratic reactions have severely impeded the clinical relevance of agents such as trovafloxacin (hepatotoxic reactions) [178], temafloxacin (haemolytic uraemic syndrome) [179], grepafloxacin (cardiotoxicity) [180], clinafloxacin, and sitafloxacin (phototoxicity) [178,181], and in some cases led to their complete withdrawal from the market. It seems rather ironic that more quinolones have left the stage than remain. Nonetheless, the increasing knowledge of the interrelationship between SAR and ADR (adverse drug reactions) is poised to guide the future development of this class of drugs with well-informed predictions. Asides the unexpected ADRs, there are anticipated side effects of FQs that can be easily explained from their structure. The ketocarbonyl group at positions-3 and 4 with which they bind to the unpaired DNA bases via magnesium ions could potentially bind to other ions as well, such as aluminum, calcium, etc., as found in antacids, thereby forming a non-absorbable complex [182–184]. Also, the piperazine at position-7 has been associated with the tendency of FQs to displace γ-aminobutyric acid (GABA) or compete with its binding at the receptor sites within the central nervous system [185]. This suggests that FQs may only be used advisedly by patients with history of convulsion.

Furthermore, the clinical utility of FQs is threatened by multifactorial mechanisms of resistance present in almost every bacterial infection that is being treated with this class of drugs. Since the primary targets of FQs are DNA gyrase and Top IV, it is not surprising that the most prevalent resistance-conferring mutations occur at the highly-conserved serine and acidic residues in the A subunit of gyrase or Top IV (Ser83 and Glu87, respectively, in *E. coli*) [5,64]. This region is known as the quinolone resistance-determining region (QRDR) and alteration(s) in target protein structure alters the FQ-binding affinity of the enzyme. Other mechanisms of resistance to FQs include overexpression of multidrug resistance (MDR) efflux pumps, modifying enzymes, and/or target-protection proteins [186]. Surprisingly, long-term evolution experiments with *E. coli* showed that selection for fitness under some conditions can cause mutations within the genes that control supercoiling even in the absence of any antibiotic selective pressure [187]. This implicates evolution in the development of quinolone resistance, suggesting that merely restricting usage might probably not curtail long-term resistance development.

Lastly, while the immunomodulatory properties of FQs are beneficial in diverse conditions and are proven not to be an in vitro artifact, caution must be taken when used during transplantation. For instance, the super-induction of IL-2 (and potential activation of natural killer cells) and stimulatory effects on bone marrow generation by activation of IL-3 and GM-CSF synthesis could be important in immune-compromised cancer patients. On the contrary, this will be detrimental in patients transplanted with solid grafts on therapy with the immunosuppressive drug cyclosporine A, with whom additional T-cell stimulation would be deleterious upon rejection [151,188].

9. Conclusions

It is clear from the foregoing that the quinolone core is a privileged scaffold of drug that was accidentally discovered in the reaction flask of an observant chemist. From antimalarial to antibiotics, they evolved speedily into what has now become a reference towards the development of an "ideal" molecule [189,190]. Beyond the classical antimicrobial activities for which they were optimized and well-known for, FQs also display non-classical mechanisms of action, including but not limited to, antiproliferative and immunomodulatory properties. This provides a working scaffold that can either be developed as an anticancer or antibiotic agent. Unfortunately, the exact mechanism(s), by which they oscillate snugly between these extended roles is currently poorly understood. Since clinically relevant FQs are relatively safe in humans, their observed antiproliferative effects at clinically achievable concentrations might indeed be peculiar to aggressively-growing tumor cells, warranting a critical appraisal of their intrinsic potentials. Correlative and mechanistic studies of this class of drugs could perhaps give insights on their structural basis of selectivity for prokaryotic topoisomerases, and their ability to induce cell cycle arrest in eukaryotic cancer cells, while sparing non-tumorigenic ones. FQs that target eukaryotic topoisomerase show the same DNA damaging properties as other topoisomerase poisons [13,14], hence, drug optimization towards exclusive targeting of other eukaryotic mechanisms, such as apoptosis [74] and enhancement of miRNA production [83], will be a major step towards derivatizing this class of drugs exclusively for antiproliferative actions. How well FQs can be optimized for these evolving roles remain an interesting adventure in drug discovery. When fully understood, the intrinsic potentials of FQs could open a new paradigm in synthetic drug discovery, especially if the desired activity can be selectively amplified to discriminate bacteria from humans, and cancer cells from normal ones.

Acknowledgments: The authors thank NSERC (DG-261311-2013) and the University of Manitoba (GETS program) for financial support.

Author Contributions: Temilolu Idowu conducted the literature review and wrote the manuscript. Frank Schweizer provided constructive feedback.

References

1. Becker, B.; Cooper, M.A. Aminoglycoside antibiotics in the 21st century. *ACS Chem. Biol.* **2013**, *8*, 105–115. [CrossRef] [PubMed]
2. Cooper, M.A. A community-based approach to new antibiotic discovery. *Nat. Rev. Drug Discov.* **2015**, *14*, 587–588. [CrossRef] [PubMed]
3. Mitscher, L.A. Bacterial topoisomerase inhibitors: Quinolone and pyridone antibacterial agents. *Chem. Rev.* **2005**, *105*, 559–592. [CrossRef] [PubMed]
4. Ball, P. Quinolone generations: Natural history or natural selection? *J. Antimicrob. Chemother.* **2000**, *46*, 17–24. [CrossRef] [PubMed]
5. Aldred, K.J.; Schwanz, H.A.; Li, G.; Mcpherson, S.A.; Turnbough, C.L.; Kerns, R.J.; Osheroff, N. Overcoming target-mediated quinolone resistance in topoisomerase IV by introducing metal-ion-independent drug–enzyme interactions. *ACS Chem. Biol.* **2013**, *8*, 2660–2668. [CrossRef] [PubMed]
6. World Health Organization (WHO). Cancer. Available online: http://www.who.int/mediacentre/factsheets/fs297/en/ (accessed on 5 September 2017).

7. Hanahan, D.; Weinberg, R.A. Hallmarks of cancer: The next generation. *Cell* **2011**, *144*, 646–674. [CrossRef] [PubMed]
8. Schmitz, F.J.; Higgins, P.; Mayer, S.; Fluit, A.; Dalhoff, A. Activity of quinolones against gram-positive cocci: Mechanisms of drug action and bacterial resistance. *Eur. J. Clin. Microbiol. Infect. Dis.* **2002**, *21*, 647–659. [PubMed]
9. Drlica, K.; Zhao, X. DNA gyrase, topoisomerase IV, and the 4-quinolones. *Microbiol. Mol. Biol. Rev.* **1997**, *61*, 377–392. [PubMed]
10. Baldwin, E.L.; Osheroff, N. Etoposide, topoisomerase II and cancer. *Curr. Med. Chem. Anticancer Agents* **2005**, *5*, 363–372. [CrossRef] [PubMed]
11. Nitiss, J.L. Targeting DNA topoisomerase II in cancer chemotherapy. *Nat. Rev. Cancer* **2009**, *9*, 338–350. [CrossRef] [PubMed]
12. Bourikas, L.A.; Kolios, G.; Valatas, V.; Notas, G.; Drygiannakis, I.; Pelagiadis, I.; Manousou, P.; Klironomos, S.; Mouzas, I.A.; Kouroumalis, E. Ciprofloxacin decreases survival in HT-29 cells via the induction of TGF-beta1 secretion and enhances the anti-proliferative effect of 5-fluorouracil. *Br. J. Pharmacol.* **2009**, *157*, 362–370. [CrossRef] [PubMed]
13. Elsea, S.H.; Osheroff, N.; Nitiss, J.L. Cytotoxicity of quinolones toward eukaryotic cells. *J. Biol. Chem.* **1992**, *267*, 13150–13153. [PubMed]
14. Elsea, S.H.; Mcguirk, P.R.; Gootz, T.D.; Moynihan, M.; Osheroffl, N. Drug features that contribute to the activity of quinolones against mammalian topoisomerase II and cultured cells: Correlation between enhancement of enzyme-mediated DNA cleavage in vitro and cytotoxic potential. *Antimicrob. Agents Chemother.* **1993**, *37*, 2179–2186. [CrossRef] [PubMed]
15. Dayam, R.; Al-Mawsawi, L.Q.; Zawahir, Z.; Witvrouw, M.; Debyser, Z.; Neamati, N. Quinolone 3-carboxylic acid pharmacophore: Design of second generation HIV-1 integrase inhibitors. *J. Med. Chem.* **2008**, *51*, 1136–1144. [CrossRef] [PubMed]
16. Stern, E.; Muccioli, G.G.; Millet, R.; Goossens, J.F.; Farce, A.; Chavatte, P.; Poupaert, J.H.; Lambert, D.M.; Depreux, P.; Hénichart, J.P. Novel 4-oxo-1,4-dihydroquinoline-3-carboxamide derivatives as new CB2 cannabinoid receptors agonists: Synthesis, pharmacological properties and molecular modeling. *J. Med. Chem.* **2006**, *49*, 70–79. [CrossRef] [PubMed]
17. Manera, C.; Benetti, V.; Castelli, M.P.; Cavallini, T.; Lazzarotti, S.; Pibiri, F.; Saccomanni, G.; Tuccinardi, T.; Vannacci, A.; Martinelli, A.; Ferrarini, P.L. Design, synthesis, and biological evaluation of new 1,8-naphthyridin-4(1*H*)-on-3-carboxamide and quinolin-4(1*H*)-on-3-carboxamide derivatives as CB_2 selective agonists. *J. Med. Chem.* **2006**, *49*, 5947–5957. [CrossRef] [PubMed]
18. Kahnberg, P.; Howard, M.H.; Liljefors, T.; Nielsen, M.; Nielsen, E.Ø.; Sterner, O.; Pettersson, I. The use of a pharmacophore model for identification of novel ligands for the benzodiazepine binding site of the GABA A receptor. *J. Mol. Graph. Model.* **2004**, *23*, 253–261. [CrossRef] [PubMed]
19. Lager, E.; Andersson, P.; Nilsson, J.; Pettersson, I.; Nielsen, E.O.; Nielsen, M.; Sterner, O.; Liljefors, T. 4-Quinolone derivatives: High-affinity ligands at the benzodiazepine site of brain GABAA receptors. Synthesis, pharmacology, and pharmacophore modeling. *J. Med. Chem.* **2006**, *49*, 2526–2533. [CrossRef] [PubMed]
20. Park, C.H.; Lee, J.; Jung, H.Y.; Kim, M.J.; Lim, S.H.; Yeo, H.T.; Choi, E.C.; Yoon, E.J.; Kim, K.W.; Cha, J.H.; et al. Identification, biological activity, and mechanism of the anti-ischemic quinolone analog. *Bioorganic Med. Chem.* **2007**, *15*, 6517–6526. [CrossRef] [PubMed]
21. Lucero, B.D.; Gomes, C.R.; Frugulhetti, I.C.; Faro, L.V.; Alvarenga, L.; De Souza, M.C.; De Souza, T.M.; Ferreira, V.F. Synthesis and anti-HSV-1 activity of quinolonic acyclovir analogues. *Bioorg. Med. Chem. Lett.* **2006**, *16*, 1010–1013. [CrossRef] [PubMed]
22. Steiner, H.; Hultmark, D.; Engström, Å.; Bennich, H.; Boman, H.G. Sequence and specificity of two antibacterial proteins involved in insect immunity. *Nature* **1981**, *292*, 246–248. [CrossRef] [PubMed]
23. Ganz, T.; Selsted, M.E.; Szklarek, D.; Harwig, S.S.; Daher, K.; Bainton, D.F.; Lehrer, R.I. Defensins. Natural peptide antibiotics of human neutrophils. *J. Clin. Investig.* **1985**, *76*, 1427–1435. [CrossRef] [PubMed]
24. Zasloff, M. Magainins, a class of antimicrobial peptides from Xenopus skin: Isolation, characterization of two active forms, and partial cDNA sequence of a precursor. *Proc. Natl. Acad. Sci. USA* **1987**, *84*, 5449–5453. [CrossRef] [PubMed]

25. Vandamme, D.; Landuyt, B.; Luyten, W.; Schoofs, L. A comprehensive summary of LL-37, the factotum human cathelicidin peptide. *Cell. Immunol.* **2012**, *280*, 22–35. [CrossRef] [PubMed]
26. Velkov, T.; Roberts, K.D.; Nation, R.L.; Thompson, P.E.; Li, J. Pharmacology of polymyxins: New insights into an "old" class of antibiotics. *Future Microbiol.* **2013**, *8*, 711–724. [CrossRef] [PubMed]
27. Bud, R. *Penicillin: Triumph and Tragedy*; Slinn, J., Ed.; Oxford University Press: Oxford, UK, 2009; ISBN 978-19-925406-4.
28. Lesher, G.Y.; Froelich, E.J.; Gruett, M.D.; Bailey, J.H.; Brundage, P.R. 1,8-Naphthyridine derivatives. A new class of chemotherapeutic agents. *J. Med. Pharm. Chem.* **1962**, *5*, 1063–1068. [CrossRef]
29. Bisacchi, G.S. Origins of the quinolone class of antibacterials: An expanded "discovery story. *J. Med. Chem.* **2015**, *58*, 4874–4882. [CrossRef] [PubMed]
30. Domagala, J.M. Structure-activity and structure-side-effect relationships for the quinolone antibacterials. *J. Antimicrob. Chemother.* **1994**, *33*, 685–706. [CrossRef] [PubMed]
31. Bertino, J.; Fish, D. The safety profile of the fluoroquinolones. *Clin. Ther.* **2000**, *22*, 798–817. [CrossRef]
32. Naber, K.G.; Hollauer, K.; Kirchbauer, D.; Witte, W. In vitro activity of gatifloxacin compared with gemifloxacin, moxifloxacin, trovafloxacin, ciprofloxacin and ofloxacin against uropathogens cultured from patients with complicated urinary tract infections. *Int. J. Antimicrob. Agents* **2000**, *16*, 239–243. [CrossRef]
33. Stein, G.E.; Goldstein, E.J.C. Fluoroquinolones and anaerobes. *Clin. Infect. Dis.* **2006**, *42*, 1598–1607. [CrossRef] [PubMed]
34. Davis, B.D. Mechanism of bactericidal action of aminoglycosides. *Microbiol. Rev.* **1987**, *51*, 341–350. [PubMed]
35. Mingeot-Leclercq, M.P.; Glupczynski, Y.; Tulkens, P.M. Aminoglycosides: Activity and resistance. *Antimicrob. Agents Chemother.* **1999**, *43*, 727–737. [PubMed]
36. Owens, R.C.; Ambrose, P.G. Clinical use of the fluoroquinolones. *Med. Clin. N. Am.* **2000**, *84*, 1447–1469. [CrossRef]
37. Oliphant, C.M.; Green, G.M. Quinolones: A comprehensive review. *Am. Fam. Physician* **2002**, *65*, 455–464. [PubMed]
38. Hooper, D.C.; Wolfson, J.S. The Fluoroquinolones: Pharmacology, clinical uses, and toxicities in humans. *Antimicrob. Agents Chemother.* **1985**, *28*, 716–721. [CrossRef] [PubMed]
39. Freifeld, A.G.; Bow, E.J.; Sepkowitz, K.A.; Boeckh, M.J.; Ito, J.I.; Mullen, C.A.; Raad, I.I.; Rolston, K.V.; Young, J.A.H.; Wingard, J.R. Clinical practice guideline for the use of antimicrobial agents in neutropenic patients. *Clin. Infect. Dis.* **2011**, *52*, e56–e93. [CrossRef] [PubMed]
40. Stein, G.E. Pharmacokinetics and pharmacodynamics of newer fluoroquinolones. *Clin. Infect. Dis.* **1996**, *23*, S19–S24. [CrossRef] [PubMed]
41. Blondeau, J.M. A review of the comparative in-vitro activities of 12 antimicrobial agents, with a focus on five new respiratory quinolones'. *J. Antimicrob. Chemother.* **1999**, *43*, 1–11. [CrossRef] [PubMed]
42. Dong, Y.; Zhao, X.; Domagala, J.; Drlica, K. Effect of fluoroquinolone concentration on selection of resistant mutants of *Mycobacterium bovis* BCG and *Staphylococcus aureus*. *Antimicrob. Agents Chemother.* **1999**, *43*, 1756–1758. [PubMed]
43. Zhanel, G.G.; Ennis, K.; Vercaigne, L.; Walkty, A.; Gin, A.S.; Embil, J.; Smith, H.; Hoban, D.J. A critical review of the fluoroquinolones. *Drugs* **2002**, *62*, 13–59. [CrossRef] [PubMed]
44. Gorityala, B.K.; Guchhait, G.; Fernando, D.M.; Deo, S.; McKenna, S.A.; Zhanel, G.G.; Kumar, A.; Schweizer, F. Adjuvants based on hybrid antibiotics overcome resistance in *Pseudomonas aeruginosa* and enhance fluoroquinolone efficacy. *Angew. Chem. Int. Ed. Engl.* **2016**, *55*, 555–559. [CrossRef] [PubMed]
45. Diggle, S.P.; Matthijs, S.; Wright, V.J.; Fletcher, M.P.; Ram Chhabra, S.; Lamont, I.L.; Kong, X.; Hider, R.C.; Cornelis, P.; Cá mara, M.; et al. The *Pseudomonas aeruginosa* 4-quinolone signal molecules HHQ and PQS play multifunctional roles in quorum sensing and iron entrapment. *Chem. Biol.* **2007**, *14*, 87–96. [CrossRef] [PubMed]
46. Zhanel, G.G.; Fontaine, S.; Adam, H.; Schurek, K.; Mayer, M.; Noreddin, A.M.; Gin, A.S.; Rubinstein, E.; Hoban, D.J. A review of new fluoroquinolones: Focus on their use in respiratory tract infections. *Treat. Respir. Med.* **2006**, *5*, 437–465. [CrossRef] [PubMed]
47. Gillespie, S.H. The role of moxifloxacin in tuberculosis therapy. *Eur. Respir. Rev.* **2016**, *25*, 19–28. [CrossRef] [PubMed]

48. Dawson, R.; Diacon, A.H.; Everitt, D.; van Niekerk, C.; Donald, P.R.; Burger, D.A.; Schall, R.; Spigelman, M.; Conradie, A.; Eisenach, K.; et al. Efficiency and safety of the combination of moxifloxacin, pretomanid (PA-824), and pyrazinamide during the first 8 weeks of antituberculosis treatment: A phase 2b, open-label, partly randomised trial in patients with drug-susceptible or drug-resistant pulmonary tuberculosis. *Lancet* **2015**, *385*, 1738–1747. [PubMed]
49. Scheld, W.M. Maintaining fluoroquinolone class efficacy: Review of influencing factors. *Emerg. Infect. Dis.* **2003**, *9*, 1–9. [CrossRef] [PubMed]
50. Pestova, E.; Millichap, J.J.; Noskin, G.A.; Peterson, L.R. Intracellular targets of moxifloxacin: A comparison with other fluoroquinolones. *J. Antimicrob. Chemother.* **2000**, *45*, 583–590. [CrossRef] [PubMed]
51. Bast, D.J.; Low, D.E.; Duncan, C.L.; Kilburn, L.; Mandell, L.A.; Davidson, R.J.; De Azavedo, J.C. Fluoroquinolone resistance in clinical isolates of *Streptococcus pneumoniae*: Contributions of type II topoisomerase mutations and efflux to levels of resistance. *Antimicrob. Agents Chemother.* **2000**, *44*, 3049–3054. [CrossRef] [PubMed]
52. Smith, H.J.; Walters, M.; Hisanaga, T.; Zhanel, G.G.; Hoban, D.J. Mutant prevention concentrations for single-step fluoroquinolone-resistant mutants of wild-type, efflux-positive, or ParC or GyrA mutation-containing *Streptococcus pneumoniae* isolates. *Antimicrob. Agents Chemother.* **2004**, *48*, 3954–3958. [CrossRef] [PubMed]
53. Fukuda, H.; Kishii, R.; Takei, M.; Hosaka, M. Contributions of the 8-methoxy group of gatifloxacin to resistance selectivity, target preference, and antibacterial activity against *Streptococcus pneumoniae*. *Antimicrob. Agents Chemother.* **2001**, *45*, 1649–1653. [CrossRef] [PubMed]
54. Kishii, R.; Takei, M.; Fukuda, H.; Hayashi, K.; Hosaka, M. Contribution of the 8-methoxy group to the activity of gatifloxacin against type II topoisomerases of *Streptococcus pneumoniae*. *Antimicrob. Agents Chemother.* **2003**, *47*, 77–81. [CrossRef] [PubMed]
55. Frémaux, A.; Sissia, G.; Geslin, P. In-vitro bacteriostatic activity of levofloxacin and three other fluoroquinolones against penicillin-susceptible and penicillin-resistant *Streptococcus pneumoniae*. *J. Antimicrob. Chemother.* **1999**, *43*, 9–14. [CrossRef] [PubMed]
56. Goldstein, E.J.; Citron, D.M.; Merriam, C.V.; Tyrrell, K.; Warren, Y. Activity of gatifloxacin compared to those of five other quinolones versus aerobic and anaerobic isolates from skin and soft tissue samples of human and animal bite wound infections. *Antimicrob. Agents Chemother.* **1999**, *43*, 1475–1479. [PubMed]
57. Poole, R.M. Nemonoxacin: First global approval. *Drugs* **2014**, *74*, 1445–1453. [CrossRef] [PubMed]
58. McKeage, K. Finafloxacin: First global approval. *Drugs* **2015**, *75*, 687–693. [CrossRef] [PubMed]
59. US FDA Highlights of Prescribing Information for Baxdela. Available online: https://www.accessdata.fda.gov/drugsatfda_docs/label/2017/208610s000,208611s000lbl.pdf (accessed on 14 September 2017).
60. Boucher, H.W.; Talbot, G.H.; Bradley, J.S.; Edwards, J.E.; Gilbert, D.; Rice, L.B.; Scheld, M.; Spellberg, B.; Bartlett, J. Bad bugs, no drugs: No ESKAPE! An update from the Infectious Diseases Society of America. *Clin. Infect. Dis.* **2009**, *48*, 1–12. [CrossRef] [PubMed]
61. Peterson, L.R. Quinolone molecular structure-activity relationships: What we have learned about improving antimicrobial activity. *Clin. Infect. Dis.* **2001**, *33*, S180–186. [CrossRef] [PubMed]
62. Shen, L.L. Molecular mechanisms of DNA gyrase inhibition by quinolone antibacterials. *Adv. Pharmacol.* **1994**, *29*, 285–304.
63. Bhanot, S.K.; Singh, M.; Chatterjee, N.R. The chemical and biological aspects of fluoroquinolones: Reality and dreams. *Curr. Pharm. Des.* **2001**, *7*, 311–335. [CrossRef] [PubMed]
64. Aldred, K.J.; McPherson, S.A.; Turnbough, C.L.; Kerns, R.J.; Osheroff, N.; Osheroff, N. Topoisomerase IV-quinolone interactions are mediated through a water-metal ion bridge: Mechanistic basis of quinolone resistance. *Nucleic Acids Res.* **2013**, *41*, 4628–4639. [CrossRef] [PubMed]
65. Pan, X.S.; Gould, K.A.; Fisher, L.M. Probing the differential interactions of quinazolinedione PD 0305970 and quinolones with gyrase and topoisomerase IV. *Antimicrob. Agents Chemother.* **2009**, *53*, 3822–3831. [CrossRef] [PubMed]
66. Oppegard, L.M.; Streck, K.R.; Rosen, J.D.; Schwanz, H.A.; Drlica, K.; Kerns, R.J.; Hiasa, H. Comparison of in vitro activities of fluoroquinolone-like 2,4-and 1,3-diones. *Antimicrob. Agents Chemother.* **2010**, *54*, 3011–3014. [CrossRef] [PubMed]

67. Malik, M.; Marks, K.R.; Mustaev, A.; Zhao, X.; Chavda, K.; Kerns, R.J.; Drlica, K. Fluoroquinolone and quinazolinedione activities against wild-type and gyrase mutant strains of *Mycobacterium smegmatis*. *Antimicrob. Agents Chemother.* **2011**, *55*, 2335–2343. [CrossRef] [PubMed]
68. Al-Trawneh, S.A.; Zahra, J.A.; Kamal, M.R.; El-Abadelah, M.M.; Zani, F.; Incerti, M.; Cavazzoni, A.; Alfieri, R.R.; Petronini, P.G.; Vicini, P. Synthesis and biological evaluation of tetracyclic fluoroquinolones as antibacterial and anticancer agents. *Bioorg. Med. Chem.* **2010**, *18*, 5873–5884. [CrossRef] [PubMed]
69. Anderson, V.E.; Osheroff, N. Type II topoisomerases as targets for quinolone antibacterials: Turning Dr. Jekyll into Mr. Hyde. *Curr. Pharm. Des.* **2001**, *7*, 337–353. [CrossRef] [PubMed]
70. El-Rayes, B.F.; Grignon, R.; Aslam, N.; Aranha, O.; Sarkar, F.H. Ciprofloxacin inhibits cell growth and synergises the effect of etoposide in hormone resistant prostate cancer cells. *Int. J. Oncol.* **2002**, *21*, 207–211. [CrossRef] [PubMed]
71. Noris, M.D.; Madafiglio, J.; Gilbert, J.; Marshall, G.M.; Haber, M. Reversal of multidrug resistance-associated protein-mediated drug resistance in cultured human neuroblastoma cells by the quinolone antibiotic difloxacin. *Med. Pediatr. Oncol.* **2001**, *36*, 177–180. [CrossRef]
72. Herold, C.; Ocker, M.; Ganslmayer, M.; Gerauer, H.; Hahn, E.G.; Schuppan, D. Ciprofloxacin induces apoptosis and inhibits proliferation of human colorectal carcinoma cells. *Br. J. Cancer* **2002**, *86*, 443–448. [CrossRef] [PubMed]
73. Hussy, P.; Maass, G.; Tümmler, B.; Grosse, F.; Schomburg, U. Effect of 4-quinolones and novobiocin on calf thymus DNA polymerase alpha primase complex, topoisomerases I and II, and growth of mammalian lymphoblasts. *Antimicrob. Agents Chemother.* **1986**, *29*, 1073–1078. [CrossRef] [PubMed]
74. Aranha, O.; Grignon, R.; Fernandes, N.; McDonnell, T.J.; Wood, D.P.; Sarkar, F.H. Suppression of human prostate cancer cell growth by ciprofloxacin is associated with cell cycle arrest and apoptosis. *Int. J. Oncol.* **2003**, *22*, 787–794. [CrossRef] [PubMed]
75. Schaeffer, A.J. The expanding role of fluoroquinolones. *Am. J. Med.* **2002**, *113*, 45S–54S. [CrossRef]
76. Simpson, K.J.; Brodie, M.J. Convulsions related to enoxacin. *Lancet* **1985**. [CrossRef]
77. De Sarro, A.; Zappala, M.; Chimirri, A.; Grasso, S.; De Sarro1, G.B. Quinolones potentiate cefazolin-induced seizures in DBA/2 mice. *Antimicrob. Agents Chemother.* **1993**, *37*, 1497–1503. [CrossRef] [PubMed]
78. Mukherjee, P.; Mandal, E.R.; Das, S.K. Evaluation of antiproliferative activity of enoxacin on a human breast cancer cell line. *Int. J. Hum. Genet.* **2005**, *5*, 57–63.
79. Melo, S.; Villanueva, A.; Moutinho, C.; Davalos, V.; Spizzo, R.; Ivan, C.; Rossi, S. Small molecule enoxacin is a cancer-specific growth inhibitor that acts by enhancing TAR RNA-binding protein 2-mediated microRNA processing. *Proc. Natl. Acad. Sci. USA* **2011**, *108*, 4394–4399. [CrossRef] [PubMed]
80. He, L.; Hannon, G.J. MicroRNAs: Small RNAs with a big role in gene regulation. *Nat. Rev. Genet.* **2004**, *5*, 522–531. [CrossRef] [PubMed]
81. Lu, J.; Getz, G.; Miska, E.A.; Alvarez-Saavedra, E.; Lamb, J.; Peck, D.; Sweet-Cordero, A.; Ebert, B.L.; Mak, R.H.; Ferrando, A.A.; et al. MicroRNA expression profiles classify human cancers. *Nature* **2005**, *435*, 834–838. [CrossRef] [PubMed]
82. Gaur, A.; Jewell, D.A.; Liang, Y.; Ridzon, D.; Moore, J.H.; Chen, C.; Ambros, V.R.; Israel, M.A. Characterization of microRNA expression levels and their biological correlates in human cancer cell lines. *Cancer Res.* **2007**, *67*, 2456–2468. [CrossRef] [PubMed]
83. Shan, G.; Li, Y.; Zhang, J.; Li, W.; Szulwach, K.E.; Duan, R.; Faghihi, M.A.; Khalil, A.M.; Lu, L.; Paroo, Z.; et al. A small molecule enhances RNA interference and promotes microRNA processing. *Nat. Biotechnol.* **2008**, *26*, 933–940. [CrossRef] [PubMed]
84. Patel, S.S.; Spencer, C.M. Enoxacin: A reappraisal of its clinical efficacy in the treatment of genitourinary tract infections. *Drugs* **1996**, *51*, 137–160. [CrossRef] [PubMed]
85. O'Brien, T.P.; Arshinoff, S.A.; Mah, F.S. Perspectives on antibiotics for postoperative endophthalmitis prophylaxis: Potential role of moxifloxacin. *J. Cataract Refract. Surg.* **2007**, *33*, 1790–1800. [CrossRef] [PubMed]
86. Brillault, J.; De Castro, W.V.; Harnois, T.; Kitzis, A.; Olivier, J.C.; Couet, W. P-glycoprotein-mediated transport of moxifloxacin in a Calu-3 lung epithelial cell model. *Antimicrob. Agents Chemother.* **2009**, *53*, 1457–1462. [CrossRef] [PubMed]

87. Espiritu, C.R.G.; Caparas, V.L.; Bolinao, J.G. Safety of prophylactic intracameral moxifloxacin 0.5% ophthalmic solution in cataract surgery patients. *J. Cataract Refract. Surg.* **2007**, *33*, 63–68. [CrossRef] [PubMed]
88. Arshinoff, S.A.; Modabber, M. Dose and administration of intracameral moxifloxacin for prophylaxis of postoperative endophthalmitis. *J. Cataract Refract. Surg.* **2016**, *42*, 1730–1741. [CrossRef] [PubMed]
89. Sobolewska, B.; Hofmann, J.; Spitzer, M.S.; Bartz-Schmidt, K.U.; Szurman, P.; Yoeruek, E. Antiproliferative and cytotoxic properties of moxifloxacin on rat retinal ganglion cells. *Curr. Eye Res.* **2013**, *38*, 662–669. [CrossRef] [PubMed]
90. Matsuura, K.; Miyoshi, T.; Suto, C.; Akura, J.; Inoue, Y. Efficacy and safety of prophylactic intracameral moxifloxacin injection in Japan. *J. Cart. Refract. Surg.* **2013**, *39*, 1702–1706. [CrossRef] [PubMed]
91. Robinson, M.J.; Martin, B.A.; Gootz, T.D.; McGuirk, P.R.; Moynihan, M.; Sutcliffe, J.A.; Osheroff, N. Effects of quinolone derivatives on eukaryotic topoisomerase II. A novel mechanism for enhancement of enzyme-mediated DNA cleavage. *J. Biol. Chem.* **1991**, *266*, 14585–14592. [PubMed]
92. Robinson, M.J.; Martin, B.A.; Gootz, T.D.; McGuirk, P.R.; Osheroff, N. Effects of novel fluoroquinolones on the catalytic activities of eukaryotic topoisomerase II: Influence of the C-8 fluorine group. *Antimicrob. Agents Chemother.* **1992**, *36*, 751–756. [CrossRef] [PubMed]
93. Isaacs, J.T.; Pili, R.; Qian, D.Z.; Dalrymple, S.L.; Garrison, J.B.; Kyprianou, N.; Björk, A.; Olsson, A.; Leanderson, T. Identification of ABR-215050 as lead second generation quinoline-3-carboxamide anti-angiogenic agent for the treatment of prostate cancer. *Prostate* **2006**, *66*, 1768–1778. [CrossRef] [PubMed]
94. Osanto, S.; van Poppel, H.; Burggraaf, J. Tasquinimod: A novel drug in advanced prostate cancer. *Future Oncol.* **2013**, *9*, 1271–1281. [CrossRef] [PubMed]
95. Mondal, E.R.; Das, S.K.; Mukherjee, P. Comparative evaluation of antiproliferative activity and induction of apoptosis by some fluoroquinolones with a human non-small cell lung cancer cell line in culture. *Asian Pac. J. Cancer Prev.* **2004**, *5*, 196–204. [PubMed]
96. Pommier, Y.; Leo, E.; Zhang, H.; Marchand, C. DNA topoisomerases and their poisoning by anticancer and antibacterial drugs. *Chem. Biol.* **2010**, *17*, 421–433. [CrossRef] [PubMed]
97. Champoux, J.J. DNA topoisomerases: Structure, function, and mechanism. *Annu. Rev. Biochem.* **2001**, *70*, 369–413. [CrossRef] [PubMed]
98. Nitiss, J.L. DNA topoisomerase II and its growing repertoire of biological functions. *Nat. Rev. Cancer* **2009**, *9*, 327–337. [CrossRef] [PubMed]
99. Pommier, Y.; Sun, Y.; Huang, S.N.; Nitiss, J.L. Roles of eukaryotic topoisomerases in transcription, replication and genomic stability. *Nat. Rev. Mol. Cell Biol.* **2016**, *17*, 703–721. [CrossRef] [PubMed]
100. Pommier, Y. Topoisomerase I inhibitors: Camptothecins and beyond. *Nat. Rev. Cancer* **2006**, *6*, 789–802. [CrossRef] [PubMed]
101. Pommier, Y. Drugging Topoisomerases: Lessons and Challenges. *ACS Chem. Biol.* **2013**, *8*, 82–95. [CrossRef] [PubMed]
102. Capranico, G.; Marinello, J.; Chillemi, G. Type I DNA Topoisomerases. *J. Med. Chem.* **2017**, *60*, 2169–2192. [CrossRef] [PubMed]
103. Drlica, K.; Malik, M.; Kerns, R.J.; Zhao, X. Quinolone-mediated bacterial death. *Antimicrob. Agents Chemother.* **2008**, *52*, 385–392. [CrossRef] [PubMed]
104. Pan, X.S.; Fisher, L.M. Targeting of DNA gyrase in *Streptococcus pneumoniae* by sparfloxacin: Selective targeting of gyrase or topoisomerase IV by quinolones. *Antimicrob. Agents Chemother.* **1997**, *41*, 471–474. [PubMed]
105. Pan, X.S.; Fisher, L.M. DNA gyrase and topoisomerase IV are dual targets of clinafloxacin action in *Streptococcus pneumoniae*. *Antimicrob. Agents Chemother.* **1998**, *42*, 2810–2816. [PubMed]
106. Fournier, B.; Zhao, X.; Lu, T.; Drlica, K.; Hooper, D.C. Selective targeting of topoisomerase IV and DNA gyrase in *Staphylococcus aureus*: Different patterns of quinolone-induced inhibition of DNA synthesis. *Antimicrob. Agents Chemother.* **2000**, *44*, 2160–2165. [CrossRef] [PubMed]
107. Kreuzer, K.N.; Cozzarelli, N.R. Escherichia coli mutants thermosensitive for deoxyribonucleic acid gyrase subunit A: Effects on deoxyribonucleic acid replication, transcription, and bacteriophage growth. *J. Bacteriol.* **1979**, *140*, 424–435. [PubMed]
108. Arnoldi, E.; Pan, X.S.; Fisher, L.M. Functional determinants of gate-DNA selection and cleavage by bacterial type II topoisomerases. *Nucleic Acids Res.* **2013**. [CrossRef] [PubMed]

109. Laponogov, I.; Veselkov, D.A.; Crevel, I.M.T.; Pan, X.S.; Fisher, L.M.; Sanderson, M.R. Structure of an "open" clamp type II topoisomerase-DNA complex provides a mechanism for DNA capture and transport. *Nucleic Acids Res.* **2013**, *41*, 9911–9923. [CrossRef] [PubMed]
110. Laponogov, I.; Sohi, M.K.; Veselkov, D.A.; Pan, X.S.; Sawhney, R.; Thompson, A.W.; McAuley, K.E.; Fisher, L.M.; Sanderson, M.R. Structural insight into the quinolone-DNA cleavage complex of type IIA topoisomerases. *Nat. Struct. Mol. Biol.* **2009**, *16*, 667–669. [CrossRef] [PubMed]
111. Vos, S.M.; Tretter, E.M.; Schmidt, B.H.; Berger, J.M. All tangled up: How cells direct, manage and exploit topoisomerase function. *Nat. Rev. Mol. Cell Biol.* **2011**, *12*, 827–841. [CrossRef] [PubMed]
112. Wohlkonig, A.; Chan, P.F.; Fosberry, A.P.; Homes, P.; Huang, J.; Kranz, M.; Leydon, V.R.; Miles, T.J.; Pearson, N.D.; Perera, R.L.; et al. Structural basis of quinolone inhibition of type IIA topoisomerases and target-mediated resistance. *Nat. Struct. Mol. Biol.* **2010**, *17*, 1152–1153. [CrossRef] [PubMed]
113. Shen, L.L.; Pernet, A.G. Mechanism of inhibition of DNA gyrase by analogues of nalidixic acid: The target of the drugs is DNA. *Proc. Natl. Acad. Sci. USA* **1985**, *82*, 307–311. [CrossRef] [PubMed]
114. Palù, G.; Valisena, S.; Ciarrocchi, G.; Gatto, B.; Palumbo, M. Quinolone binding to DNA is mediated by magnesium ions. *Proc. Natl. Acad. Sci. USA* **1992**, *89*, 9671–9675. [CrossRef] [PubMed]
115. Shen, L.L.; Mitscher, L.A.; Sharma, P.N.; O'Donnell, T.J.; Chu, D.W.; Cooper, C.S.; Rosen, T.; Pernet, A.G. Mechanism of inhibition of DNA gyrase by quinolone antibacterials: A cooperative drug-DNA binding model. *Biochemistry* **1989**, *28*, 3886–3894. [CrossRef] [PubMed]
116. Shen, L.L.; Baranowski, J.; Pernet, A.G. Mechanism of inhibition of DNA gyrase by quinolone antibacterials: Specificity and cooperativity of drug binding to DNA. *Biochemistry* **1989**, *28*, 3879–3885. [CrossRef] [PubMed]
117. Shen, L.L.; Kohlbrenner, W.E.; Weigl, D.; Baranowski, J. Mechanism of quinolone inhibition of DNA gyrase. Appearance of unique norfloxacin binding sites in enzyme-DNA complexes. *J. Biol. Chem.* **1989**, *264*, 2973–2978. [PubMed]
118. Yoshida, H.; Bogaki, M.; Nakamura, M.; Yamanaka, L.M.; Nakamura, S. Quinolone resistance-determining region in the DNA gyrase gyrB gene of *Escherichia coli*. *Antimicrob. Agents Chemother.* **1991**, *35*, 1647–1650. [CrossRef] [PubMed]
119. Blower, T.R.; Williamson, B.H.; Kerns, R.J.; Berger, J.M. Crystal structure and stability of gyrase-fluoroquinolone cleaved complexes from *Mycobacterium tuberculosis*. *Proc. Natl. Acad. Sci. USA.* **2016**, *113*, 1706–1713. [CrossRef] [PubMed]
120. Leo, E.; Gould, K.A.; Pan, X.S.; Capranico, G.; Sanderson, M.R.; Palumbo, M.; Fisher, L.M. Novel symmetric and asymmetric DNA scission determinants for *Streptococcus pneumoniae* topoisomerase IV and gyrase are clustered at the DNA breakage site. *J. Biol. Chem.* **2005**, *280*, 14252–14263. [CrossRef] [PubMed]
121. Kwok, Y.; Zeng, Q.; Hurley, L.H. Structural insight into a quinolone-topoisomerase II-DNA complex. Further evidence for a 2:2 quinobenzoxazine-mg^{2+} self-assembly model formed in the presence of topoisomerase II. *J. Biol. Chem.* **1999**, *274*, 17226–17235. [CrossRef] [PubMed]
122. Kathiravan, M.K.; Khilare, M.M.; Nikoomanesh, K.; Chothe, A.S.; Jain, K.S. Topoisomerase as target for antibacterial and anticancer drug discovery. *J. Enzyme Inhib. Med. Chem.* **2013**, *28*, 419–435. [CrossRef] [PubMed]
123. Tewey, K.M.; Rowe, T.C.; Yang, L.; Halligan, B.D.; Liu, L.F. Adriamycin-induced DNA damage mediated by mammalian DNA topoisomerase II. *Science* **1984**, *226*, 466–468. [CrossRef] [PubMed]
124. Liu, L.F. DNA topoisomerase poisons as antitumor drugs. *Annu. Rev. Biochem.* **1989**, *58*, 351–375. [CrossRef] [PubMed]
125. Walker, J.V.; Nitiss, J.L. DNA topoisomerase II as a target for cancer chemotherapy. *Cancer Investig.* **2002**, *20*, 570–589. [CrossRef]
126. Goto, T.; Wang, J.C. Yeast DNA topoisomerase II is encoded by a single-copy, essential gene. *Cell* **1984**, *36*, 1073–1080. [CrossRef]
127. Wyckoff, E.; Natalie, D.; Nolan, J.M.; Lee, M.; Hsieh, T. Structure of the Drosophila DNA topoisomerase II gene. Nucleotide sequence and homology among topoisomerases II. *J. Mol. Biol.* **1989**, *205*, 1–13. [CrossRef]
128. Nitiss, J.L. Investigating the biological functions of DNA topoisomerases in eukaryotic cells. *Biochim. Biophys. Acta Gene Struct. Expr.* **1998**, *1400*, 63–81. [CrossRef]
129. Yang, X.; Li, W.; Prescott, E.D.; Burden, S.J.; Wang, J.C. DNA topoisomerase IIβ and neural development. *Science* **2000**, *287*, 131–134. [CrossRef] [PubMed]

130. Wang, J.C. Cellular roles of DNA topoisomerases: A molecular perspective. *Nat. Rev. Mol. Cell Biol.* **2002**, *3*, 430–440. [CrossRef] [PubMed]
131. Mandell, G.L.; Coleman, E. Uptake, transport, and delivery of antimicrobial agents by human polymorphonuclear neutrophils. *Antimicrob. Agents Chemother.* **2001**, *45*, 1794–1798. [CrossRef] [PubMed]
132. Carryn, S.; Van Bambeke, F.; Mingeot-Leclercq, M.P.; Tulkens, P.M. Comparative intracellular (THP-1 macrophage) and extracellular activities of beta-lactams, azithromycin, gentamicin, and fluoroquinolones against *Listeria monocytogenes* at clinically relevant concentrations. *Antimicrob. Agents Chemother.* **2002**, *46*, 2095–2103. [CrossRef] [PubMed]
133. McClendon, A.K.; Rodriguez, A.C.; Osheroff, N. Human topoisomerase IIalpha rapidly relaxes positively supercoiled DNA: Implications for enzyme action ahead of replication forks. *J. Biol. Chem.* **2005**, *280*, 39337–39345. [CrossRef] [PubMed]
134. D'arpa, P.; Beardmore, C.; Liu, L.F. Involvement of nucleic acid synthesis in cell killing mechanisms of topoisomerase poisons. *Cancer Res.* **1990**, *50*, 6919–6924. [PubMed]
135. Andoh, T.; Ishida, R. Catalytic inhibitors of DNA topoisomerase II. *Biochim. Biophys. Acta* **1998**, *1400*, 155–171. [CrossRef]
136. Hsiung, Y.; Elsea, S.H.; Osheroff, N.; Nitiss, J.L. A mutation in yeast TOP2 homologous to a quinolone-resistant mutation in bacteria. Mutation of the amino acid homologous to Ser83 of *Escherichia coli* gyrA alters sensitivity to eukaryotic topoisomerase inhibitors. *J. Biol. Chem.* **1995**, *270*, 20359–20364. [CrossRef] [PubMed]
137. Gruger, T.; Nitiss, J.L.; Maxwell, A.; Zechiedrich, E.L.; Heisig, P.; Seeber, S.; Pommier, Y.; Strumberg, D. A mutation in *Escherichia coli* DNA gyrase conferring quinolone resistance results in sensitivity to drugs targeting eukaryotic topoisomerase II. *Antimicrob. Agents Chemother.* **2004**, *48*, 4495–4504. [CrossRef] [PubMed]
138. Gabrielli, B.; Brooks, K.; Pavey, S. Defective cell cycle checkpoints as targets for anti-cancer therapies. *Front. Pharmacol.* **2012**. [CrossRef] [PubMed]
139. Schaad, U.B. Will fluoroquinolones ever be recommended for common infections in children? *Pediatr. Infect. Dis. J.* **2007**, *26*, 865–867. [CrossRef] [PubMed]
140. Kohlbrenner, W.E.; Wideburg, N.; Weigl, D.; Saldivar, A.; Chu, D.T. Induction of calf thymus topoisomerase II-mediated DNA breakage by the antibacterial isothiazoloquinolones A-65281 and A-65282. *Antimicrob. Agents Chemother.* **1992**, *36*, 81–86. [CrossRef] [PubMed]
141. Permana, P.A.; Snapka, R.M.; Shen, L.L.; Chu, D.T.; Clement, J.J.; Plattner, J.J. Quinobenoxazines: A class of novel antitumor quinolones and potent mammalian DNA topoisomerase II catalytic inhibitors. *Biochemistry* **1994**, *33*, 11333–11339. [CrossRef] [PubMed]
142. Tomita, K.; Tsuzuki, Y.; Shibamori, K.; Tashima, M.; Kajikawa, F.; Sato, Y. Synthesis and structure-activity relationships of novel 7-substituted antitumor agents. Part 1. *J. Med. Chem.* **2002**, *45*, 5564–5575. [CrossRef] [PubMed]
143. Tsuzuki, Y.; Tomita, K.; Shibamori, K.I.; Sato, Y.; Kashimoto, S.; Chiba, K. Synthesis and structure-activity relationships of novel 7-substituted 1,4-dihydro-4-oxo-1-(2-thiazolyl)-1,8-naphthyridine-3-carboxylic acids as antitumor agents. Part 2. *J. Med. Chem.* **2004**, *47*, 2097–2109. [CrossRef] [PubMed]
144. Golub, A.G.; Yakovenko, O.Y.; Bdzhola, V.G.; Sapelkin, V.M.; Zien, P.; Yarmoluk, S.M. Evaluation of 3-carboxy-4(1*H*)-quinolones as inhibitors of human protein kinase CK2. *J. Med. Chem.* **2006**, *49*, 6443–6450. [CrossRef] [PubMed]
145. Meggio, F.; Pinna, L.A. One-thousand-and-one substrates of protein kinase CK2? *FASEB* **2003**, *17*, 349–368. [CrossRef] [PubMed]
146. Tauber, S.C.; Nau, R. Immunomodulatory properties of antibiotics. *Curr. Mol. Pharmacol.* **2008**, *1*, 68–79. [PubMed]
147. Kanoh, S.; Rubin, B.K. Mechanisms of action and clinical application of macrolides as immunomodulatory medications. *Clin. Microbiol. Rev.* **2010**, *23*, 590–615. [CrossRef] [PubMed]
148. Guchhait, G.; Altieri, A.; Gorityala, B.; Yang, X.; Findlay, B.; Zhanel, G.G.; Mookherjee, N.; Schweizer, F. Amphiphilic tobramycins with immunomodulatory properties. *Angew. Chem. Int. Ed. Engl.* **2015**, *54*, 6278–6282. [CrossRef] [PubMed]
149. Roche, Y.; Fay, M.; Gougerot-Pocidalo, M.A. Effects of quinolones on interleukin 1 production in vitro by human monocytes. *Immunopharmacology* **1987**, *13*, 99–109. [CrossRef]

150. Riesbeck, K.; Andersson, J.; Gullberg, M.; Forsgren, A. Fluorinated 4-quinolones induce hyperproduction of interleukin 2. *Proc. Natl. Acad. Sci. USA* **1989**, *86*, 2809–2813. [CrossRef] [PubMed]
151. Riesbeck, K. Immunomodulating activity of quinolones: Review. *J. Chemother.* **2002**, *14*, 3–12. [CrossRef] [PubMed]
152. Dalhoff, A.; Shalit, I. Immunomodulatory effects of quinolones. *Lancet Infect. Dis.* **2003**, *3*, 359–371. [CrossRef]
153. Nau, R.; Eiffert, H. Modulation of release of proinflammatory bacterial compounds by antibacterials: Potential impact on course of inflammation and outcome in sepsis and meningitis. *Clin. Microbiol. Rev.* **2002**, *15*, 95–110. [CrossRef] [PubMed]
154. Nau, R.; Eiffert, H. Minimizing the release of proinflammatory and toxic bacterial products within the host: A promising approach to improve outcome in life-threatening infections. *FEMS Immunol. Med. Microbiol.* **2005**, *44*, 1–16. [CrossRef] [PubMed]
155. Turner, M.D.; Nedjai, B.; Hurst, T.; Pennington, D.J. Cytokines and chemokines: At the crossroads of cell signalling and inflammatory disease. *Biochim. Biophys. Acta Mol. Cell Res.* **2014**, *1843*, 2563–2582. [CrossRef] [PubMed]
156. Baggiolini, M. Chemokines and leukocyte traffic. *Nature* **1998**, *392*, 565–568. [CrossRef] [PubMed]
157. Laing, K.J.; Secombes, C.J. Chemokines. *Dev. Comp. Immunol.* **2004**, *28*, 443–460. [CrossRef] [PubMed]
158. Nitsche, D.; Schulze, C.; Oesser, S.; Dalhoff, A.; Sack, M. Impact of different classes of antimicrobial agents on plasma endotoxin activity. *Arch. Surg.* **1996**. [CrossRef]
159. Gollapudi, S.V.; Chuah, S.K.; Harvey, T.; Thadepalli, H.D.; Thadepalli, H. In vivo effects of rufloxacin and ciprofloxacin on T-cell subsets and tumor necrosis factor production in mice infected with Bacteroides fragilis. *Antimicrob. Agents Chemother.* **1993**, *37*, 1711–1712. [CrossRef] [PubMed]
160. Thadepalli, H.; Gollapudi, S.V.; Chuah, S.K. Therapeutic evaluation of difloxacin (A-56619) and A-56620 for experimentally induced *Bacteroides fragilis*-associated intra-abdominal abscess. *Antimicrob. Agents Chemother.* **1986**, *30*, 574–576. [CrossRef] [PubMed]
161. Thadepalli, H.; Hajji, M.; Perumal, V.K.; Chuah, S.K.; Gollapudi, S. Evaluation of temafloxacin in a rat model of intra-abdominal abscess. *J. Antimicrob. Chemother.* **1992**, *29*, 687–692. [CrossRef] [PubMed]
162. Thadepalli, H.; Reddy, U.; Chuah, S.K.; Thadepalli, F.; Malilay, C.; Polzer, R.J.; Hanna, N.; Esfandiari, A.; Brown, P.; Gollapudi, S. In vivo efficacy of trovafloxacin (CP-99,217), a new quinolone, in experimental intra-abdominal abscesses caused by *Bacteroides fragilis* and *Escherichia coli*. *Antimicrob. Agents Chemother.* **1997**, *41*, 583–586. [PubMed]
163. Thadepalli, H.; Chuah, S.K.; Reddy, U.; Hanna, N.; Clark, R.; Polzer, R.J.; Gollapudi, S. Efficacy of trovafloxacin for treatment of experimental Bacteroides infection in young and senescent mice. *Antimicrob. Agents Chemother.* **1997**, *41*, 1933–1936. [PubMed]
164. King, A.; May, J.; French, G.; Phillips, I. Comparative in vitro activity of gemifloxacin. *J. Antimicrob. Chemother.* **2000**, *45*, 1–12. [CrossRef] [PubMed]
165. Riesbeck, K.; Sigvardsson, M.; Leanderson, T.; Forsgren, A. Superinduction of cytokine gene transcription by ciprofloxacin. *J. Immunol.* **1994**, *153*, 343–352. [PubMed]
166. Riesbeck, K.; Forsgren, A. Commentary on ciprofloxacin-dependent superinduction of IL-2 synthesis and thymidine uptake. *Transplantation* **1998**, 1282–1283.
167. Abdel-Aziz, M.; Park, S.E.; Abuo-Rahma, G.D.; Sayed, M.A.; Kwon, Y. Novel N-4-piperazinyl-ciprofloxacin-chalcone hybrids: Synthesis, physicochemical properties, anticancer and topoisomerase I and II inhibitory activity. *Eur. J. Med. Chem.* **2013**, *69*, 427–438. [CrossRef] [PubMed]
168. Idowu, T.; Samadder, P.; Arthur, G.; Schweizer, F.M. Amphiphilic modulation of glycosylated antitumor ether lipids results in a potent triamino scaffold against epithelial cancer cell lines and BT474 cancer stem cells. *J. Med. Chem.* **2017**. [CrossRef] [PubMed]
169. Idowu, T.; Samadder, P.; Arthur, G.; Schweizer, F. Design, synthesis and antitumor properties of glycosylated antitumor ether lipid (GAEL)-chlorambucil-hybrids. *Chem. Phys. Lipids* **2016**, *194*, 139–148. [CrossRef] [PubMed]
170. Ogunsina, M.; Samadder, P.; Idowu, T.; Arthur, G.; Schweizer, F. Replacing D-glucosamine with Its L-enantiomer in glycosylated antitumor ether lipids (GAELs) retains cytotoxic effects against epithelial cancer cells and cancer stem cells. *J. Med. Chem.* **2017**, *60*, 2142–2147. [CrossRef] [PubMed]
171. Silva, H.; Valério Barra, C.; França da Costa, C.; de Almeida, M.V.; César, E.T.; Silveira, J.N.; Garnier-Suillerot, A.; Silva de Paula, F.C.; Pereira-Maia, E.C.; Fontes, A.P.S. Impact of the carbon chain

length of novel platinum complexes derived from N-alkyl-propanediamines on their cytotoxic activity and cellular uptake. *J. Inorg. Biochem.* **2008**, *102*, 767–772. [CrossRef] [PubMed]
172. Sánchez-Martín, R.; Campos, J.M.; Conejo-García, A.; Cruz-López, O.; Báñez-Coronel, M.; Rodríguez-González, A.; Gallo, M.A.; Lacal, J.C.; Espinosa, A. Symmetrical bis-quinolinium compounds: New human choline kinase inhibitors with antiproliferative activity against the HT-29 cell line. *J. Med. Chem.* **2005**, *48*, 3354–3363. [CrossRef] [PubMed]
173. Teicher, B.A. Next generation topoisomerase I inhibitors: Rationale and biomarker strategies. *Biochem. Pharmacol.* **2008**, *75*, 1262–1271. [CrossRef] [PubMed]
174. Carew, J.S.; Giles, F.J.; Nawrocki, S.T. Histone deacetylase inhibitors: Mechanisms of cell death and promise in combination cancer therapy. *Cancer Lett.* **2008**, *269*, 7–17. [CrossRef] [PubMed]
175. Azéma, J.; Guidetti, B.; Dewelle, J.; Le Calve, B.; Mijatovic, T.; Korolyov, A.; Vaysse, J.; Malet-Martino, M.; Martino, R.; Kiss, R. 7-((4-Substituted)piperazin-1-yl) derivatives of ciprofloxacin: Synthesis and in vitro biological evaluation as potential antitumor agents. *Bioorg. Med. Chem.* **2009**, *17*, 5396–5407. [CrossRef] [PubMed]
176. Shalit, I.; Kletter, Y.; Weiss, K.; Gruss, T.; Fabian, I. Enhanced hematopoiesis in sublethally irradiated mice treated with various quinolones. *Eur. J. Haematol.* **2009**, *58*, 92–98. [CrossRef]
177. Shi, Y.; Liu, C.H.; Roberts, A.I.; Das, J.; Xu, G.; Ren, G.; Zhang, Y.; Zhang, L.; Yuan, Z.R.; Tan, H.S.W.; Das, G.; Devadas, S. Granulocyte-macrophage colony-stimulating factor (GM-CSF) and T-cell responses: What we do and don't know. *Cell Res.* **2006**, *16*, 126–133. [CrossRef] [PubMed]
178. Ball, P.; Mandell, L.; Niki, Y.; Tillotson, G. Comparative tolerability of the newer fluoroquinolone antibacterials. *Drug Saf.* **1999**, *21*, 407–421. [CrossRef] [PubMed]
179. Blum, M.D.; Graham, D.J.; McCloskey, C.A. Temafloxacin syndrome: Review of 95 cases. *Clin. Infect. Dis.* **1994**, *18*, 946–950. [CrossRef] [PubMed]
180. Stahlmann, R. Clinical toxicological aspects of fluoroquinolones. *Toxicol. Lett.* **2002**, *127*, 269–277. [CrossRef]
181. Ball, P. Quinolone-induced QT interval prolongation: A not-so-unexpected class effect. *J. Antimicrob. Chemother.* **2000**, *45*, 557–559. [CrossRef] [PubMed]
182. Uivarosi, V. Metal complexes of quinolone antibiotics and their applications: An update. *Molecules* **2013**, *18*, 11153–11197. [CrossRef] [PubMed]
183. Turel, I. The interactions of metal ions with quinolone antibacterial agents. *Coord. Chem. Rev.* **2002**, *232*, 27–47. [CrossRef]
184. Shimada, J.; Shiba, K.; Oguma, T.; Miwa, H.; Yoshimura, Y.; Nishikawa, T.; Okabayashi, Y.; Kitagawa, T.; Yamamoto, S. Effect of antacid on absorption of the quinolone lomefloxacin. *Antimicrob. Agents Chemother.* **1992**, *36*, 1219–1224. [CrossRef] [PubMed]
185. Owens, R.C.; Ambrose, P.G. Antimicrobial safety: Focus on fluoroquinolones. *Clin. Infect. Dis.* **2005**, *41*, S144–S157. [CrossRef] [PubMed]
186. Redgrave, L.S.; Sutton, S.B.; Webber, M.A.; Piddock, L.J.V. Fluoroquinolone resistance: Mechanisms, impact on bacteria, and role in evolutionary success. *Trends Microbiol.* **2014**, *22*, 438–445. [CrossRef] [PubMed]
187. Crozat, E.; Philippe, N.; Lenski, R.E.; Geiselmann, J.; Schneider, D. Long-term experimental evolution in *Escherichia coli*. XII. DNA topology as a key target of selection. *Genetics* **2005**, *169*, 523–532. [CrossRef] [PubMed]
188. Riesbeck, K.; Gullberg, M.; Forsgren, A. Evidence that the antibiotic ciprofloxacin counteracts cyclosporine-dependent suppression of cytokine production. *Transplantation* **1994**, *57*, 267–272. [CrossRef] [PubMed]
189. Lipinski, C.A.; Lombardo, F.; Dominy, B.W.; Feeney, P.J. Experimental and computational approaches to estimate solubility and permeability in drug discovery and development settings. *Adv. Drug Deliv. Rev.* **2001**, *46*, 3–26. [CrossRef]
190. O'Shea, R.; Moser, H.E. Physicochemical properties of antibacterial compounds: Implications for drug discovery. *J. Med. Chem.* **2008**, *51*, 2871–2878. [CrossRef] [PubMed]

17

Antimicrobial Silver in Medicinal and Consumer Applications: A Patent Review of the Past Decade (2007–2017)

Wilson Sim [1], Ross T. Barnard [1,2], M.A.T. Blaskovich [3] and Zyta M. Ziora [3,*]

[1] School of Chemistry & Molecular Biosciences, The University of Queensland, Brisbane, QLD 4072, Australia; wilson.sim@uq.net.au (W.S.); rossbarnard@uq.edu.au (R.T.B.)
[2] ARC Training Centre for Biopharmaceutical Innovation, The University of Queensland, Brisbane, QLD 4072, Australia
[3] Institute of Molecular Bioscience, The University of Queensland, Brisbane, QLD 4072, Australia; m.blaskovich@imb.uq.edu.au
* Correspondence: z.ziora@imb.uq.edu.au

Abstract: The use of silver to control infections was common in ancient civilizations. In recent years, this material has resurfaced as a therapeutic option due to the increasing prevalence of bacterial resistance to antimicrobials. This renewed interest has prompted researchers to investigate how the antimicrobial properties of silver might be enhanced, thus broadening the possibilities for antimicrobial applications. This review presents a compilation of patented products utilizing any forms of silver for its bactericidal actions in the decade 2007–2017. It analyses the trends in patent applications related to different forms of silver and their use for antimicrobial purposes. Based on the retrospective view of registered patents, statements of prognosis are also presented with a view to heightening awareness of potential industrial and health care applications.

Keywords: antibiotic resistance; antimicrobial activity; medicinal silver; patents; silver; silver nanoparticles; synergism

---

1. Introduction

Silver is a soft and shiny transition metal which is known to have the highest reflectivity of all metals [1]. Among its many useful properties, silver it recognized to have antimicrobial activity. Silver is known to be biologically active when it is dispersed into its monoatomic ionic state (Ag^+), when it is soluble in aqueous environments [2]. This is the same form which appears in ionic silver compounds such as silver nitrate and silver sulfadiazine, which have been frequently used to treat wounds [3]. Another form of silver is its native nanocrystalline form (Ag^0). The metallic (Ag^0) and ionic forms can also appear loosely associated with other elements such as oxygen or other metals and can form covalent bonds or coordination complexes [3].

To date, there are three known mechanisms by which silver acts on microbes. Firstly, silver cations can form pores and puncture the bacterial cell wall by reacting with the peptidoglycan component [4]. Secondly, silver ions can enter into the bacterial cell, both inhibiting cellular respiration and disrupting metabolic pathways resulting in generation of reactive oxygen species [5]. Lastly, once in the cell silver can also disrupt DNA and its replication cycle [6] (Figure 1). A recently published review includes more details about the bactericidal mechanisms of silver, along with methods of silver nanoparticle preparation [7]. Throughout history, silver has consistently been used to restrict the spread of human disease by incorporation into articles used in daily life. The earliest recorded use of silver for therapeutic purposes dates back to the Han Dynasty in China *circa.* 1500 B.C.E [8]. Silver vessels and plates were frequently used during the Phoenician, Macedonian, and Persian empires [9]. Families of the higher socioeconomic classes during the middle-ages were so acquainted with the usage of silver that they developed bluish skin discolorations known as *argyria*, an affliction which may have led to the term 'blue blood' to describe members of the aristocracy [10]. Modern medicine utilizes medical grade forms of silver, such as silver nitrate, silver sulfadiazine, and colloidal silver [11].

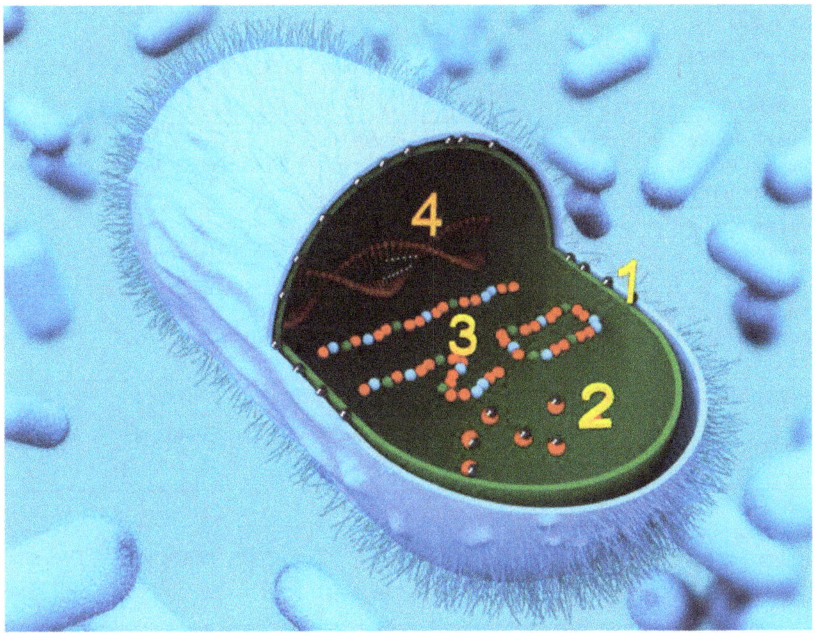

Figure 1. Silver's action on a bacterial cell. 1. Silver can perforate the peptidoglycan cell wall. 2. Silver inhibits the cell respiration cycle. 3. Metabolic pathways are also inhibited when in contact with silver. 4. Replication cycle of the cell is disrupted by silver particles via interaction with DNA.

The discovery of antibiotics in the early 20th century led to a cessation in the development of silver as an antimicrobial agent. However, the development of increasing levels of bacterial resistance to most antibiotics in recent years has led to reexamination of the potential of this ancient remedy [7,12] including studies with patients using colloidal silver and antibiotics [13]. This review aims to demonstrate the wide and ever-expanding applications of silver in medicine, health care, and other daily life activities, with a focus on the patents registered during the past decade. A similar patent review was published in Expert Opinion on Therapeutic Patents in 2005 [14], covering patents compiled from 2001–2004. The current review extends to the years 2007–2017. An analysis of the growth of patents describing antimicrobial silver applications is presented throughout this review, along with commentary of selected examples demonstrating some of the more interesting applications. Our analysis has separated these discussions of the use of silver into four general categories: Medical applications, personal care products, domestic household products, and agricultural/industrial applications.

2. Discussion

2.1. Antimicrobial Silver for Clinical and Medical Usage

This section presents a selection of some of the most interesting and unique patented products which utilize silver for their bactericidal action in the medical field, including therapies based on silver's antimicrobial properties. The product numbers referred to in this section correspond to those listed in Table 1.

Table 1. List of patented medical grade products and medically related products containing silver as an antimicrobial agent.

No.	Patent Title	Brief Product Description	Patent Number	Filing Date	Ref.
1	Ready to use medical device with instant antimicrobial effect	A medical apparatus packaging designed to activate a bioactive silver coating and other bactericidal elements upon opening of package.	US20150314103A1	5 November 2015	[15]
2	Use of silver-containing layers at implant surfaces	The method of coating medical implants with various forms of silver for infection prevention.	US20130344123A1	4 March 2013	[16]
3	Medical needles having antibacterial and painless function	Surgical needles coated with silver nanoparticles for the prevention of infection.	WO2006088288A1	5 January 2006	[17]
4	Fracture-setting nano-silver antibacterial coating	A method to coat invasive medical instruments with silver nanoparticles.	CN203128679U	3 April 2013	[18]
5	Antimicrobial closure element and closure element applier	The coating of the internal structure of a vascular portal device and the interior of its applicator.	US20080312686A1	9 June 2008	[19]
6	Bone implant and systems that controllably release silver	A specially designed bone implant which allows surgeons to control the release of silver ions.	WO2012064402A1	19 May 2012	[20]
7	Nanometer silver antibacterial biliary duct bracket and preparation method thereof	A biliary duct implant bracket made from plastic coated uniformly with silver nanoparticles to prevent biofilm formation at site of implant.	CN102485184A	3 December 2010	[21]
8a	Antimicrobial coatings on building surfaces	A coating with antimicrobial silver applied to the interior surface of a building's exterior wall.	US7641912B1	5 January 2010	[22]
8b			US8282951B2	9 October 2012	[23]
9a	Silver nanoparticle dispersion formulation	A topical gel to treat dermal infections with 1% w/w silver nanoparticles as active ingredient.	WO2007017901A2	16 February 2007	[24]
9a			EP3359166A1	15 August 2018	[25]
10	Antimicrobial silver hydrogel composition for the treatment of burns and wounds	An aqueous gel with a range of silver salt as its active ingredient made for the treatment of wounds specifically caused by burns.	WO20120282348A1	5 May 2011	[26]
11	Polysaccharide fibers for wound dressings	The method of coating wound dressing with a gel matrix where silver can be immobilized and applied to a wound to aid healing.	WO2013050794A1	5 December 2012	[27]
12	Antimicrobial, silver-containing wound dressing for continuous release	Wound dressing capable of releasing silver ions to aid healing upon contact with fluids from the wound.	US20070286895A1	24 August 2007	[28]
13	Nano-silver wound dressing	A wound dressing with enhanced antimicrobial properties for improved scarring.	US20070293799A1	9 December 2008	[29]
14a	Metal containing materials	Silver containing materials for treatment of bacterial conditions.	US8425880B1	23 April 2013	[30]
14b			US7255881B2	14 August 2007	[31]
15	Dental Uses of Silver Hydrosol	Silver suspended in aqueous gel used to reduce infection risks of dental procedures.	US9192626B2	24 November 2015	[32]
16	Antimicrobial silver nanoparticle additive for polymerizable dental materials	Denture material made with the addition of silver nanoparticles for additional antimicrobial effect.	US20070213460A1	13 September 2007	[33]
17	Silver ion coated products for dental and other body restoration objects	Silver coating with antimicrobial, antifouling and deodorant properties	US20180245278A1	30 August 2018	[34]

Surface coatings incorporating silver are a common application. One new approach is a method for producing ready packed medical apparatus which sterilizes itself upon the opening of the package, by creating a vapor that activates a silver-containing hydrophilic surface coating (Product No. 1). The antimicrobial properties of silver have been highly valued in medical application where implanted devices are coated with silver nanoparticles for the antimicrobial effects, but manufacturers need to be aware that this application is claimed in a patent application (Product No. 2) with a very broad claim 1: "An article that is implantable in an animal, the article comprising a microparticulate silver-containing antimicrobial layer stably adhered upon at least one surface of the article." However, the application does not appear to have progressed towards granting. Invasive surgical tools such as medical grade needles (Product No. 3) can also be coated with silver nanoparticles as described in its related patent (Product No. 4). Medical devices that are directly introduced into the human body that contain silver include vascular catheters (Product No. 5), bone implants (Product No. 6), and biliary duct brackets (Product No. 7). Another topical application of antimicrobial silver has incorporated it into coatings applied to the interior surface of a building's exterior wall (Products No. 8a and 8b).

Another general use is for topical treatments. Numerous topical gels with different formulations of silver have been patented. Silver was first used to treat burn wounds in the form of 0.5% silver nitrate solution and silver sulfadiazine cream in 1960 [35]. However, this was impractical as the dressings required rehydration every couple of hours. To overcome this limitation silver nanoparticle-based gels and silver salt-based gels have been developed (Products No. 9a, 9b and 10), with all approaches still considered novel.

Silver based wound dressings have greatly improved in efficacy compared to standard dressings, and more complex dressings have been developed. New knowledge in burn wound management led to the discovery of a method to immobilize silver nanoparticles on a gel-support matrix which is attached to a wound dressing (Product No. 11). A recently commercialized wound dressing allows a prolonged use of the dressing for up to 7 days or until saturation, without reapplication (Figure 2). It is made possible through its design, which slowly releases silver ions upon contact with wound exudates. Its highly absorbent padding is also coated with a layer of silicone which is aimed to reduce pain during removal and reapplication of the dressing. (Product No. 12). The use of silver with wound dressings is known to reduce scarring and such formulations are widely used (Product No.13). Silver-based wound dressings are available under brand names with different compositions, such as Mepilex® Ag, Acticoat™, Aquacel®, Flaminal®, Allevyn® Ag, and Biatain® Ag, SILVERCEL™. Other products containing a silver component, not specifically developed for wound healing, have been patented for treatment of bacterial infection (Products No. 14a and 14b).

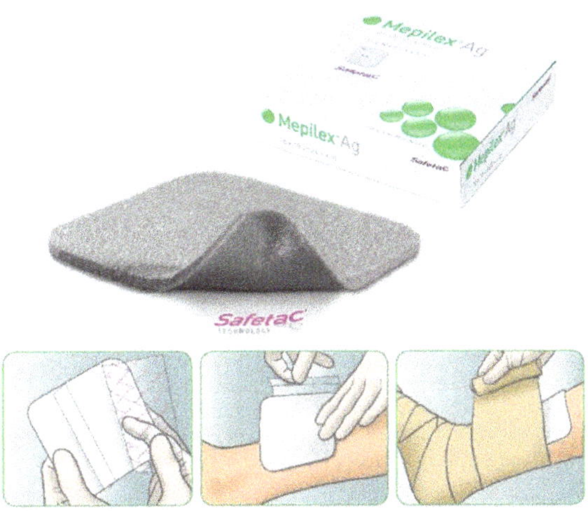

Figure 2. Mepilex® Ag with instructions for application. Images used with permission of Mölnlycke Health care, Sweden.

Silver has also been applied across the dental field. Silver has been the key component in dental amalgam fillings for more than one hundred years. However, its antimicrobial properties were not patented. Silver is used in the prevention of infection during and after dental surgery (Product No. 15). Dental support fixtures made out of silver and denture materials, and other body restoration objects, having silver nanoparticles as additives can reduce bacterial infections, especially during first few months of installation (Products No. 16 and 17).

2.2. *Antimicrobial Silver in Personal Care Products*

This section presents grooming products and devices which utilize silver for its sanitizing effects, summarized in Table 2. Hygiene and grooming products such as shavers (Product No. 18), toothbrushes (Product No. 19) and sanitary pads (Product No. 20) are frequently employed under adverse conditions where they encounter the bacteria microbiome, but are relied upon to be sanitary. One example of such usage is by the German public company "Beiersdorf AG" which has products incorporating silver for its added antimicrobial properties. They have applied silver over a wide range of products from shower gels and deodorants to first aid bandages (Figure 3).

Table 2. List of patented personal-care products containing silver as an antimicrobial agent.

No.	Patent Title	Brief Product Description	Patent Number	Filing Date	Ref.
18	Cosmetic and /or medical device for antimicrobial treatment of human skin with silver particles	Technology in which shaving devices can deposit silver ions unto skin in place of traditional antiseptic medium.	DE102012224176A1	26 June 2014	[36]
19	Antimicrobial thermoplastic polyurethane for toothbrush and preparation method for antimicrobial thermoplastic polyurethane	Addition of silver nanoparticles into plastic materials which are used to manufacture bristles of tooth brushes.	CN103254401A	28 April 2013	[37]
20	Sanitary towel capable of removing peculiar smell and manufacturing method thereof	Infusion of silver nanoparticles into fibers of sanitary pads which prevents the growth of odor causing microbes on menstrual discharges.	CN102961778A	21 November 2012	[38]
21	Solid oil cosmetics containing antimicrobial Ag zeolites and aluminum chlorohydrate	Deodorants and topical creams for the prevention of odor causing bacteria.	JP2013071914A	22 April 2013	[39]
22	Antimicrobial agents containing fine silver particle-carrying polypeptides and daikon radish fermentation products, and cosmetics containing them	The invention of a cosmetic lotion preservative consisting of silver nanoparticles.	JP2010059132A	18 March 2010	[40]
23	Functional cosmetic including nano silver	Addition of silver nanoparticles into manufactured cosmetics for its antimicrobial effect which aids in the prevention of acne and pimples.	KR20070119971A	21 December 2007	[41]
24	Antimicrobial contact lenses and methods for their production	Contact lenses manufactured from materials infused with silver nanoparticles for antimicrobial effects.	US20030044447A1	6 March 2003	[42]
25a	Silver-containing antimicrobial fabric	Textile material manufactured from fibers embedded with silver nanoparticles.	US20050037057A1	17 February 2005	[43]
25b			US7754625B2	13 July 2010	[44]
25c			WO2018160708	7 September 2018	[45]
26	Breast pump assemblies having an antimicrobial agent	Suction cup segment of device coated with silver ion exchange resin to prevent possible microbial contamination into breast milk.	US20080139998A1	12 June 2008	[46]
27	Nano-silver inorganic antibacterial nutritional hair dye	Hair colorant having additional silver nanoparticles as preservatives.	CN104224617A	27 August 2014	[47]

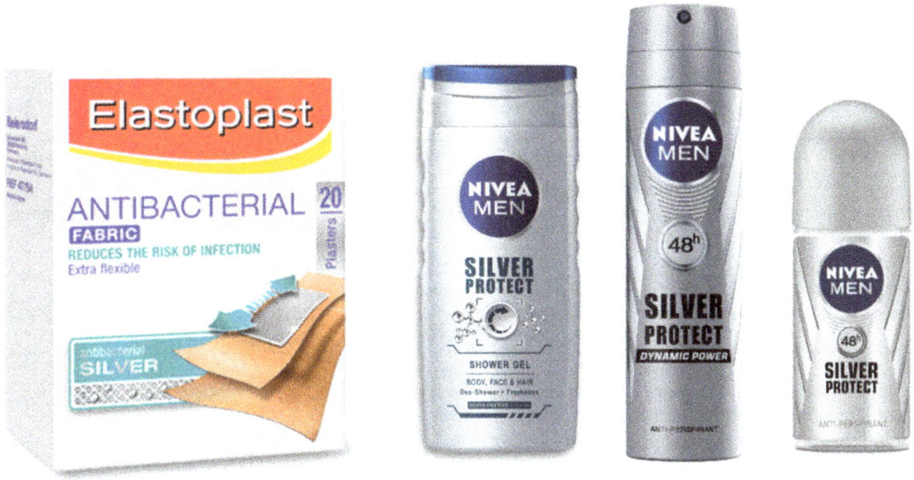

Figure 3. Commercial utilization of silver in consumer product lines, including Elastoplast (First aid bandages) and NIVEA (Shower gels and deodorants) for enhanced antimicrobial properties. *Images used with permission of Beiersdorf AG, Germany.*

Since using silver to treat skin infections is common, researchers in dermatology frequently resort to silver for treating conditions related to bacterial colonization, such as body odors (Product No. 21), acne outbreaks (Product No. 22), eczema and rash (Product No. 23).

A range of other personal health products have also added silver to improve their hygienic capacities, including contact lenses (Product No. 24), antimicrobial fabric garments (Products No. 25a, 25b and 25c), breast pump assemblies (Product No. 26), and hair dye (Product No. 27).

Most cosmetic products come in the form of cream, aqueous lotions, or hydrogel medium. It is observed that most manufacturers favor the incorporation of silver colloids into their products as they do not precipitate and separate, with the added benefit of acting as a preservative. Colloidal silver is defined as a mixture of silver ions and silver nanoparticles suspended in an aqueous medium. They are usually synthesized by electrolysis using a set of silver cathodes [48]. Colloidal silver was first used in 1891 by a surgeon named B.C Crede to sterilize wounds [9]. The use of silver grew in popularity between 1900 to the 1940s. Subsequently, antibiotics supplanted the use of silver [9]. Today, many products are offered not only as colloidal silver solutions, but also as personal devices suitable for home use, that synthesize colloidal silver. However, the commercialization of colloidal silver has been accompanied by inconsistencies in colloidal silver production and properties, as well as cases of unexpected side effects. Therefore, the Food and Drug Administration (FDA) has excluded any commercialized colloidal silver that claims health benefits without scientific evidence [49]. Similar action has been taken by the Therapeutic Goods Administration (TGA) in Australia [49] and the European Commission (EC) [50]. The commercial sales of colloidal silver are not banned, but claims of health benefits without scientific support are not permitted.

2.3. Antimicrobial Silver in Domestic Products

The antimicrobial applications of silver started in ancient times in domestic products like silver plates and pitchers [9]. With that in mind, there continue to be domestic applications of silver, particular for surface treatments (Table 3).

Silver is widely incorporated into surface coatings of electrical goods such as automated bathtubs (Product No. 28), laundry washing machines (Product No. 29), air purifiers with silver filters (Product No. 30) and refrigerators (Product No. 31), to produce 'bacteria-free' products. Application of silver nanoparticles to other household objects with frequent handling such as keyboards (Product No. 32), bath safety aids (Product No. 33), and bathroom safety handles (Product No. 34). Special stand-alone products such as containers for meat or water/wine/milk storage (Products No. 35a and 35b) are useful applications where bacterial contamination may present a health issue.

Table 3. List of patented home-use products containing silver as an antimicrobial agent.

No.	Patent Title	Brief Product Description	Patent Number	Filing Date	Ref.
28	Automatic cleaning system for bathtub or piping	A cleaning system attached to a Silver ion generator which flows through hot water inlet pipe which sanitizes bathtubs as a self-cleaning function.	JP2009268576A	19 November 2009	[51]
29	Clothes washing machine	Laundry washing machine consisting of a silver ion generator which will be released during each wash cycle.	US20080041117A1	21 February 2008	[52]
30	Air purifier, useful for neutralizing bad smells	An electronic air cleaning device which draws unclean air through an immobilized silver filter killing any airborne odor causing bacteria.	DE102007040742A1	3 March 2009	[53]
31	Antibiotic method for parts of refrigerator using antibiotic substance	Distribute silver ions within the fridge to slow the spoilage of food spoilage.	US7781497B2	24 March 2010	[54]
32	Submersible keyboard	A waterproof and washable keyboard with key caps made from plastic embedded with silver ions.	US20090262492A1	22 October 2009	[55]
33	Bactix silver-based antimicrobial additive in bath aids	Bath safety aids made from silver impregnated polymers for long lasting antimicrobial effects.	US20130029029A1	31 January 2013	[56]
34	Bacteria-resistant grab bar	Disability support bar paddings made out of silicone rubber impregnated with silver nanoparticles as antimicrobial additives.	US20100148395A1	17 December 2008	[57]
35a	Antimicrobial reusable plastic or glass container	Collapsible food storage containers mainly for meat or water/wine/ milk storage in kitchen composing of an antimicrobial silver fabric as its bottom inner layer.	US20070189932A1	10 February 2006	[58]
35b			WO2018137725A1	2 August 2018	[59]
36	Nano-silver antibacterial gloves	Domestic latex gloves impregnated with silver nanoparticles and other antimicrobial elements.	CN202738872U	20 February 2013	[60]
37	Natural silver disinfectant compositions	General surface cleaner containing soluble silver salt for added antimicrobial effect.	US20100143494A1	10 June 2010	[61]
38	Antiseptic solutions containing silver chelated with polypectate and EDTA	Laundry liquid having aqueous suspension of colloidal silver as additive for its antimicrobial properties.	US7311927B2	25 December 2007	[62]

Despite the many beneficial innovations in the use of silver as an antimicrobial agent, its application in cleaning products and disposable tools such as gloves (Product No. 36), disinfectant wipes (Product No. 37), and cleaning detergent (Product No. 38) may have negative environmental impacts. Cleaning products, once used, usually end up in sewage treatment systems, and eventually the environment. This is a concern for silver nanoparticles, as there are currently no effective methods for filtering out silver nanoparticles. The release of large amount of silver products into the environment may lead to disturbances of the microbiological ecosystem, and potentially lead to bacterial resistance to silver [63]. Consequently, alternative methods of sanitization should be considered such as the application of alcohol or bleach which are sufficient for domestic purposes, or employing 'fixed' silver containing surfaces that reduce the risk of environmental release.

Apart from being a threat to beneficial environmental bacteria, another issue to be addressed is the possible longer-term reduction of the potency of silver in killing microbes. Since the discovery of antibiotics, the efficacy of antibiotics has been compromised by over-prescription and over-usage, leading to the current antibiotic crisis. The presence of low levels of antibiotics in the environment fosters the generation of multiple drug resistant strains [64]. Silver is not immune to the generation of bacterial resistance, with several reports in recent years [65,66]. This history suggests a need for a systemic reassessment of the usage of silver in domestic products, so that it is not used too extravagantly, or released haphazardly.

2.4. Antimicrobial Silver in Agricultural and Industrial Products

Silver has also been used for a variety of agricultural and industrial products. In industry, large scale water purification can be made cost effective by using colloidal silver for purification as it is needed only in small quantities and can purify large quantities of water, though potential environmental risk needs to be considered [67]. For agriculture use, silver has been incorporated in nylon ropes that are used to tie down plants, cover them with netting, and for various other applications. These ropes normally decay after time due to bacterial biofilm formation, so the silver prevents this decomposition [68]. Agricultural use of silver products must be carefully assessed to avoid any impact on the microbial flora and symbiosis. The growth of healthy crop plants relies heavily upon the formation of symbiotic microbes around the roots such as nitrifying bacteria and mycorrhiza [69]. Studies have shown that the contact of bioactive silver to nitrifying bacteria impedes the formation of symbiotic channels [70].

Table 4 presents patented industry and agricultural related products utilizing silver as an antimicrobial agent. An example of agricultural use is Product No. 39 which uses Ag (I) and Ag (II) to treat infections in plants, while Products No. 40 and 41 with coating of a single rope strand with silver to prolong resistance to biofilm formation. Silver coatings can be beneficial in industrial machines which require a completely sterile environment to manufacture food or medical grade products, employing silver in the parts that come in direct contact with the products (Product No. 42). Machinery parts are usually designed for prolonged periods and incorporating silver particles into these materials provides an effective means of isolation and retention of silver so that it is not released into the environment easily.

Table 4. List of patented industry and agricultural related products utilizing silver as an antimicrobial agent.

No.	Patent Title	Brief Product Description	Patent Number	Filing Date	Ref.
39	Method and compositions for treating plant infections	Method of applying high valency silver to treat infection in plants of the *Rosaceae* family.	US20120219638A1	21 November 2011	[71]
40	Silver yarn, plied yarn silver yarn, functional fabric using same, and method for producing	Strong weather resistant rope for agricultural purposes made with polyester and silver-plated fiber yarn to prevent growth of biofilms.	CN102439205A	2 May 2012	[72]
41	Silver coated nylon fibers and associated methods of manufacture and use	The method and manufacture of industrialized antimicrobial fabric woven from nylon fibers impregnated with silver.	US20100166832A1	1 July 2010	[68]
42	Rolling apparatus having plastic parts containing antibacterial and antifungal silver (oxides)	Industry scale food grade rollers made from silver impregnated plastic for better hygiene and disease prevention.	JP2005201385A	28 July 2005	[73]
43	An antimicrobial food package	Food grade polymer containers with interiors coated with silver nanoparticles to prolong food freshness.	WO2014001541A1	28 June 2013	[74]
44	Rotationally molded plastic refuse container with microbial inhibiting inner surface and method	Industry scale plastic garbage container interiorly lined with silver nanoparticles for improved waste treatment.	US20080185311A1	7 August 2008	[75]
45a	Sustained silver release composition for water purification	Water filtration unit containing immobilized silver nanoparticles for water purification purposes.	WO2012140520A8	23 March 2012	[76]
45b			US20180186667A1	5 July 2018	[77]
46	Method for Producing Antimicrobial Agent Micro-Particle	An industry cleaning liquid having silver nanoparticles as its active ingredients.	JP2007161649A	28 June 2007	[78]

Polymers are extremely versatile and when impregnated with silver nanoparticles, they can be used for numerous applications, such as mass-produced food storage containers (Product No. 43) and industrial scale waste bins (Product No. 44). Sterility in the food and therapeutics industry is crucial, so the incorporation of silver into manufacturing equipment in contact with consumer products can be regarded as an appropriate usage. However, in the case of daily used food containers, frequent usage of silver may not be ideal as there is a risk of accumulation in the human body if the silver leaches, potentially leading to similar side effects as were observed in the middle ages when silver utensils were frequently used [9].

Products No. 45a and 45b describes a water filtration unit containing immobilized silver nanoparticles for water purification purposes. The invention and manufacture of industrial cleaning solutions containing silver (Product No. 46) is a potentially widespread application, as there is a need for instant effective sanitization to prevent bacterial transmission. However, precautions must be observed to prevent environmental release.

2.5. Overview of Patent Literature from 2007–2017

In the previous sections, applications of antibacterial silver in a variety of fields were discussed. This section presents an overview of silver-related patents on a global level for the purpose of understanding the trends, major applications as well as major contributors. Methods by which the data sets were obtained are reported in Section 3.

Tracking the number of patents disclosing antimicrobial applications of silver for each year over the past decade, as summarized in Figure 4, shows that there has been a steady upward trajectory in the number of silver patent applications in recent years. The increase may have reached a plateau in 2016/17, but it will be necessary to consider data from 2018 and onwards to confirm this hypothesis.

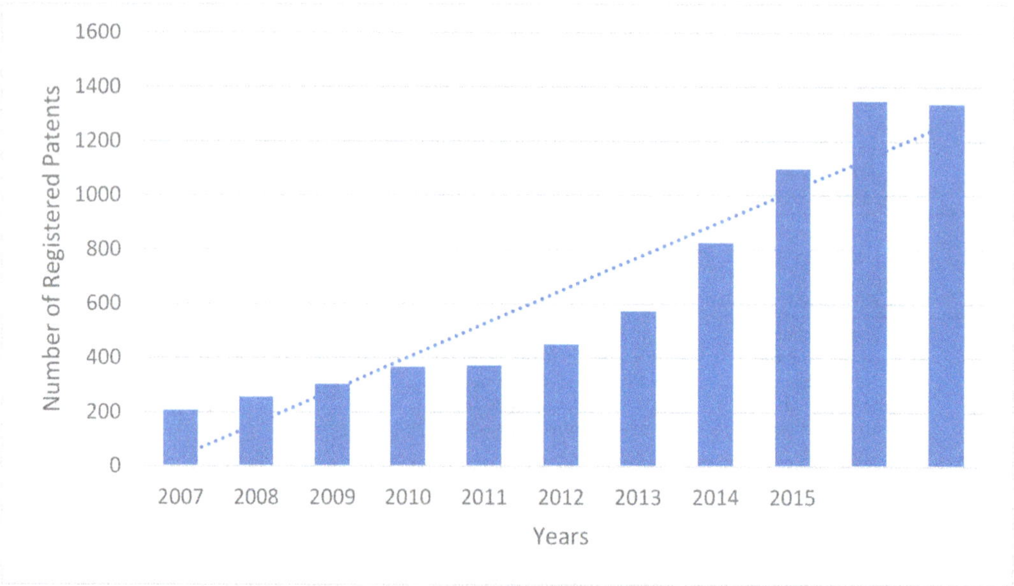

Figure 4. Trend analysis of yearly number of patent registrations involving antimicrobial silver applications over the past decade.

The data obtained from Figure 4 can be further dissected to reveal patents registered under each language, as shown in Figure 5. This can be linked to a deduction of the country of origin of these patents. This analysis demonstrates that patents claiming antimicrobial silver products are predominantly contributed by Asian countries, with China (55%), Korea (7%), and Japan (8%) comprising 70% of the chart. Patents registered in English compose 25% while another 5% are various European language patent registrations. It has been speculated that since the FDA and EMA have reduced influence in the Asian countries [49], this opens up opportunities in Asia for innovations with antimicrobial silver. Indeed, there is some basis for this speculation given the large number of silver related patents being registered in Asian languages, but additional research will be needed to establish the causes of this phenomenon. One of the potential reasons explaining the more substantial contribution of Asian countries in patented silver related innovations and consumer products is the fast-track approval pathway for new drugs in China, supported by consumer trials that are significantly cheaper than in other countries, which can be performed on higher number of participants. There is also a Chinese government strategy to commercialize non-Chinese ideas in China and financially support innovators who are willing to patent their ideas in China, with a preference to procure products whose IP is owned or registered in China. Finally, the database search may produce multiple results for a single patent that are particularly difficult to detect for Chinese applications because Chinese individuals' names typically have only three or two characters [79].

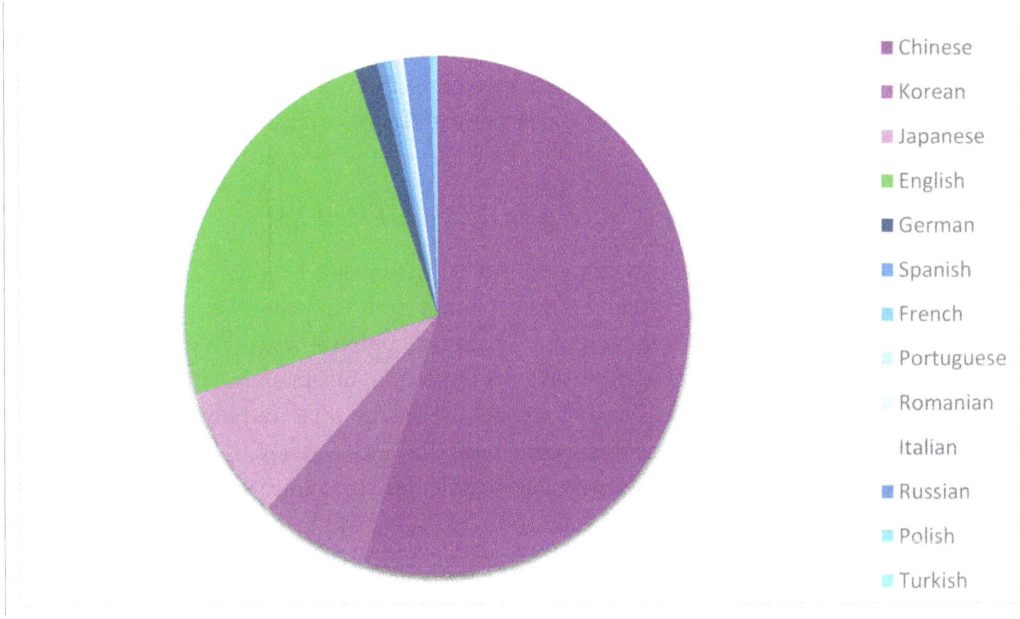

Figure 5. Analysis of language of patent registrations involving antimicrobial silver over the past decade with major contribution of Chinese (55%), English (25%), Korean (7%), Japanese (8%), and others (5%).

We have also assessed the application of silver according to its field of use. Based on the analysis from Figure 6, only about 20% of the patents in each year claimed medical uses of silver. This could mean that approximately about 80% of the patented silver applications are for other usages, such as domestic, agricultural and industrial usage. If this trend continues, there is potential for damage to the ecosystem if the non-medical uses result in release to the environment. This could lead to a worrisome situation where bacteria evolve resistance to silver, one of few promising alternatives to current classes of antibiotics.

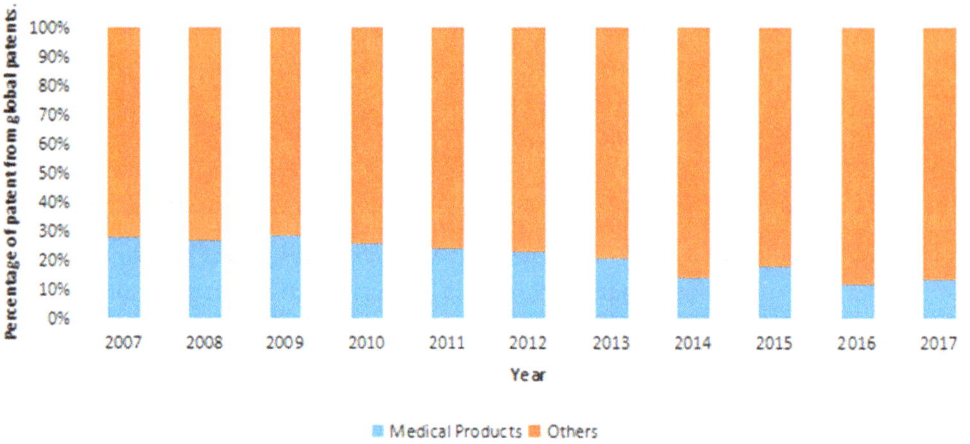

Figure 6. Total patents registered globally for silver used in the medical field compared to all other applications.

3. Materials and Methods

The patent analysis data and trend chart were generated through search results obtained from the scientific publication database, SciFinder® by the American Chemical Society. It was accessed through the University of Queensland Library portal. Results generated were accurate as of 15 June 2018.

3.1. Dataset 1—Application of Antibacterial Silver from the Global Perspective

The keywords used to generate this search were "antibacterial + silver" and "silver + medical" that narrowed down the number of silver related patents to those presenting the word "silver" in the title and describing only silver components. Therefore, patents with the general terms such as "metal nanoparticles" covering all nanomaterials with potential antibacterial applications like silver, platinum, gold, palladium, copper, zinc, and other metals, are not included here. Result limiters used were publication years (2007–2017) and document type (Patent). Search results yielded 5054 hits of exact words and concepts related to its words. No duplicates were found throughout the result set. The full result was analyzed by publication year and was sorted out by natural order to reflect results in yearly order. Obtained results were used to generate a bar chart as Figure 5 by using Microsoft Word chart sketching function.

3.2. Dataset 2—Application of Antibacterial Silver from a Regional Perspective

The keywords used to generate this search were as for Dataset 1, "antibacterial + silver". Result limiters used were publication years (2007–2017) and document type (Patent). Search results yielded 5054 hits of exact words and concepts related to its words. No duplicates were found throughout the result set. The full result was analyzed by language and was sorted out by frequency of region. Results obtained were used to generate the pie chart (Figure 6) by using the Microsoft Word chart sketching function.

3.3. Dataset 3—Application of Antibacterial Silver in the Medical Field

The keywords used to generate this search were "silver + medical". Result limiters used were publication years (2007–2017) and document type (Patent). Search results yielded 1310 hits of exact words and concept related to its words. No duplicates were found throughout the result set. The full result was analyzed by publication year and was sorted out by natural order to reflect results in yearly order. Results obtained were tabulated against dataset 1 to in order to obtain a 100% stacked bar chart presented at Figure 6 by using Microsoft Word chart sketching function.

4. Conclusions

The use of silver for its antimicrobial properties is increasing in numerous fields, including the medical, consumer, agricultural and industrial sectors. In just over 10 years, nearly 5000 new applications have been registered. The majority of the patents are from Asian countries, with Chinese language applications representing more than 50% of the global total, followed by Korean and Japanese language filings. Only about 20% of patents are registered in English.

While the potential benefits of silver are attracting increased attention, a number of publications have pointed out potential adverse effects from the overuse of silver, such as ecosystem disturbance [80], and bacterial resistance to silver [81]. Since our "armory" of antibiotics has been depleted by the rise in antimicrobial resistance, silver represents a new hope, but mindful use must be considered at an early stage to prevent a repetition of past mistakes.

We suggest that the application and commercialization of silver related products should be critically reassessed to avoid, or at least minimize, these adverse effects. In particular, while incorporation of silver products in an enclosed environment is justifiable, products which are expected to release silver into the environment should be avoided. There is ample evidence [82] that there can be adverse long-term effects from consumption or exposure to silver, so silver products should only be used in circumstances where (1) there is an absolute need for it, such as a medical intervention, and (2) in modes where silver is immobilized and containable.

Author Contributions: W.S. and Z.M.Z. designed and wrote the manuscript, Z.M.Z. coordinated the writing progress. All authors discussed the results and commented on the manuscript with the input from R.T.B. and M.A.T.B.

Funding: This research received no external funding.

References

1. National Institute of Standards and Technology. *CRC Handbook of Chemistry and Physics*, 81st ed.; Lide, D.R., Ed.; CRC Press: Boca Raton, FL, USA, 2000; p. 2556. ISBN 0-8493-0481-4.
2. Hoffman, R.K.; Surkiewicz, B.F.; Chambers, L.A.; Phillips, C.R. Bactericidal action of movidyn. *Ind. Eng. Chem.* **1953**, *45*, 2571–2573. [CrossRef]
3. Fong, J.; Wood, F. Nanocrystalline silver dressings in wound management: A review. *Int. J. Nanomed.* **2006**, *1*, 441–449. [CrossRef]
4. Jung, W.K.; Koo, H.C.; Kim, K.W.; Shin, S.; Kim, S.H.; Park, Y.H. Antibacterial activity and mechanism of action of the silver ion in staphylococcus aureus and escherichia coli. *Appl. Environ. Microbiol.* **2008**, *74*, 2171–2178. [CrossRef] [PubMed]
5. Morones-Ramirez, J.R.; Winkler, J.A.; Spina, C.S.; Collins, J.J. Silver enhances antibiotic activity against gram-negative bacteria. *Sci. Transl. Med.* **2013**, *5*, 190ra181. [CrossRef] [PubMed]
6. Yakabe, Y.; Sano, T.; Ushio, H.; Yasunaga, T. Kinetic studies of the interaction between silver ion and deoxyribonucleic acid. *Chem. Lett.* **1980**, *9*, 373–376. [CrossRef]
7. Möhler, J.S.; Sim, W.; Blaskovich, M.A.T.; Cooper, M.A.; Ziora, Z.M. Silver bullets: A new lustre on an old antimicrobial agent. *Biotechnol. Adv.* **2018**, *36*, 1391–1411. [CrossRef] [PubMed]
8. Yamada, K. The two phases of the formation of ancient medicine. In *The Origins of Acupuncture and Moxibustion, The Origins of Decoction*; International Research Center for Japanese Studies: Kyoto, Japan, 1998; p. 154.
9. Alexander, J.W. History of the medical use of silver. *Surg. Infect. (Larchmt)* **2009**, *10*, 289–292. [CrossRef] [PubMed]
10. Davies, O. *They Didn't Listen, They Didn't Know How*; AuthorHouse: Bloomington, IN, USA, 2013; p. 805.
11. Hill, W.R.; Pillsbury, D.M. *Argyria: The Pharmacology of Silver*; Williams & Wilkins Company: Philadelphia, PA, USA, 1939; p. 188.

12. Möhler, J.S.; Kolmar, T.; Synnatschke, K.; Hergert, M.; Wilson, L.A.; Ramu, S.; Elliott, A.G.; Blaskovich, M.A.T.; Sidjabat, H.E.; Paterson, D.L.; et al. Enhancement of antibiotic-activity through complexation with metal ions—Combined ITC, NMR, enzymatic and biological studies. *J. Inorg. Biochem.* **2017**, *167*, 134–141. [CrossRef] [PubMed]
13. Ooi, M.L.; Richter, K.; Bennett, C.; Macias-Valle, L.; Vreugde, S.; Psaltis, A.J.; Wormald, P.-J. Topical colloidal silver for the treatment of recalcitrant chronic rhinosinusitis. *Front. Microbiol.* **2018**, *9*. [CrossRef] [PubMed]
14. Melaiye, A.; Youngs, W.J. Silver and its application as an antimicrobial agent. *Expert. Opin. Ther. Pat.* **2005**, *15*, 125–130. [CrossRef]
15. Hannon, D.; Gilman, T.H. Ready to Use Medical Device with Instant Antimicrobial Effect. US20150314103A1, 5 November 2015.
16. Ostrum, R.; Hettinger, J.; Krchnavek, R.; Caputo, G.A. Use of Silver-Containing Layers at Implant Surfaces. US20130344123A1, 26 December 2013.
17. Yang, W.-D. Medical Needles Having Antibacterial and Painless Function. WO2006088288A1, 24 August 2006.
18. Li, Y. Fracture-Setting Nano-Silver Antibacterial Coating. CN203128679U, 14 August 2013.
19. Ellingwood, B.A. Antimicrobial Closure Element and Closure Element Applier. US20080312686A1, 18 December 2008.
20. Dehnad, H.; Chopko, B.; Chirico, P.; McCORMICK, R. Bone Implant and Systems that Controllably Releases Silver. WO2012064402A1, 19 May 2012.
21. Linghu, E.; Wang, K.; Wang, Y.; Yang, J. Nanometer Silver Antibacterial Biliary Duct Bracket and Preparation Method Thereof. CN102485184A, 6 June 2012.
22. Redler, B.M. Antimicrobial Coatings for Treatment of Surfaces in a Building Setting and Method of Applying Same. US7641912B1, 5 January 2010.
23. Redler, B.M. Antimicrobial Coatings for Treatment of Surfaces in a Building Setting and Method of Applying Same. US8282951B2, 9 October 2012.
24. Omray, P. Silver Nanoparticle Dispersion Formulation. WO2007017901A2, 16 February 2007.
25. Meledandri, C.J.; Schwass, D.R.; Cotton, G.C.; Duncan, W.J. Antimicrobial Gel Containing Silver Nanoparticles. EP3359166A1, 15 August 2018.
26. Yates, K.M.; Proctor, C.A.; Atchley, D.H. Antimicrobial Silver Hydrogel Composition for the Treatment of Burns and Wounds. WO2012151438A1, 8 November 2012.
27. Miraftab, M. Polysaccharide Fibres for Wound Dressings. WO2013050794A1, 11 April 2013.
28. Bowler, P.; Parsons, D.; Walker, M. Wound Dressing. US20070286895A1, 13 December 2007.
29. Ma, R.-H.; Yu, Y.-H. Nano-Silver Wound Dressing. US20070293799A1, 20 December 2007.
30. Lyczak, J.B.; Thompson, K.; Turner, K. Metal-Containing Materials for Treatment of Bacterial Conditions. US8425880B1, 23 April 2013.
31. Gillis, S.H.; Schechter, P.; Stiles, J.A.R. Metal-Containing Materials. US7255881B2, 14 August 2007.
32. Willoughby, A.J.M.; Moeller, W.D. Dental Uses of Silver Hydrosol. US9192626B2, 24 November 2015.
33. Ruppert, K.; Grundler, A.; Erdrich, A. Antimicrobial Nano Silver Additive for Polymerizable Dental Materials. US20070213460A1, 13 September 2007.
34. Ukegawa, S. Silver-Ion Coated Object Obtained by Microwave Irradiation and a Method for Coating a Silver-Ion Onto a Target Object. US20180245278A1, 30 August 2018.
35. Nherera, L.M.; Trueman, P.; Roberts, C.D.; Berg, L. A systematic review and meta-analysis of clinical outcomes associated with nanocrystalline silver use compared to alternative silver delivery systems in the management of superficial and deep partial thickness burns. *Burns* **2017**, *43*, 939–948. [CrossRef] [PubMed]
36. Banowski, B.; Garnich, F.; Simmering, R.; Device, I.E. Handset, for Performing Cosmetic and Medical Treatment for Human Skin, Has Application Surface Contacted with To-Be-Treated Skin Zone and Silver Portion, Which is Provided for Delivering Antimicrobial Silver Ions. DE102012224176A1, 26 June 2014.
37. Su, J.; Wang, D. Antimicrobial Thermoplastic Polyurethane for Toothbrush and Preparation Method for Antimicrobial Thermoplastic Polyurethane. CN103254401A, 4 March 2015.
38. Zhao, H. Sanitary Towel Capable of Removing Peculiar Smell and Manufacturing Method Thereof. CN102961778A, 13 March 2013.
39. Hasegawa, S. Solid Oily Cosmetic. JP2013071914A, 22 April 2013.
40. Miyata, S.; Kakihara, H.; Takahashi, F.; Nagaoka, H.; Kubota, T.; Ueda, G. Antimicrobial Agent. JP2010059132A, 18 March 2010.

41. Jang, H.C. Functional Cosmetic Including Nano Silver. KR20070119971A, 21 December 2007.
42. Zanini, D.; Alli, A.; Ford, J.; Steffen, R.; Vanderlaan, D.; Petisce, J. Antimicrobial Contact Lenses and Methods for their Production. US20030044447A1, 6 March 2003.
43. Schuette, R.; Kreider, J.; Goulet, R.; Wiencek, K.; Sturm, R.; Canada, T. Silver-Containing Antimicrobial Fabric. US20050037057A1, 17 February 2005.
44. Hendriks, E.P.; Trogolo, J.A. Wash-Durable and Color Stable Antimicrobial Treated Textiles. US7754625B2, 13 July 2010.
45. Hutt Pollard, E.A.; Morham, S.; Brown, D.E.; Kray, J.S. Systems and Processes for Treating Textiles with an Antimicrobial Agent. WO2018160708, 7 September 2018.
46. Silver, B.H. Breastpump Assemblies Having Silver-Containing Antimicrobial Compounds. US20080139998A1, 12 June 2008.
47. Wang, X. Nano-Silver Inorganic Antibacterial Nutritional Hair Dye. CN104224617A, 24 December 2014.
48. Panáček, A.; Kvítek, L.; Prucek, R.; Kolář, M.; Večeřová, R.; Pizúrová, N.; Sharma, V.K.; Nevěčná, T.J.; Zbořil, R. Silver colloid nanoparticles: Synthesis, characterization, and their antibacterial activity. *J. Phys. Chem. B.* **2006**, *110*, 16248–16253. [CrossRef] [PubMed]
49. Rulemaking History for OTC Colloidal Silver Drug Products. Available online: https://www.fda.gov/drugs/developmentapprovalprocess/developmentresources/over-the-counterotcdrugs/statusofotcrulemakings/ucm071111.htm (accessed on 27 September 2018).
50. Hartemann, P.; Hoet, P.; Proykova, A.; Fernandes, T.; Baun, A.; De Jong, W.; Filser, J.; Hensten, A.; Kneuer, C.; Maillard, J.-Y.; et al. Nanosilver: Safety, health and environmental effects and role in antimicrobial resistance. *Mater. Today* **2015**, *18*, 122–123. [CrossRef]
51. Sasaki, H. Automatic Bathtub Washing System. JP2009268576A, 19 November 2009.
52. Lee, Y.S. Clothes Washing Machine. US20080041117A1, 21 February 2008.
53. Nuernberger, C.; Nienaber, R.D. Air Purifier, Useful for Neutralizing Bad Smells, Preferably for Air Purification in Refrigerators, and for Controlling Bad Smells E.G. In Textiles and Vacuum Cleaners, Comprises a Silver Zeolite with a Nanoparticulate Metallic Silver. DE102007040742A1, 5 March 2009.
54. Kim, H.-K. Antibiotic Method for Parts of Refrigerator using Antibiotic Substance. US7781497B2, 24 August 2010.
55. Whitchurch, B.W.; Vaillancourt, D.; Jack, P.C.I.; Chen, W.; Huang, J. Submersible Keyboard. US20090262492A1, 22 October 2009.
56. Davis, W. Bactix Silver-Based Antimicrobial Additive in Bath Aids. US20130029029A1, 31 January 2013.
57. Gifford, S. Bacteria-Resistant Grab Bar. US20100148395A1, 17 June 2010.
58. Glenn, J.; Vogt, K.; Bridges, D. Antimicrobial Reusable Plastic Container. US20070189932A1, 16 August 2007.
59. Molnár, M. Vessel with Transparent Antimicrobial Silver Coating. WO2018137725A1, 2 August 2018.
60. Wang, X.; Gao, S. Nano-Silver Antibacterial Gloves. CN202738872U, 20 February 2013.
61. Scheuing, D.R.; Szekres, E.; Bromberg, S. Natural Silver Disinfectant Compositions. US20100143494A1, 10 June 2010.
62. Miner, E.O.; Eatough, C.N.; Miner, E.O.; Eatough, C.N. Antiseptic Solutions Containing Silver Chelated with Polypectate and Edta. US7311927B2, 25 December 2007.
63. Yu, S.-J.; Yin, Y.-G.; Liu, J.-F. Silver nanoparticles in the environment. *Environ. Sci. Process. Impacts* **2012**, *15*, 78–92. [CrossRef]
64. Stewart, P.S.; Costerton, J.W. Antibiotic resistance of bacteria in biofilms. *Lancet* **2001**, *358*, 135–138. [CrossRef]
65. Muller, M. Bacterial silver resistance gained by cooperative interspecies redox behavior. *Antimicrob. Agents Chemother.* **2018**, *62*, e00672. [CrossRef] [PubMed]
66. Elkrewi, E.; Randall, C.P.; Ooi, N.; Cottell, J.L.; O'Neill, A.J. Cryptic silver resistance is prevalent and readily activated in certain gram-negative pathogens. *J. Antimicrob. Chemother.* **2017**, *72*, 3043–3046. [CrossRef] [PubMed]
67. Oyanedel-Craver, V.A.; Smith, J.A. Sustainable Colloidal-Silver-Impregnated Ceramic Filter for Point-of-Use Water Treatment. *Environ. Sci. Technol.* **2008**, *42*, 927–933. [CrossRef] [PubMed]
68. Ingle, E.M.; Fisher, B.J.; Finney, J.W. Silver Coated Nylon Fibers and Associated Methods of Manufacture and Use. US2010166832A1, 1 July 2010.
69. Hayat, R.; Ali, S.; Amara, U.; Khalid, R.; Ahmed, I. Soil beneficial bacteria and their role in plant growth promotion: A review. *Ann. Microbiol.* **2010**, *60*, 579–598. [CrossRef]

70. Choi, O.; Hu, Z. Size dependent and reactive oxygen species related nanosilver toxicity to nitrifying bacteria. *Environ. Sci. Technol.* **2008**, *42*, 4583–4588. [CrossRef] [PubMed]
71. Olson, M.E.; Harding, M.W. Method and Compositions for Treating Plant Infections. US20120219638A1, 30 August 2012.
72. Song, Y.S.; Kim, M.H.; Won, M.H. Silver Yarn, Plied Yarn Silver Yarn, Functional Fabric Using Same, and Method for Producing Same. CN102439205A, 2 May 2012.
73. Yabe, S. Rolling Device. JP2005201385A, 28 July 2005.
74. Morris, M.; Kerry, J.; Cruz, M.; Cummins, E. An Antimicrobial Food Package. WO2014001541A1, 3 January 2014.
75. Maggio, R.A.; Pearson, R.C. Rotationally Molded Plastic Refuse Container with Microbial Inhibiting Inner Surface and Method. US20080185311A1, 7 August 2008.
76. Pradeep, T.; Chaudhary, A.; Sankar, M.U.; Rajarajan, G. Anshup Sustained Silver Release Composition for Water Purification. WO2012140520A8, 7 November 2013.
77. Pradeep, T.; Chaudhary, A.; Sankar, M.U.; Rajarajan, G. Sustained Silver Release Composition for Water Purification. US20180186667A1, 5 July 2018.
78. Takahashi, H.; Arakawa, H. Method for Producing Antimicrobial Agent Micro-Particle. JP2007161649A, 28 June 2007.
79. He, Z.-L.; Tong, T.W.; Zhang, Y.; He, W. A database linking chinese patents to china's census firms. *Sci Data* **2018**, *5*, 180042. [CrossRef] [PubMed]
80. Tlili, A.; Jabiol, J.; Behra, R.; Gil-Allué, C.; Gessner, M.O. Chronic exposure effects of silver nanoparticles on stream microbial decomposer communities and ecosystem functions. *Environ. Sci. Technol.* **2017**, *51*, 2447–2455. [CrossRef] [PubMed]
81. Gugala, N.; Lemire, J.; Chatfield-Reed, K.; Yan, Y.; Chua, G.; Turner, R. Using a chemical genetic screen to enhance our understanding of the antibacterial properties of silver. *Genes* **2018**, *9*, 344. [CrossRef] [PubMed]
82. Drake, P.L.; Hazelwood, K.J. Exposure-related health effects of silver and silver compounds: A review. *Ann. Occup. Hyg.* **2005**, *49*, 575–585. [PubMed]

Permissions

All chapters in this book were first published in ANTIBIOTICS, by MDPI; hereby published with permission under the Creative Commons Attribution License or equivalent. Every chapter published in this book has been scrutinized by our experts. Their significance has been extensively debated. The topics covered herein carry significant findings which will fuel the growth of the discipline. They may even be implemented as practical applications or may be referred to as a beginning point for another development.

The contributors of this book come from diverse backgrounds, making this book a truly international effort. This book will bring forth new frontiers with its revolutionizing research information and detailed analysis of the nascent developments around the world.

We would like to thank all the contributing authors for lending their expertise to make the book truly unique.

They have played a crucial role in the development of this book. Without their invaluable contributions this book wouldn't have been possible. They have made vital efforts to compile up to date information on the varied aspects of this subject to make this book a valuable addition to the collection of many professionals and students.

This book was conceptualized with the vision of imparting up-to-date information and advanced data in this field. To ensure the same, a matchless editorial board was set up. Every individual on the board went through rigorous rounds of assessment to prove their worth. After which they invested a large part of their time researching and compiling the most relevant data for our readers.

The editorial board has been involved in producing this book since its inception. They have spent rigorous hours researching and exploring the diverse topics which have resulted in the successful publishing of this book. They have passed on their knowledge of decades through this book. To expedite this challenging task, the publisher supported the team at every step. A small team of assistant editors was also appointed to further simplify the editing procedure and attain best results for the readers.

Apart from the editorial board, the designing team has also invested a significant amount of their time in understanding the subject and creating the most relevant covers. They scrutinized every image to scout for the most suitable representation of the subject and create an appropriate cover for the book.

The publishing team has been an ardent support to the editorial, designing and production team. Their endless efforts to recruit the best for this project, has resulted in the accomplishment of this book. They are a veteran in the field of academics and their pool of knowledge is as vast as their experience in printing. Their expertise and guidance has proved useful at every step. Their uncompromising quality standards have made this book an exceptional effort. Their encouragement from time to time has been an inspiration for everyone.

The publisher and the editorial board hope that this book will prove to be a valuable piece of knowledge for researchers, students, practitioners and scholars across the globe.

List of Contributors

Dimitri Chérier, Sean Giacomucci, Delphine Patin, Ahmed Bouhss, Thierry Touzé, Didier Blanot, Dominique Mengin-Lecreulx and Hélène Barreteau
Institute for Integrative Biology of the Cell (I2BC), CEA, CNRS, Univ Paris-Sud, Université Paris-Saclay, Gif-sur-Yvette 91198, France

Jude Ajuebor, Colin Buttimer, Sara Arroyo-Moreno, Emma M. Gabriel, Jim O'Mahony and Aidan Coffey
Department of Biological Sciences, Cork Institute of Technology, Bishopstown, Cork T12 P928, Ireland

Nina Chanishvili
Eliava Institute of Bacteriophages, Microbiology and Virology, Tbilisi 0160, Georgia

Olivia McAuliffe
Teagasc, Moorepark Food Research Centre, Fermoy, Cork P61 C996, Ireland

Horst Neve and Charles Franz
Department of Microbiology and Biotechnology, Max Rubner-Institut, DE-24103 Kiel, Germany

Aidan Coffey
Alimentary Pharmabiotic Centre, University College, Cork T12 YT20, Ireland

Des Field, Inès Baghou, R. Paul Ross and Colin Hill
School of Microbiology, University College Cork, Cork T12 YT20, Ireland

Mary C. Rea
Teagasc Food Research Centre, Moorepark, Fermoy, Co., Cork P61 C996, Ireland

Mary C. Rea, R. Paul Ross and Colin Hill
APC Microbiome Institute, University College Cork, Cork T12 YT20, Ireland

Gillian E. Gardiner
Department of Science, Waterford Institute of Technology, Waterford X91 K0EK, Ireland

Janet Y. Nale, Andrew Millard and Martha R. J. Clokie
Department of Infection, Immunity and Inflammation, University of Leicester, Leicester LE1 9HN, UK

Tamsin A. Redgwell
School of Life Sciences, University of Warwick, Coventry CV4 7AL, UK

David F. Driscoll
Stable Solutions LLC, Goleta, CA 93117, USA

Daniel Carter, André Charlett, Stefano Conti, Julie V. Robotham, Alan P. Johnson, Tom Fowler and Neil Woodford
National Infection Service, Public Health England, London NW9 5EQ, UK

David M. Livermore
Norwich Medical School, University of East Anglia, Norwich NR4 7TJ, UK

Mike Sharland
Paediatric Infectious Diseases Research Group, St George's University of London, Cranmer Terrace, London SW17 0RE, UK

Susan Hopkins
Antimicrobial Resistance Programme, Public Health England, London NW9 5EQ, UK

Philip Burgess and Stephen Dobra
Health Protection Analytical Team, Department of Health, Richmond House, 79 Whitehall, London SW1A 2NS, UK

Liang-Chun Wang, Madeline Litwin, Zahraossadat Sahiholnasab, Wenxia Song and Daniel C. Stein
Department of Cell Biology and Molecular Genetics, University of Maryland College Park, College Park, MD 20904, USA

Michael J. Love, Dinesh Bhandari, Renwick C. J. Dobson and Craig Billington
Biomolecular Interaction Centre and School of Biological Sciences, University of Canterbury, Christchurch 8041, New Zealand

Dinesh Bhandari and Craig Billington
Institute of Environmental Science and Research, Christchurch 8041, New Zealand

Renwick C. J. Dobson
Department of Biochemistry and Molecular Biology, University of Melbourne, Melbourne 3052, Australia

Beatriz Suay-García and María Teresa Pérez-Gracia
Área de Microbiología, Departamento de Farmacia, Instituto de Ciencias Biomédicas, Facultad de Ciencias de la Salud, Universidad CEU Cardenal Herrera, C/ Santiago Ramón y Cajal, 46115 Alfara del Patriarca, Valencia, Spain

Inés Urbiztondo, Lars Bjerrum and Gloria Córdoba
The Research Unit for General Practice and Section of General Practice, Department of Public Health, University of Copenhagen, 1353 Copenhagen, Denmark

Lidia Caballero
Dr. Pedro Baliña Hospital, Public Health Ministry, Posadas 3300, Misiones, Argentina

Miguel Angel Suarez
Policlínica Central de la Caja Nacional de Salud, La Paz 15000, Bolivia

Monica Olinisky
Department of Family and Community Medicine, Faculty of Medicine, University of the Republic, Montevideo 11600, Uruguay

Roberto Chulluncuy, Carlos Espiche, Jose Alberto Nakamoto and Pohl Milón
Centro de Investigación e Innovación, Faculty of Health Sciences, Universidad Peruana de Ciencias Aplicadas—UPC, Lima L-33, Peru

Jose Alberto Nakamoto
Facultad de Ciencias y Filosofía Alberto Cazorla Talleri, Universidad Peruana Cayetano Heredia—UPCH, Lima L-31, Peru

Attilio Fabbretti
Laboratory of Genetics, Department of Biosciences and Veterinary Medicine, University of Camerino, 62032 Camerino, Italy

Montserrat Lopez-Carrizales, Karla Itzel Velasco and Fidel Martinez-Gutierrez
Laboratorio de Microbiología, Universidad Autónoma de San Luis Potosí, San Luis Potosí, CP 78210, Mexico

Claudia Castillo
Laboratorio de Células Neurales Troncales, CIACYT-Facultad de Medicina, Universidad Autónoma de San Luis Potosí, San Luis Potosí, CP 78210, Mexico

Andrés Flores and Martín Magaña
Hospital Central Dr. Ignacio Morones Prieto, San Luis Potosí, CP 78290, Mexico

Gabriel Alejandro Martinez-Castanon
Facultad de Estomatología, Universidad Autónoma de San Luis Potosí, San Luis Potosí, CP 78290, Mexico

Ziyad Al-Kass, Anders Johannisson and Jane M. Morrell
Clinical Sciences, Swedish University of Agricultural Sciences (SLU), SE-75007 Uppsala, Sweden

Ziyad Al-Kass
Department of Surgery and Theriogenology, College of Veterinary Medicine, University of Mosul, Mosul 41002, Iraq

Joachim Spergser
Institute of Microbiology, Vetmeduni Vienna, 1210 Vienna

Christine Aurich, Juliane Kuhl and Kathrin Schmidt
Centre for Artificial Insemination and Embryo Transfer, Vetmeduni Vienna, 1210 Vienna, Austria

Sara Blaabjerg, Daniel Maribo Artzi and Rune Aabenhus
The Research Unit for General Practice and Section of General Practice, University of Copenhagen, 1014 Copenhagen K, Denmark

Tahl Zimmerman and Salam A. Ibrahim
Food Microbiology and Biotechnology Laboratory, Food and Nutritional Sciences Program, North Carolina A and T State University, 1601 East Market Street, Greensboro, NC 27411, USA

Temilolu Idowu and Frank Schweizer
Department of Chemistry, University of Manitoba, Winnipeg, MB R3T 2N2, Canada

Frank Schweizer
Department of Medical Microbiology and Infectious Diseases, University of Manitoba, Winnipeg, MB R3T 1R9, Canada

Wilson Sim and Ross T. Barnard
School of Chemistry and Molecular Biosciences, The University of Queensland, Brisbane, QLD 4072, Australia

Ross T. Barnard
ARC Training Centre for Biopharmaceutical Innovation, The University of Queensland, Brisbane, QLD 4072, Australia

M. A. T. Blaskovich and Zyta M. Ziora
Institute of Molecular Bioscience, The University of Queensland, Brisbane, QLD 4072, Australia

Index

www.ingramcontent.com/pod-product-compliance
Lightning Source LLC
Chambersburg PA
CBHW080511200326
41458CB00012B/4171
9781632417909